The

PLACEBO
EFFECT
and
HEALTH

"*The Placebo Effect and Health* is written with style and humor that makes it not just accessible to nonexpert readers but captures them with a fascinating account of important issues in medical research and treatment. Dr. Thompson completes that account with, what is for me a particularly compelling part of the book, the implications of the placebo effect for one of the most pressing social and economic questions of our time—the effectiveness and efficiency of the health-care system. This is a book that I would recommend to everyone who is interested or involved in health care."

Gordon Thiessen
Former Governor of the Bank of Canada

"Some issues in medicine are crucially important yet associated with more myths than clarity. Placebo, I think, is one of them. Grant Thompson's book aims at demystifying the subject. He has succeeded admirably. This book is as fascinating as it is informative—a truly good read for everyone with an interest in health care."

Edzard Ernst, MD, PhD, FRCP
Complementary Medicine,
Peninsula Medical School, Exeter (England)

"This readable overview of some of the salient research on placebo effects and their implications for health-care delivery is for and about practicing physicians. Dr. Thompson extols the virtues of evidence-based medicine and champions the nature of the patient-physician relationship as the most critical element in promoting placebo effects, an essential feature of good medical care."

Robert Ader, PhD, MD
Distinguished University Professor,
Dept. of Psychiatry, University of Rochester, NY

"Grant Thompson, a world leader in gastroenterology, an excellent clinician, and a superb writer, is in the best position to put this effect into proper perspective. Using both a historical and up-to-date scientific perspective, Dr. Thompson clarifies the mystery of the placebo while addressing its implications for pharmaceutical trials, complementary and alternative medicine, and for the patient and health-care provider in daily care. Highly recommended."

Douglas A. Drossman, MD
Codirector, UNC Center for Functional GI and Motility Disorders,
University of North Carolina at Chapel Hill

"While technical advances and super-specialization have lead to dramatic improvements in care for some acute illnesses, much of medicine deals with patients with more mundane, chronic fluctuating illnesses, for whom caring is as important as attempting to cure.

"Grant Thompson's book highlights the important role the placebo effect has in the management of chronic relapsing diseases and draws our attention to this neglected but vital aspect of the healing process, which depends more on the doctor's manner than his prescription. It also discusses the changes in medical practice, which are threatening to diminish this potent component of the healing process.

"He argues that the placebo effect is not 'the enemy' but our friend and should be maximized to harness our therapeutic efficacy.

"These are wise words based on a wealth of experience and careful research, drawing the attention of the busy physician to vital aspects of medical care. It also emphasizes how recent changes in medical practice threaten to erode one of the most important aspects of the doctor's art, namely the placebo effect. An essential read for all who aim to heal."

R. C. Spiller
Professor of Gastroenterology,
University of Nottingham (UK)

"Advances in medical technologies are often paralleled by increases in public expectations and the presumption of cures. But individuals who suffer chronic conditions know otherwise and must place their hopes elsewhere—on healing. In this fascinating account of the placebo, Grant Thompson explores the nature of healing. In fact, in the hands of a caring clinician, the 'placebo effect' might better be called the 'healing effect.' As we live longer in an age of rising health-care costs, patients, physicians, and health-care administrators would be well served by finding ways to put this healing effect, as so clearly explained by Dr. Thompson, into practice."

Nancy J. Norton
President, International Foundation for Functional Gastrointestinal Disorders

"Dr. Thompson's timely discussion appears as increasing pressures on physicians threaten their most powerful therapy, the placebo effect. In explaining its potential to augment all forms of health care, he corrects common misunderstandings and points out how an opposite, nocebo effect on people's health can occur. The book should reassure physicians that, despite rapid technological advances, the importance of their interaction with patients is paramount. Dr. Thompson guides the reader through the principles and limitations of evidence-based medicine by clearly explaining health-care research. By linking his topic to health-care systems, he should convince laypeople and health practitioners and administrators that improving health care cannot be accomplished without preserving the placebo effect. This engaging, comprehensive account should have wide appeal."

George F. Longstreth, MD
Kaiser Permanente Medical Care Plan, San Diego

"Grant Thompson is clear and concise in the information he provides, full of integrity in addressing the three themes of his book, providing us with a sound understanding that it is not so much just the placebo itself, but rather the 'placebo effect' that is influenced by the relationship between the patient and the physician. Understanding placebo effects are important in our appreciation of evidence-based medicine, our appreciation of why certain health policies should or shouldn't be developed, and knowing when and how to apply medical evidence in the perspective of the art of caring. This book will be a reminder to all of us that while the science needs to be sound, the art of medicine must always include caring for and caring about people."

Alan B. R. Thomson, MD
Professor of Medicine,
University of Alberta

BOOKS BY DR. W. GRANT THOMPSON

The Irritable Gut
Baltimore: University Park Press, 1979.

Gut Reactions
New York: Plenum, 1989.

The Angry Gut: Coping with Colitis and Crohn's Disease
New York: Plenum, 1993.

With K. W. Drossman, J. E. Richter, N. J. Talley, E. Corazziari, and
W. E. Whitehead.
Functional Gastrointestinal Disorders
Boston: Little, Brown, 1994;
2nd ed., McLean, VA: Degnon Press, 2000.

The Ulcer Story
New York: Plenum, 1996.

With K. W. Heaton.
Fast Fact: Irritable Bowel Syndrome
Oxford: Health Press, 1999; 2nd ed., 2003.

The

PLACEBO
EFFECT
and
HEALTH

Combining Science &
Compassionate Care

W. GRANT
THOMPSON, MD

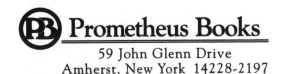

Prometheus Books
59 John Glenn Drive
Amherst, New York 14228-2197

Published 2005 by Prometheus Books

Inquiries should be addressed to
Prometheus Books
59 John Glenn Drive
Amherst, New York 14228–2197
VOICE: 716–691–0133, ext. 207
FAX: 716–564–2711
WWW.PROMETHEUSBOOKS.COM

09 08 07 06 05   5 4 3 2 1

Library of Congress Cataloging-in-Publication Data

Thompson, W. Grant.
    The placebo effect and health : combining science and compassionate care /
W. Grant Thompson.
        p. cm.
    Includes bibliographical references and index.
    ISBN 1–59102–275–4 (pbk. : alk. paper)
    1. Placebo (Medicine). 2. Physician and patient.
    [DNLM: 1. Placebo Effect. 2. Evidence-Based Medicine. 3. Physician-Patient
Relations. WB 330 T471p 2005] I. Title.

R726.5.T488 2005
615.5—dc22

2005006906

Printed in the United States of America on acid-free paper

To

Jacob

Ava

Ryan

&

Gillian

ACKNOWLEDGMENTS

Many people helped me in the preparation of this book. My daughter Jennifer Maxwell read an early manuscript and checked the proofs. Gordon Thiessen, former governor of the Bank of Canada, kindly read it as well, offering many helpful suggestions and reining in my rhetorical excesses. Collaboration with Kenneth Heaton over many years provided experience with the British National Health Service. George Longstreth (California), Douglas Drossmen (North Carolina), Michel Delvaux (France), Enrico Corrazziari (Italy), Stefan Müller-Lissner (Germany), and John Kellow (Australia) helped me understand health care in other countries in a way the written word could not convey. Diane and Tom Mountain of Victoria, British Columbia, helped me with some of the material. My editor Linda Regan was an encouraging but stringent editor. Jeremy Sauer was painstaking with the proofs. The work would be impossible without the loving support of my wife, Sue, who is not only my best fan but also my most demanding critic. Of course, any faults are mine.

CONTENTS

INTRODUCTION

I have three objectives in writing this book. The first is to explore the *placebo effect* and explain how it plays a role in the repertoire of every healer. The second is to demonstrate how the placebo has permitted researchers to gather medical evidence through *randomized clinical trials*. This evidence enables doctors to apply *evidence-based medicine* to their practices. The third objective is to explain how these two phenomena, the placebo effect and evidence-based medicine, are essential to good medical care. Though the interaction of these three themes is neglected in current national health debates, I will make the case that they are indispensable components of good care, and of vital interest to all citizens.

Many misunderstand the placebo, partly because it falls under the intellectual purview of many disciplines, and some are hostile to the idea (see table 2-2). Each discipline contributes its own terminology, which is addressed in the glossary at the end of this book. The first two chapters in part 1 describe the evolution of the meaning of "placebo" and its vital role in treatment since prehistory. Chapter 3 reviews some facts and myths about placebos. The facts are disconnected, yet constitute a nascent discipline, or body of scientific study. By this point, the reader will appreciate that the subject of part 1 is the "placebo effect," not the placebo itself. Chapters 4 and 5 are devoted to the nature of the placebo effect and the elements that promote it. A therapeutic effect includes three main components: the benefit of the treatment itself, the natural history of the illness being treated, and the placebo effect. When an individual receives a treatment, these components are so blended that one cannot estimate their relative contribution. Chapter 4 introduces the notion of the doctor as placebo. The character, personality, compassion, and authority of the healer are essential to the placebo effect. The doctor/patient, or healer/ill person, relationship is an important determinant of the success of any treatment. Chapter 6 introduces the *nocebo effect*. If the placebo effect of a successful therapeutic encounter is a force for good, it follows that bad things may result from an unsuccessful one. Whether voodoo death, a disaffected patient, or an adverse encounter leading to litigation, a nocebo effect is the unhappy alter ego of the placebo effect.

Harmful treatments that healers believed to be effective figure prominently in the history of healing. The only explanations for this can be the tendency of the body to heal despite the treatment (*natural history*), and the placebo effect. Part 2 discusses the implications of placebo and nocebo effects in modern treatments. Some treatments are obviously beneficial, but others are not. The scientific way to prove a treatment's efficacy is to submit it to a randomized clinical trial comparing outcomes in subjects receiving the treatment to outcomes in subjects receiving a control treatment, usually a placebo. Randomized clinical trials are described in chapter 7, and the application of the evidence gained from such trials is explained in chapter 8. While randomized clinical trials can validate some drug therapies and refute others, the testing of surgical, psychologic, and alternate therapies presents special problems that are addressed in the next three chapters. Since the character and personality of the healer are so important to placebo and nocebo effects, chapter 12 further examines the doctor as a placebo. Clinical trial investigators have long had an interest in the "placebo responder," sometimes seeing him as an obstacle to the demonstration of a treatment's efficacy. In chapter 13, we learn that the placebo responder is everyman. At some times in our lives, we are all susceptible. Part 2 ends with a discussion of the ethics of placebos. Is it right to deliberately give an ill person an inert treatment? What are the ethical implications of using placebos in clinical trials?

Part 3 explores the vital importance of placebo effects and evidence-based medicine to successful health-care policy. Placebo/nocebo effects depend upon doctor/patient relationships and are important determinants of health outcomes. Chapter 15 discusses the managers, bureaucrats, economists, lawyers, reporters, ethicists, advocates, and others who increasingly seek to insert themselves between doctor and patient, threatening the integrity of their therapeutic interaction. For many illnesses, there are several therapeutic options. Many are fanciful and thrive on the placebo effect. Chapter 16 explores how society should be reassured that treatments are safe. As third parties increasingly underwrite treatments, they need to know that they are not only safe but also effective. Therefore, proponents of therapies must assume the burden of proof, and the authorities of any successful health-care system must deploy information technology to ensure that medical evidence is readily available to doctors. Each developed nation has evolved its own health-care system. All are undergoing financial stresses and are under pressure to reform. Chapter 17 briefly describes some of these systems and their unique national debates. The chapter urges that these debates address the provision of adequate doctor/patient interaction, particularly in primary care, and the promotion of medical evidence as the basis of medical decision making. In developed countries, many doctors are dissatisfied with their working conditions. Chapter 18 suggests some ways that doctors can help themselves. Central to their happiness and success is a reaffirmation of the values that likely drew them to the profession in the first place—due attention to the healing power of a good doctor/patient relationship on one hand, and the judicious deployment of medical evidence on the other.

The three themes of this book flow from one another. The placebo effects of therapeutic encounters require study in their own right but also necessitate sophisticated clinical trials of most treatment and diagnostic interventions. Further, the placebo effect and medical evidence should be critical considerations in deciding how a society should deliver health care. My purpose is not to define what the best system would look like or specify what changes should be made. Rather it is to alert the reader to these issues, since they seldom are discussed publicly. The demand for medical care seems bottomless. Experts and politicians seek reduced costs but more bureaucracy, less administration but more regulation, fewer invasions of privacy but more transparency, risk management but quality assurance, shorter waiting lists but more surgery, and better gatekeepers but more choice. Lost among these contradictions are the two core elements of good medical care, the caring doctor/patient interface, and the efficient and wise deployment of medical evidence to medical care. Any medical-care system that fails to embrace these complementary treatment essentials is doomed to suboptimal results and unhappy patients. Then, no amount of money or regulation will fix it.

***

I have been a general practitioner, gastroenterologist, academic physician, clinical researcher, medical writer, clinical-trials consultant, and medical educator. I have trained or practiced in three Canadian provinces and in the United States and Great Britain. In addition, my research interests have taken me around the world, permitting me glimpses of health-care issues in many places. Just ahead of the baby boom, I am increasingly a patient. In each role, I have encountered the placebo effect. An early 1970s lecture by Howard Brody introduced me to the placebo as a vehicle for providing meaning for patients' suffering and to the study of placebo effects as a discipline. Since then, I have followed the placebo through medical and other literature, and have come to understand its great relevance to medical care. Many disciplines claim placebos as their own territory. This makes it a special challenge for a student of any one discipline to address the three themes of this book. I write from the viewpoint of my own disciplines, tempered by the thoughts of many others, whose works are cited in the notes.

W. Grant Thompson
Ottawa, Ontario
April 3, 2005

PART 1

THE PLACEBO EFFECT

The meaning of *placebo* has metamorphosed from a treatment meant more to please than cure, to an inert pill or other device given to patients in the placebo control group of a randomized clinical trial. Placebo effects are part of every treatment, and along with nature's tendency to ameliorate, account for the existence of many otherwise useless medicines or procedures. There are sufficient data to consider the study of placebos as an emerging scientific discipline. We know some of the factors that are likely to induce a placebo effect—that much depends upon the circumstances of the patient, and the authority, character, and personality of the practitioner or healer. Conversely, bad doctor/patient interactions can be harmful and cause "nocebo" effects. Part 1 describes the placebo and its history, emphasizing that it is the placebo's *effect* that is important, not the device. Indeed beneficial placebo effects occur in the absence of a placebo, and in conjunction with almost all treatments. This part also explores how to exploit the placebo effect and avoid nocebo effects.

***

A PubMed search retrieved 101,541 citations for "placebo." Google turned up over seven million, Yahoo! nearly five million. No reviewer can hope to capture them all, so this is not a systematic review. Nevertheless, material gathered over thirty years and presented here should convince readers that "yes, there is a placebo effect," and that it can and should be employed by all who profess to heal.

CHAPTER 1

WHAT IS A PLACEBO?

Placebo: "I shall please."

ROMAN CATHOLIC VESPERS OF THE DEAD

Before the advent of modern, "evidence-based" medicine, physicians commonly employed sugar pills or other harmless nostrums as treatment. They sensed intuitively that the giving of medicine helped ill people feel better. There was little thought as to whether these conferred actual benefit or, as Voltaire put it, "amused the patient until he got well." Thomas Jefferson justified placebos as "a pious fraud." Because of the implied deceit and an increasingly informed populace, the use of placebos as a treatment has fallen into disrepute. Physicians and pharmacists no longer secrete sugar pills in their desk drawer. Meanwhile, the term *placebo* has been applied anew to the dummy medications or procedures used as the controls for clinical trials that are designed to test treatments. This new meaning is unfortunate since such controls embrace no deceit and the consenting subjects are informed. To understand placebos we must comprehend this distinction. We also need to distinguish *placebo* from *placebo effect*.

THE TERM *PLACEBO*

"Placebo" is the first person future indicative of the Latin *placere*, "to please."[1] The word *placebo* translates to "I will please," "I shall please," or "I shall be pleasing." "Placebo Domino in regione vivorum" begins the vespers for the dead, which translates into "I will please the Lord in the land of the living." In the fourteenth century *placebo* referred to a hired mourner at a funeral. The executors of an unpopular grandee's estate might recruit mourners to chant suitable religious and secular sentiments at his funeral. Hence, "placebos" became flatterers or sycophants. Chaucer used the word in this sense in *The Canterbury Tales*: "Flattereres been the develes chapelynes, that syngen ever placebo. I rekene flaterye among the vyces. . . ."[2]

In *The Merchant's Tale*,[3] the principal character, an elderly man called "January," is addressed with false praise by a fawning acquaintance called "Placebo." Here Chaucer meant sycophant. Later dictionaries such as those of Elisha Coles in 1676 or Samuel Johnson in 1755 do not include the word.

The meaning of the placebo has undergone a long metamorphosis from its medieval context to its ambivalent meaning today. Table 1-1 illustrates some dictionary definitions over the last two centuries. In 1785 a medical dictionary described placebo as "a commonplace method of medicine," and by 1811, it was a medicine "given more to please than benefit the patient." Note the subtle change from "a commonplace method of medicine" to seemingly pejorative references to flattery and eventually "humoring the patient." Later versions employ the words gratify, soothe, and flatter. Modern dictionaries speak of faith and of psychological effects.

TABLE 1-1
Dictionary Definitions of Placebos

Source	Year	Definition of Placebo
New Medical Dictionary	1785	A commonplace method of medicine.
Hooper's Medical Dictionary	1811	An epithet given to any medicine adapted more to please than to benefit the patient.
Dunglison; Dictionary of Medical Science	1874	"I will please" (from placeo)—A medicine usually prescribed rather to satisfy the patient rather than with any expectation of its effecting a cure.

Medical Lexicon	1881	Name for a medicine given by a doctor to a patient simply to satisfy the patient's mind; usually of a harmless nature e.g. water coloured with cochineal (dried insects used as dye).
Standard Dictionary of the English Language	1895	Any harmless substance as bread pills given to soothe a patient's anxiety rather than as a remedy.
Century Dictionary	1900	A medicine adapted rather to pacify than to benefit the patient.
Chalmers Twentieth-Century Dictionary	1911	A medicine given more to humour or gratify a patient than to exercise any curative effect.
Pepper, O.H.P. (Quoted by Stewart Wolf)[4]	1948	The giving of a placebo ... seems to be a function of the physician which, like certain functions of the body is not to be mentioned in polite society.
Stedman's Medical Dictionary	1953	An indifferent substance in the form of a medicine, given for the moral or suggestive effect.
Oxford English Dictionary	1953	A medicine given to humour rather than to cure the patient.
American Pocket Medical Dictionary	1953	An inert substance given as a medication.
Britannica World Language	1960	Any harmless substance given to humour a patient or as a test in controlled experiments. Anything said to flatter or please.

Webster's 3rd New International Dictionary	1971	An inert medicament or preparation given for its psychological effect esp. to satisfy a patient or act as a control in an experimental series.
Taber's Medical Dictionary	1971	1. Inactive substance given to satisfy patient's demand for medicine. 2. Also used in the controlled studies of drugs. The placebo is given to a group of patients, and the drug being tested is given to a similar group; then the results obtained in the two groups are compared. Also, something tending to soothe or gratify.
Brewer's Dictionary of Phrase and Fable	1981	An innocuous medicine designed to humour a patient, and which may have a beneficial psychological and physical effect.
Collins Dictionary of Medicine	1992	1. A pharmacologically inactive substance made up in a form apparently identical to an active drug that is under trial. 2. A harmless preparation prescribed to satisfy a patient who does not require active medication.
Oxford Concise Medical Dictionary	1999	A medicine that is ineffective but may help relieve a condition because a patient has faith in its powers. New drugs are tested against placebos in clinical trials: the drug effect compared with the placebo response which occurs even in the absence of any pharmacologically active substance in the placebo.

Dorland's Medical Dictionary, 29th edition	2001	Any dummy medical treatment; originally a medical preparation having no specific pharmacological activity against the patient's illness or complaint given solely for the psychophysiological effects of the treatment; more recently, a dummy treatment administered to a control group in a controlled clinical trial in order that the specific and non-specific effects of the experimental treatment can be distinguished—i.e. the experimental treatment must produce better results than the placebo in order to be considered effective. *Active placebo, impure placebo*: A substance having pharmacological properties that are not relevant to the condition being treated.

The Latin verb *placere* has also come into use in English via the French word *plaisir*, meaning to please. *Please*, *placate*, and *placid* are derived from this word and hint at the pleasing, pacifying functions of placebos in prescientific medicine. *Placebo* thus acquired a nonmedical use as something tending to soothe or gratify. As medicine became more science based, the deliberate use of placebo treatment came to be considered unethical. By 1945 the giving of placebos was described as "a function of the physician that like certain body functions should not be mentioned in polite company."[5] After World War II, the sense of the word changed dramatically as *placebos* came to be "the control treatment in a clinical trial." Today, medical students and others may understand this meaning rather than earlier ones, but both continue in common use.

PLACEBOS AS TREATMENT

A. K. Shapiro and E. Shapiro describe three categories of placebo therapy (see table 1-2).[6] The first is the deliberate use of inert substances or procedures to treat an illness. Within living memory, physicians, pharmacists, and others maintained a supply of inert pills or "elixirs" to give patients who seemed to require some treatment when a "real" therapy was unavailable or unnecessary. This practice was deemed paternalistic, even deceitful, and is seldom if ever employed now.

TABLE 1-2
Three Categories of Placebo Therapy

Category	Examples	Characteristics
Prescription of inert or inactive treatment	Sugar pill	Healer aware Patient deceived "Paternalistic"
Inadequate dose Inappropriate use "Impure" placebos	Homeopathy Low-dose antispasmodics Vitamins for bodybuilding	Healer may or may not be aware Patient deceived
Treatment erroneously believed to be effective	Many "alternative" treatments Antibiotics for colds	Both healer and patient deceived

A more common placebo category is the use of inappropriate drugs or ineffective dosages of drugs. The latter is characteristic of homeopathy (see chapter 11). Sometimes, doctors consciously or unconsciously use "harmless" doses of drugs as pacifiers. Examples are the use of anticholinergic drugs for gut "spasm" in doses that avoid side effects (indeed any effect), or the too-late use of antihistamines during an asthma attack. Inappropriate use of drugs includes the employment of vitamins for other than nutrition purposes, such as bodybuilding or cold prevention. Another might be the prescription of antibiotics (used against bacteria) for a viral infection such as a cold. The Shapiros euphemistically called such treatments *active* or *impure* placebos.[7]

By far the most common category of placebo use is the deployment of treatments that are erroneously believed to be effective by both healer and patient. This practice is as old as healing itself. Shapiro and

Shapiro provocatively declare that the history of medicine is the history of the placebo response.[8] Many "alterative" therapies fit this category. I will cite other examples throughout this book. Suffice it for now to point to the 1827 importation into France of thirty-three million leeches for treatment purposes. Doctors and patients believed them to be effective so they had exhausted the domestic supply!

When a doctor deliberately prescribes an inactive treatment, the patient is deceived (category 1). When a doctor erroneously prescribes an ineffective drug or dose, both are deceived (category 3). In the prescribing of "impure" placebos, both possibilities exist (category 2).

PLACEBOS IN SCIENCE

Our medical forebears deliberately prescribed inert medication or fanciful devices, knowing intuitively that this made patients feel better. The placebo effect was not approached scientifically, nor was its reality fully appreciated until the advent of controlled clinical trials in the 1930s. If a doctor believes that his treatment is effective, it is more likely to be so, and transient "cures" and their enthusiastic exponents litter the history of medicine. As Sir William Osler wryly observed a century ago, "One should treat as many patients as possible with a new drug while it still has the power to heal."[9]

In our own time, examples of treatments that have failed to sustain their early enthusiasm include dietary fiber to prevent arteriosclerosis (hardening of the arteries), licorice extract to treat gastric ulcers, exotic diet regimens to lose weight, and megavitamins to treat almost everything.

Placebo Effect in Clinical Trials

Figure 1-1 illustrates a hypothetical modern, randomized, double-blind, placebo-controlled clinical trial of a drug developed to treat a chronic painful disease. Such trials provide the scientific basis of rational therapy. Data from properly performed trials are the basis of *evidence-based medicine*. They permit doctors to make therapeutic decisions that help most patients whose medical status fits the conditions of an appropriate trial.

RELIEF OF CHRONIC PAIN

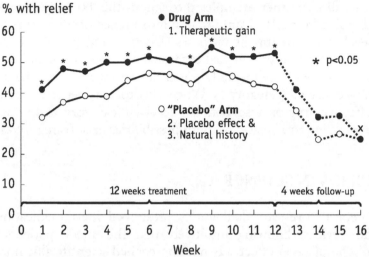

Figure 1-1: Randomized, placebo-controlled trial of a drug in the treatment of a chronic painful condition that illustrates the components of a therapeutic response. The difference between the "relief of symptoms" in the *drug* and "*placebo*" patients is the *therapeutic gain*—in eleven of the twelve weeks, the drug relieved the pain "significantly" better than placebo ($p < .05$). The gain of 10–12 percent seems superficially disappointing. However, it is typical of the therapeutic gains of many drugs approved by regulatory authorities.

Notice the improvement in the "placebo" patients (about 40 percent). Note also that when the drug and placebo are discontinued, the number of subjects experiencing "relief of symptoms" drops dramatically (X), but not to zero. The drop to X may represent the loss of the *placebo effect* in both groups of patients, and the therapeutic gain in the drug-treated patients. *The natural history* of painful conditions is for the pain to fluctuate in intensity. Therefore, the approximately 25 percent end of follow-up improvement over baseline (X) may indicate where the improved subjects would have been had no treatment been given (see text). These two influences, placebo effect and natural improvement (or deterioration), are at work in every successful therapeutic encounter.

Obviously, these powerful improvement tendencies are present in subjects given the test drug as well as those given a placebo. Indeed, were a drug's benefit limited to the therapeutic gain of 10–12 percent, its clinical value would be unimpressive. Healers instinctively utilize these helpful assets: the likelihood of natural improvement and the force of their therapeutic personality to coax maximum benefit from treatment. The natural history of a disease (except when downhill as in terminal cancer) and the placebo effect are exploited in most successful treatments. In many disorders, these two factors may be the most powerful components of a treatment's success. (This illustration will be referred to in future chapters.)[10]

Though we will discuss clinical trials in chapter 7, here we focus on the role of the placebo. Briefly, three features of a randomized, controlled clinical trial are

(1) All entered subjects have a similar illness and are equally likely to fall in either the control (placebo) group or the treatment group (randomization);
(2) The endpoint and measurment of treatment success or failure are decided in advance; and
(3) All engaged parties are unaware (blinded) as to whether an individual subject is receiving the drug to be tested or an inert replica, the so-called placebo. This is a double-blind test.

In the study illustrated in figure 1-1, all the entered subjects had the chronic painful disease under study and weekly recorded whether they had achieved "relief of pain." In random order, each patient was assigned to one of two groups. Those in one group received the drug to be tested and the other an inert substance known as the placebo. Doctors and patients were unaware (blinded) as to which treatment was given. The illustration demonstrates that most weeks, during the treatment period, more patients had pain relief on the drug than on the placebo. The difference between the two is the *therapeutic gain*. Without this difference, it must be concluded that the drug has no (beneficial) effect.

However, in both groups most of the observed improvement was apparently *not* due to the drug. This effect, imprecisely called the *placebo response*, has two main components, the *placebo effect* and the *natural history of the disease*. Since pain intensity tends to fluctuate, some of the study patients would have improved with no treatment at all. In the figure, notice that when the drug is stopped the benefit falls to a point X but not to the baseline. Also, notice the decline in benefit to a similar level (X) when the placebo is stopped. It is tempting to suggest that this fall represents the loss of the placebo effect, and that X represents the subjects' likely status if no treatment had been given (i.e., the improvement attributable to the natural course of the disease). However, it is impossible to say from such a study how much of this nondrug improvement was due to natural history and how much to the therapeutic encounter, that is, the placebo effect. Nonetheless, such data are the most compelling scientific evidence of a placebo effect. Sometimes the term "nonspecific effects" describes other components of the *placebo response* described above. The term is meaningless. Since ill-defined circumstances of treatment and the doctor/patient relationship are inseparable, I shall treat nonspecific effects as part of the *placebo effect*. Indeed, I shall argue that the doctor/patient relationship and the therapeutic circumstances are vital, perhaps necessary determinants of the placebo effect.

Consider the therapeutic equation:

Treatment benefit = Therapeutic gain + Natural history of
illness + Placebo effect

Where

- *Therapeutic gain* = the effect on a patient's symptom or pathological abnormality by the treatment itself, which may be a drug, a diet, a device, a procedure, or a psychological treatment;
- *Natural history* = the state of a patient's symptom or pathological abnormality that would exist at the end of the trial if no treatment were given; and
- *Placebo effect* = a beneficial effect on a patient's symptoms or pathological abnormality that is accounted for neither by the properties of the treatment itself, nor by the natural history of the symptom or disease. This includes so-called nonspecific effects, and has been termed the *true placebo effect*.[11]

Sometimes, investigators refer to the improvement of those in the group taking a placebo as the *placebo response*, and the improving subjects as *placebo responders*. However, this use of "placebo response" includes natural history and other time effects as well as the true placebo effect.[12]

Time Effects

There are other considerations. While many chronic painful disorders have a fluctuating course of relapses and remissions, the exact pattern in an individual is unpredictable. *Regression to the mean* refers to the tendency of an initial symptom severity measure to change toward a mean value during a trial.[13] In other words, patients visit the doctor or enter a clinical trial at a time when their symptoms are active or severe. Subsequently, these symptoms tend to lessen so that whatever intervention has occurred may seem to be beneficial. Conversely, asymptomatic subjects with a chronic painful condition are bound to become symptomatic as they also regress toward the mean. Such subjects would be unsuitable for a treatment trial since some will naturally worsen during the study. However, inclusion of initially symptom-free subjects would be appropriate if investigators were testing a maintenance treatment designed to *prevent* symptoms from occurring. (See chapter 13 for other changes during treatment that may alter the outcome.)

DEFINITION OF A *PLACEBO*

No definition of *placebo* is entirely satisfactory. As illustrated in table 1-1, the meaning has changed many times since Chaucer's day. P. C. Gotzsche has argued that *placebo* cannot be defined in a logically consistent way and leads to contradictions.[14] For example, how can an inert substance have an effect? Nevertheless, we need a starting point if we are to deal rationally with this phenomenon. In this spirit the following definitions will do for now, if we recognize that they are flawed.

> [A]ny therapy prescribed knowingly or unknowingly by a healer, or used by a layman, for its therapeutic effect on a symptom or disease, but which actually is ineffective or not specifically effective for the symptom or disorder being treated.[15]

More important than the placebo is the *placebo effect*. Gotzsche provides the most intellectually satisfying definition of this effect:

> [T]he difference in outcome between a placebo treated group and an untreated group in an unbiased experiment.

Unfortunately, a truly unbiased experiment may be impossible to design. The two groups would clearly and obviously be treated differently—one with a pill or device with expectations of benefit, the other with nothing. Knowing he was in a trial and receiving no treatment could alter a subject's subsequent behavior and responses. "No treatment" is not a placebo treatment. Changing "no treatment" to a placebo changes the dynamic because the subject is getting a "treatment" even if he is unaware of its "inertness."

Howard Brody's definition of the placebo effect is more clinically satisfying:

> [A] change in a patient's illness attributable to the symbolic import of the treatment rather than a specific pharmacologic or physiologic property.[16]

Note that no placebo pill or device is implied here, just the action and circumstances of a healer treating a patient. These definitions imply that the true placebo effect is independent of the natural history of the disease under treatment.

Say "placebo," and most readers immediately think of sugar pills. However, *any* therapy can incorporate placebo effects. Injections, surgery, diet therapy, and herbal medicine may generate them. Throughout history, countless since-discredited devices, procedures, and activities were used for their placebo effects. Moreover, as Brody's definition implies, a placebo effect may even occur with none of these. Indeed, it is the *effect* that is important, not the placebo itself. The sugar pill, the saline injection, or the sham procedure are merely vehicles or symbols.

SUMMARY

Placebos have been employed since the first healer practiced his art, and even today, placebo effects are integral components of any therapy. The meaning of *placebo* has evolved often over eight centuries, yet still defies precise definition. The placebo itself is powerless. Clinical trials best demonstrate placebo effects, but it is difficult to separate their activity from natural changes in the disease or symptom being treated. Any device or practice presented as treatment, or even no physical treatment at all, may elicit a placebo effect. While it is necessary to allude to placebos, the subject of interest is the placebo *effect*.

CHAPTER 2

HISTORY OF PLACEBOS

"[U]ntil recently, the history of medical treatment is
essentially the history of the placebo effect."

A. K. SHAPIRO AND E. SHAPIRO (1999)[1]

Placebos are the oldest treatments that are prescribed by the second-oldest profession. Doubtless, the offerings of the oldest profession have placebo effects, too! Since the beginning of history, important people in societies, whom we might now recognize as healers or doctors, gave treatments to the ill. With very few exceptions, we know that these treatments had no intrinsic healing power—indeed, we have found that many were very harmful. What all these treatments had in common was that the persons receiving them, and usually the healer himself, believed they might do some good.

HEALING IN PRIMITIVE SOCIETIES[2]

Primitive societies needed to explain the natural world and the social interactions within their societies. Lacking knowledge, they were unable to explain the natural disasters that befell them, such as droughts, floods, lightning, and apocalyptic events such as earthquakes and hurricanes. Moreover, life was brutish and short—death ever-present and inexplicable. Yet as rational beings, primitive peoples knew something of cause and effect. They could understand injury from a fall, or death in battle. They knew some success depended on their own efforts at hunting, gathering, and later agriculture. Yet much of their experience was unavoidable and terrifying. Among the disasters that stalked them were disease and death. These, too, must have a cause. The two forces, a terrifying natural world and the need to explain it, led almost all early societies to believe that spirits or ghosts were somehow responsible. The spirits were part of an imaginary environment created to explain the natural world. Whether the spirits were inside the body, lurking in the forests or residing in the heavens, they were fearsome and must be appeased. Given the creativity of men and women, it is not surprising that primitive worldviews and the spirits themselves took many forms. Ceremonies to appease the spirits occurred in almost all recorded cultures and tribes, and were prompted by imagination and faith rather than science. These ancient rituals and practices reverberate in modern cultures and religions, and, of course, in the healing arts.

Since it was beyond the capabilities of individuals to deal with the spirits, almost all societies evolved powerful personages known to anthropologists as *shamans*, *medicine men*, or other titles, depending upon the tribe or culture (table 2-1). In most cases, they were concerned with tribal affairs such as rainmaking, hunting fortunes, planting rites, and even in planning wars, but here, we are concerned only with their roles as medicine men. In many societies, the power and influence of the medicine man or woman exceeded that of the tribal chief.

TABLE 2-1
Names of Healers in Some Cultures

Healer	Tribe or Culture
Shaman	Siberia (also adopted for the description of similar people in other cultures)
Medicine Man	North American Indians
Ganga	Zulus
Bablawo	Afro-Cuban Santeria
Angahak	Inuit
Curandero	Mexico

What these preliterate healers had in common was a tribe or society vulnerable to disease and early death, ignorance of pathology, a fearful clientele who believed in their powers to heal, and a vivid imagination with which to confront the menacing natural world. Among societies, the healers' methods, rituals, and symbols attest to the limitlessness of the human imagination, and their range and variability fill texts of medical anthropology. What is important to our discussion is that the medicine men held positions as healers in their societies similar to those of the healing professions in ours. Early physicians used methods, rituals, and symbols not unlike those of our primitive ancestors. Modern equivalents are white coats, diplomas, medical instruments, and antiseptic smells. Only the evolution of medical science, beginning with the Enlightenment occurring in the seventeenth and eighteenth centuries and culminating in evidence-based medicine, distinguishes the modern doctor from the ancient shaman.

Medicine today has two fundamental components. The first is based on science. Great discoveries such as the circulation of the blood, vaccination, anesthesia, antisepsis, and the microbial basis of infectious diseases transformed medicine from the magical and fanciful treatments of Hippocrates and Galen to actions based upon an understanding of pathology. This understanding was a necessary prelude to the effective prevention and treatment of disease. Yet some ancient and harmful treatments persisted well into the twentieth century. In his 1923 book *The Medicine Man*,[3] J. L. Maddox describes the shamans and sorcery of primitive societies. This work cited therapeutic agencies such as prayer, incantation, conjuration, and bloodletting that have been employed throughout history. Ironically, he states that bloodletting was (in 1923) applied by "the most progressive of physicians in cases of apoplexy [stroke], pneumonia, typhoid fever and other complaints," where it in reality could do nothing but harm! In truth, the only rational use for therapeutic bloodletting was to temporarily relieve the pressure on the heart in congestive heart failure, and that use was rendered obsolete by the development of effective diuretics after World War II. Thus, Maddox acknowledges the shamans of our own culture. Like their primitive counterparts, these professionals ignored science in their treatments, relying on faith and unknowingly on the placebo effect to overcome bloodletting's harmful effects.

Maddox believed that the medicine man or shaman in preliterate societies possessed certain qualities.[4] In some cases, the office was hereditary, for example, among the Zulus of South Africa. Among the Navahos, the youngest son was chosen because, compared to others, he had more intellect and a better memory. Analogous to modern medicine or religion is "the call" in which an individual is deemed to have been chosen for his profession. Such people were believed to be in touch with their ancestors and often demonstrated this by peculiar behaviors. Ambitious parents pushed their offspring forward. (How many modern doctors were created thus?) Sometimes after the loss of a child, the next born was put forward for spiritual office. Physical attributes might denote special powers. Individuals with these charac-teristics included albinos, twins, eunuchs, the blind, and those born by breech delivery. People who had narrow escapes from death also impressed primitive societies. Those who were insane, or who had convulsions or meaningful dreams may have seemed possessed, or invested with a certain charisma that equipped them to deal with spirits. As an extension of this, some priests feigned fits or took hallu-cinogens to symbolize their contact with the supernatural. Others, like those at Delphi, were considered to have great intellect and inspired sufficient awe to become sages for illness and other matters.

A shaman's training often required long periods of solitude and abstinence, including celibacy. During this time, older medicine men passed on the secrets of sorcery and magic, and taught the elaborate rituals that accompanied their treatments. Often a special ritual marked the installation of a newly qualified shaman into office. These activities have their equivalents in a modern doctor's training and ini-tiation into professional societies. We may take a disdainful view of the naïveté of the shaman's qualifications, but we cannot ignore the importance of a doctor's stature. The symbolism and rituals of modern medicine, the long training and personal denial of the chosen few, the formalities of graduation and certification, and even the white coat contribute to that stature. The doctor's image as an authoritative figure has healing potential—the power to relieve anxiety and give hope that illness can be conquered.

ANCIENT REMEDIES

The treatments employed in early civilizations were many and often sophisticated. Some treatments, like acupuncture, bloodletting, leeches, faith healing, and Freudian psychiatry, have great cultural or literary meaning. Some survive to this day. Shapiro points out that the Chinese emperor Huang Ti mentions more than two thousand drugs and sixteen thousand prescriptions used without change for twenty-five hundred years. They had traditions that could not be supplanted. These, along with the remedies of ancient Sumeria, Babylon, Egypt, India, Greece, and many others, account for an almost infinite number of archaic treatment possibilities that could exist only because people believed they alleviated symptoms and suffering. Hippocratic medicine included more than two hundred remedies. The pharmacopoeia of his Roman successor Galen contained eight hundred twenty remedies (galenicals) that dominated European medicine for fifteen hundred years and only vanished with the appearance of medical science in the nineteenth century. While insisting on the infallibility of his treatments, Galen had the foresight to add these words to his formulary, "He cures most successfully in whom the people have the most confidence." The history of medicine is indeed the history of the placebo response.

MODERN ATTITUDES[5]

Earlier, we traced the evolution of the meaning of *placebo* from "I shall please," through professional mourners, synchophants, inert pills "to please the patient," and ending with dummy pills to control for "non-specific" effects in clinical trials (see table 1–1). For only the last two hundred years has the word had medical connotations. Nevertheless, it seems certain that almost all ancient remedies were placebos at best. Twentieth-century pharmacopoeias still listed many of these traditional cure-alls, and they have fallen only slowly into disuse.

Prior to World War II, the deliberate use of inert pills was part of everyday medicine. Thomas Jefferson might have condoned the use of placebos, but to the modern ethical physician, the practice is "a great deceiver, a misrepresenter, a creator of illusions."[6] Now, most physicians associate *placebos* with clinical trials. However, rejection of placebos need not sacrifice ethical employment of the placebo effect with effective therapy.

As a result of its tortuous past, the term *placebo* evokes diverse, yet strongly held, responses from students of various disciplines, and the societies from which they spring (see table 2-2). Some of these firmly held views close rather than open doors of understanding. For the scientist, the placebo is incredible. It cannot be touched or measured, and appears to confound the scientific method. Placebo effects cannot be captured and examined in a laboratory. Briefly elated by the news that *endorphins* mediated the effects of placebos,[7] scientists returned to incredulity, unable to explain how an inert substance or sham procedure could activate endorphins in the first place.

TABLE 2-2
Attitudes Toward Placebos[8]

Scientists	"incredible"
Trialists	"obstacle"
Philosophers	"undefinable"
Ethicists	"culpable"
Charlatans	"convertible" ($)
Politicians, Administrators	"incomprehensible"
Psychologists	"inevitable"
Physicians	"indispensable"

Contemporary physicians, students, and others can be forgiven if they associate placebos only with clinical trials. Indeed, these trials have made the word respectable. Moreover, a survey of modern medical texts, including *Harrison's Principles of Internal Medicine*, discovers no entry under *placebo* or *placebo effect*. If the word appears, it is only to acknowledge a drug's evaluation in a placebo-controlled clinical trial.

In clinical trials of chronic painful conditions, the placebo response (including placebo effect and natural history) is 20 to 70 percent with a mean of about 45 percent. Those conducting such trials often consider this phenomenon to be an obstacle—an artifact that obscures the true value of a treatment under study.[9] Clinical trial investigators have attempted to weed out so-called placebo responders through a pretrial test period in which prospective subjects who respond to the placebo are removed from the trial. However, this procedure fails to reduce the placebo response among those who remain in the trial. Moreover, the deliberate selection of placebo nonresponders introduces a bias that impedes the generalizability of the trial's results.[10] When marketing a drug, pharmaceutical representatives tend to play down the placebo effect. They explain that the data from trials would show the benefit of the drug to a greater advantage if the effect could be eliminated. This attitude is incorrect and counterproductive. The natural tendency of most disease is to improve in time. Beyond that, placebo effects are important to the "success" of any treatment and deserve to be exploited rather than denied.

Philosophers also find placebos confounding:[11] "A placebo is inert! How can an inert substance have an effect?" Surely, *placebo effect* is an oxymoron! They conclude that it is impossible to define a placebo, and like scientists, they despair to explain them. Trained in Cartesian logic and accustomed to exploring natural and tangible problems, many physicians also struggle to understand the intangible placebo.

The use of placebos sparks ethical debates. These center upon the notion that, while well intended, the placebo effect rests on paternalism and deceit. As we shall explore later, this is an oversimplification. Placebos may benefit people without deceit, even in our politically correct and need-to-know environment.

Conundrums to some, placebos are opportunities to many. Charlatans thrive on the placebo effect and would vanish without it. Of course, most of those proposing medical or so-called alternative therapies are not charlatans. They firmly believe in the effectiveness of their ministrations, thereby further enhancing the placebo effects.

Administrators manage health-care programs in ignorance of this effect. Yet health-care decisions made without considering the benefit of effective doctor/patient relationships ignore an important determinant of successful medical care. If health policy decisions fail to take the potential of the placebo effect into account, they risk eliciting harmful or *nocebo* effects. Escalating costs and health-care management problems may owe more to this phenomenon than is appreciated.

Even psychologists, who should best understand placebos, seldom mention them. Whatever the view, the placebo effect exists, and understanding it is important to modern medicine. Wise doctors know that it is a factor in every treatment and an essential part of their daily work. These ideas recur in the chapters that follow.

SUMMARY AND CONCLUSIONS

Placebos are the oldest treatments. Initially intuitive and paternalistic, the placebo concept has entered the twenty-first century with self-conscious uncertainty and a diaspora of attitudes. Once simply a "method of medicine" among other treatments (few of which were effective), the placebo became a device to satisfy patients, and later a deceit worthy of disdain. Meanwhile, the word *placebo* was hijacked to describe a "control" in a therapeutic trial, thereby substantially shifting its meaning. Throughout, placebos have "lurked in the shadows of biomedical understanding."[12] Does the placebo effect explain a mechanism in the psychophysiological sense, or does a placebo simply provide "meaning" for the ill and for society? Many believe the answer is both.[13]

CHAPTER 3

PLACEBO RESEARCH: SOME FACTS AND MYTHS

I have explained the origin of the word *placebo*, and described the history of treatments that we now know have no intrinsic therapeutic benefit, yet exploit the placebo effect. Placebos can be any therapeutic device from the lowly sugar pill to sham surgery. Even effective treatments exert placebo effects beyond their inherent healing power. It is not the placebo that is important, but rather the *placebo effect* that is generated when any treatment is presented to a patient. Nevertheless, we have little systematic knowledge of placebo effects—only a medley of seemingly unrelated facts accompanied by enduring and meddlesome myths. The facts are arresting but incomplete. Perhaps some contain the seeds of our greater understanding. The myths betray the mystique of the placebo effect and confuse rather than clarify our understanding.

THE STUDY OF PLACEBOS

The scientific study of the placebo effect poses formidable challenges. Not the least of these are the negative attitudes of some scientists toward placebos (see table 2-1), and the apparent indifference of those who ought to make the most use of the placebo effect, that is, practitioners of the healing arts and managers of health-care programs. Anecdotes and the tendency of the symptoms naturally to change confound our understanding of placebo effects. Finally, ethical considerations must govern placebo research.

The Influence of the Anecdote

The placebo effect on the subjective experiences of illness is greater than on objective manifestations of disease. A child with a broken arm may find a measure of pain relief through the sympathy of a comforting parent, but no observable improvement in the fracture itself. There are many widely circulated anecdotes of miracle cancer cures from many sorts of treatments by many types of healers. However, few of these survive scrutiny by independent observers, and the "cures" are never repeated in any predictable way. How can we explain the few? Often the diagnosis was in error. If there was no cancer after all, any treatment might look like a cure! Another possible explanation is the innate unpredictability of all biological processes, including cancer. Respected researchers state they have never seen the spontaneous cure of cancer or other life-threatening disease they could attribute to a placebo effect. The enthusiastic but unverifiable convictions of some that they have discovered the cure for cancer can be a cruel hoax if it causes victims to make futile, painful, and expensive choices in their treatment. (Some examples appear in chapter 16.)

Anecdotal examples of miracle cures abound in the popular press. Typical headlines are: "The Doctor Gave Him Only 6 Months, but Dr. Jones' Diet Gave Him a Lifetime"; or "Conventional Medicine Failed, but Faith in Acupuncture Saved Her." Missing from such reports are the cured patient's pathological details and the stories of similar cases where the same treatment failed. Nonetheless, making a person *feel* better is an important accomplishment even if the disease process itself is unchecked. There can be a substantial placebo effect on the pain from arthritis or coronary heart disease without demonstrable improvement in the affected joints or heart. The greatest placebo successes occur in the treatment of chronic painful conditions with no observable disease, such as headache, backache, and the irritable bowel syndrome.

Healing is a topic where the anecdote serves us ill. Individual stories prove little and have great capacity to mislead. If we are to understand treatment, and the contributions of faith, positive thinking, or other human attributes, two cohorts of similarly afflicted patients should be studied: a treated group and a control group. It is unscientific and deceitful for a healer to publicize a single, miraculous cure, when many thousands of others can hope for no measurable benefit from his ministrations. Nevertheless, the true miracle is that, without deceit, those same thousands can be given hope and encouragement—valuable commodities when one is seriously ill. If given without misrepresentation in a positive and caring manner, most treatments may help many patients. There are important distinctions between the dispensation of hope rather than deceit, as there are between the caring and the charlatan.

Confounding Natural History

The phenomenon that most bedevils our understanding of the effect of placebo effects is the natural history of the disease being treated. Most conditions may improve, at least temporarily. From trial data, it is impossible to determine how much of the observed improvement in patients receiving "inert" pills is due to the placebo effect and how much represents the natural history of their disease. Some say this answer would be forthcoming if all clinical trials included a third group randomized to receive no treatment at all. They explain the difference between the improvement on placebo and on nothing should surely be the true placebo effect. This would be true if this no-treatment group were subject only to the natural history of the disease. However, selection into a trial and the verbal, investigative, and monitoring interventions during the trial ensure that the subsequent course is not "natural." (The next chapter discusses comparisons of placebo-treated and no-treatment patients in clinical trials.)

When a person with a chronic painful condition is treated with a painkilling drug, his subsequent improvement is the sum of the unknown contributions of pharmacological effect, placebo effect, and the natural course of the pain. In an individual, the relative importance of these is impossible to know. A treatment could have a negative effect, yet the patient experiences less pain because the placebo and natural history effects were sufficiently positive to overcome the harm. Why else would our ancestors adopt bloodletting, drastic purges, and arsenic pills, when we now know that their potential for harm outweighs any possible benefit?

The Ethical Challenge

In clinical trials, the withholding of treatment that might benefit a patient is a legitimate concern. Placebos are unjustified if there is an *effective* drug for the disease for which a new drug is being tested, especially if withholding the effective one might harm the patient. Then, the already-proven drug may serve as the control or comparison for the new one. For some disorders, experts may determine that no treatment is sufficiently effective to serve as a "gold standard." When there is no acceptable alternative treatment, placebo controls face no ethical proscription.

When faced with practical and ethical difficulties, clinical investigators often turn to animal research. Animal experiments might help evaluate the pharmacology of drugs, trace neural pathways, and identify chemical transmitters. However, such experiments can do little to help us understand the natural history of human symptoms. Lacking the intellectual and linguistic characteristics that characterize humanity, animals are infertile soil for the study of placebo effects. (For more on the ethical implications of placebo use, see chapter 14.)

FACTS ABOUT PLACEBOS

The Mode of Administration

A placebo is a vehicle used by a healer to elicit a placebo effect. We have discussed the practical and philosophical paradoxes of an inert substance or activity having a treatment effect. Nevertheless, it appears that nature and the circumstances of the placebo's administration can influence the degree of a therapy's effect. In short, *how* may be more important than *what*!

A placebo administered by a doctor appears to be more powerful than one given by a nurse or a clerk. A placebo (or any medicine) sent in the mail, devoid of human interaction, is least effective. In trials, the more frequently the patient visits the physician during the study period, the greater the placebo effect.[1] The more attention paid to a patient when he first visits the doctor for a symptom, the more satisfactory will be the result.[2]

The presentation of inert treatments can convey or symbolize healing power. A placebo injection is more powerful than a placebo pill. A large pill is more effective than a small pill,[3] but a very small pill is better than a regular-sized pill. To demonstrate some nonpharmacological effects, medical students in a pharmacology class were enrolled in the following experiment.[4] In a lecture, the students were prepared to expect either stimulant or sedative effects. They then were divided into four groups, each receiving one or two inert pills that were either pink or blue. Thirty percent of the students noted mood changes. The blue pills sedated and the pink pills excited. Two pills had a greater effect than one. This observation was not an accident. S. P. Buckalew and K. E. Coffield found that capsules were more effective than tablets, and that white was associated with painkilling and yellow with stimulant and antidepressant effects.[5] K. Shapira and associates found that that yellow pills are best for depression and green ones for anxiety.[6]

Thus, the appearance of an inert treatment can symbolically convey the notion of healing, and affect the recipient's response. The symbolism embodied in a surgical procedure, psychotherapy, or even acupuncture can heal (see chapters 9–11). Some claim these phenomena are due to salesmanship or mysticism, but it is a rare person who is forever immune to the symbolism of treatment, with or without a pill.

Endorphins and the Relief of Pain

Placebo pain relief (analgesia) can be blocked by the narcotic antagonist *naloxone*, giving rise to the notion that placebos can relieve pain by releasing *endorphins* (natural opium-like substances in the body).[7] In light of this information, should we shout "eureka" and celebrate the solution of the placebo mystery? We should not! Despite its promise to confirm a scientist's dream that all human phenomena have physical or chemical explanations, the endorphin story falls short. Activation of the body's opiate activity may relieve pain, but it is unlikely to affect other symptoms such as nausea, constipation, itching, trembling, depression, and others. To be sure, there are myriad neurons, receptors, and transmitters in the nervous system that might act on other symptoms as endorphins do on pain.[8] The gut hormone cholecystokinin, neurotransmitters such as serotonin, and catacholamines are possible candidates. However, there is little information bearing on their possible role in the placebo effect.

There has been some improvement in our understanding of how placebo effects occur. Italian investigators carefully implanted electrodes into individual brain cells of the subthalamic nucleus of eleven patients with Parkinson's disease.[9] These patients had relief of muscular rigidity following apomorphine administration. Subsequently, they were given a saline infusion as treatment along with verbal suggestions of muscle improvement, and subsequently six demonstrated less muscular rigidity. Unlike in the five unimproved patients, activity in their subthalamic neurons decreased. In this case, placebo administration into a brain cell mimicked the therapeutic effects of effective medication such as L-Dopa.

Recent functional magnetic resonance imaging (fMRI) experiments have found that placebo analgesia is related to decreased brain activity in pain-sensitive regions of the brain known as the thalamus, insula, and anterior cingulate cortex.[10] Pain relief was also associated with increased activity in the prefrontal cortex (where thinking occurs) during anticipation of pain, suggesting that placebos act on pain-sensitive areas of the brain to alter the painful experience. These experiments suggest a physiological mechanism for the placebo effect.

Even supposing the biochemical mediation or brain pathways of symptom relief were elucidated, we would still need to understand how the giving of a placebo could activate such a process. With or without endorphins, by what means can the therapeutic employment of an inert substance, fanciful device, or empathetic encounter set endorphins or other mediators in motion? Do placebos alter sensory pain transmission, or do they alter expectations?

Disclosure and the Placebo Effect

Perhaps surprisingly, placebos can be effective even if the subject is aware of their nature.[11] In one study, pre- and postoperative instruction and encouragement of surgical patients reduced narcotic requirements by half and lessened the required hospital stay.[12] Not so surprisingly, patients must be aware they are receiving treatment in order to benefit fully. Following chest surgery, when pain from the chest incision (thoracotomy) was severe, forty-two patients were given morphine through their intravenous lines.[13] Twenty-one of them were told when the injection occurred, while the injection was concealed from the others. Pain relief was greatest in those who were aware they were receiving treatment. This information suggests the importance of the manner in which a healer administers care, rather than the particular vehicle or symbol she employs. Indeed, she can achieve the effect with no placebo at all. Disclosure could make the use of placebos ethical, but good doctor/patient interactions could eliminate the need for them altogether.

The Case for Disease Benefits

While placebo effects can powerfully heal symptoms, and make ill people feel better, there is little proof that they alter disease processes in humans. Rats immunosuppressed by the drug cyclophosphamide in saccharine water become immunosuppressed again when the saccharine is subsequently administered alone.[14] This and other animal experiments suggest that physiologic responses to inert treatments can be conditioned. Conditioning is difficult to demonstrate in people. The evidence that a placebo effect can lower blood pressure is mixed. If a placebo is substituted for an antihypertensive drug, the blood pressure remains lower than if the drug were simply stopped.[15] Some studies report an improvement in blood pressure in patients receiving placebos during trials of antihypertensive drugs. However, there may be other factors at work. The person taking the blood pressure may get better at it, or the patient himself may be anxious at first and have a spuriously high initial pressure (*white coat effect*). Using intra-arterial pressure measurements as controls, investigators have found that an apparent reduction of blood pressure by placebo treatment was not so.[16]

A review of trials of various treatments for angina pectoris (chest pain due to heart disease) determined that placebos sometimes appear to improve objective measures such as exercise tolerance, electrocardiographic abnormalities, and nitroglycerine requirements. Skeptics would urge caution here. Angina, like many conditions, follows an irregular course, and spontaneous remission rates occur.[17] Sometimes, the chest pain may be due to something else. Experience may improve a patient's motivation and skill in the performance of the exercise tests designed to assess treatment outcomes.

There are data to support the notion that mood and personality can have physical effects. In the elderly, depression after the loss of a spouse may hasten death.[18] Depression reduces a person's immunity and resistance to infection. Even stool size appears to be subject to such influences. In one study, positive, outgoing personality traits were associated with high stool output—perhaps the mark of an extrovert.[19] By improving mood, a placebo treatment might alter physiology. However, it is doubtful that placebo treatments have curative power for serious anatomic disease. In many diseases, spontaneous remissions do occur. Relief of anxiety may reduce some of the chemical mediators responsible for hypertension. We can imagine that an optimistic attitude, faith, or even paternalistic encouragement can improve the outcome of any condition. Nevertheless, subjective symptoms are more susceptible to placebo effects than objective pathology.

Surgery as Placebo

The placebo response is not unique to medicine. Surgery is also a powerful symbol of healing. How else can one explain the apparent improvement of symptoms following removal of a normal gall bladder or appendix? Chapter 9 includes examples of operations widely believed to relieve pain that in blinded studies performed no better than a sham incision. Many of these studies show that about a third of both the surgically treated and the sham-operated patients improved, and that the benefit appeared to last three months.

Is Placebo Therapy a Form of Psychotherapy?

Psychological therapy is very difficult to evaluate because it is nearly impossible to devise a suitable control treatment. Can one demonstrate a psychiatric placebo effect? One editorialist suggested that psychotherapy might itself be a placebo.[20]

Psychotherapeutic procedures include not only formal psychotherapy as practiced by Freud and his disciples, but also cognitive therapy in which a trained therapist attempts to improve the way a patient views his symptoms, and hypnotism, which relies on suggestion. In each case, the treatment is a human interaction greatly influenced by the therapist's personality, conviction, and enthusiasm. These issues make it difficult to design randomized, controlled trials of psychotherapy treatments. How can a therapist's enthusiasm for a test treatment be fairly applied to the control? An alternative is to compare the test therapy with an established one. Since most available treatments are themselves untested, the trial would be a comparison of two unknowns. (We take up this argument again in chapter 10.)

MYTHS ABOUT PLACEBOS

Extinction

From surgical data alluded to above, many believe that the placebo effect becomes extinct by three months.[21] The three-month benefit is common after sham operations. Inadvertent removal of a normal gall bladder is said to improve unrelated functional abdominal pain for about that time. However, in trials of treatments for panic,[22] angina,[23] and rheumatoid arthritis,[24] placebo effects continue up to thirty months. In a yearlong clinical trial of a treatment for a chronic bowel problem, the placebo effect was sustained throughout.[25] It is another myth to attribute a lingering improvement after placebo therapy solely to the placebo effect. It may have more to do with the natural history of the treated condition.

The Placebo Responder

In the 1950s Henry Beecher attempted to identify "placebo responders."[26] He failed! (See chapter 13.) The placebo effect is uninfluenced by intelligence or any test of susceptibility. Individuals may respond differently in different circumstances. The phenomenon is even demonstrable in volunteers. The placebo effect is greatest for minor illnesses, when stress has a role, and when the symptoms fluctuate. Adherence (compliance) is also important—failure to take the placebo pills lessens their effect. Some claim that analytical thinking may inhibit the placebo effect.

Some investigators, citing trial and surgical data, once believed that about one-third of people are "placebo responders." In clinical trials, they employed initial placebo "run-in periods" to identify the responders and exclude them from the subsequent trial. However, there is no evidence that this creates a less susceptible study group. From time to time, individuals vary in their placebo responsiveness.

K. B. Thomas described the "temporarily dependent patient" whose illness is neither physical nor psychological yet responds to a "positive" treatment approach.[27] On any occasion, it is impossible to predict when an individual will experience a placebo benefit. Circumstances, mood, patient/doctor interaction, and the disease itself may influence the response. The placebo responder is a mythical figure.

It seems logical that a fluctuating, nonstructural, benign condition like functional dyspepsia (upper abdominal pain without pathology) might be more susceptible to a placebo benefit than a structural condition like a peptic ulcer, which has similar symptoms plus a "crater" in the lining of the stomach. Nevertheless, in the placebo arms of clinical trials of ulcer drugs, about a third of peptic ulcers heal in four to six weeks. Ulcers also wax and wane, so we cannot be certain how much healing would occur without placebo treatment. As always, the natural history and regression to the mean are important. Sometimes "placebo responders" are simply due to get better.

The Hawthorne Effect

The "Hawthorne effect" describes an improvement in performance that results from the mere circumstance of "being studied." In a Western Electric manufacturing plant named Hawthorne, worker productivity improved when illumination was increased, but paradoxically did so again when the lighting was decreased. The explanation (since questioned)[28] was that the attention paid to the subjects by the investigators made the difference, not the lighting. Such attention undoubtedly influences a person's expectation of treatment and the notion of a "Hawthorne effect" survives. While the original conclusions may be myth, it seems very likely that close observation during a clinical trial can alter symptoms. Therefore, what is observed in a control group is not "natural" history.

"Unable to Demonstrate Benefit Because of High Placebo Response Rate"

It is a feature of the clinical trial business that the therapeutic gain often appears small in relation to the placebo and natural history effects. The trial noted in figure 1-1 is a good example. The usual regulatory hurdle requires that this gain is statistically significant—that is, that statistical tests show that the drug effect is greater than that of placebo. Critics often ask if this statistical significance translates into "clinical significance." In other words, is the observed statistical difference of any importance to patients? There are statistical devices to help determine this, but it is more a matter of judgment. Contemplating a seemingly small therapeutic gain, treatment advocates often lament that the many subjects responding to the placebo obscure the real benefits of their product.

This is another myth. The reason for blinded placebo controls is to level the playing field and ensure that a treatment's benefit is not exaggerated by the otherwise-unknown contributions of placebo effect and natural history. Under the circumstances of a properly designed study, these contributions should be identical in the treatment and placebo arms. The placebo effect is not the enemy. It is in everyone's interest to encourage it with every treatment.

CONCLUSION

Anecdotes, capricious disease progression, and ethical restraints hamper research into placebo effects. Any attempt to compare treatments to "no treatment" without blinding exposes a study to bias. Nevertheless, placebo effects exist and can result from effective healer/patient interaction. Placebo benefit is possible even when the subject knows that the treatment is inert or ineffective. *How* a treatment is given is sometimes more important than *what* is given. The interaction between the healer and the sufferer seems vital, but symbolism is also important. Even mundane considerations, such as the color and size of a pill, the mode of its delivery, the effects of previous treatments, and the frequency of doctor visits conspire to determine placebo effects. In contrast to these facts, several placebo myths have crept into the medical vernacular. An inert pill is not itself responsible for the placebo effect. Neither the longevity of the placebo effect nor the identification of "placebo responders" is predictable. The placebo effect does not obscure treatment benefits; rather, it should enhance them.

CHAPTER 4

THE PLACEBO EFFECT

"The doctor who fails to have a placebo effect on his
patients should become a pathologist."

J. N. BLAU (1985)[1]

A placebo is commonly thought to be a thing: that is, a pill, a device, or a procedure that is employed by a healer to help an ill person. However, it is more instructive to think of a placebo's *effect*: that is, the effect of a treatment that goes beyond its intended pharmacological or physiological activity. A. K. Shapiro and E. Shapiro said that the history of medical treatment is the history of the placebo effect because most medical treatments employed before the mid-twentieth century are now known to be ineffective.[2] The results of modern clinical trials provide a scientific basis for much of what contemporary doctors do. Nevertheless, for many diseases, there are few certified treatment options. Alternative therapies and much of conventional medicine rely on placebo effects. Before we explore this subject further, we must revisit the therapeutic equation.

THERAPEUTIC EQUATION

As explained earlier, the apparent effect of any treatment is expressed by the equation:

Treatment benefit = Therapeutic gain + Natural history of
illness + Placebo effect

Where

- *Therapeutic gain* = the effect on a patient's symptom or pathological abnormality by the treatment itself, which may be a drug, a diet, a device, a procedure, or a psychological treatment;
- *Natural history* = the state of a patient's symptom or pathological abnormality that would exist at the end of the trial if no treatment were given; and
- *Placebo effect* = a beneficial effect on a patient's symptoms or pathological abnormality that is not accounted for by the properties of the treatment itself, nor by the natural history of the symptom or disease. This includes so-called nonspecific effects, and has been termed the *true placebo effect*.[3]

These three components of a treatment's effects should be kept in mind as we consider the following.

THE CASE AGAINST PLACEBOS

Some recent reviews argue against any placebo effect.[4] They criticize the conclusions of a controversial paper by Henry Beecher in 1955 entitled *The Powerful Placebo*.[5] Beecher enthusiastically endorsed the notion that by modifying subjective responses to a symptom, placebos have beneficial effects on patients. In his article, Beecher cited fifteen studies where, in 35 percent of subjects, symptoms such as headache, cough, wound pain, or seasickness were "satisfactorily relieved by placebo." He suggested that placebo treatments might act "on the reaction or processing component of suffering as opposed to their effect on the original sensation." He went on to say that placebos are most effective when a patient's stress is greatest.

However, Beecher made no allowance for the natural history of the symptoms under study. In a 1997 critique of Beecher's paper, G. S. Kienle and H. Kiene describe these and other characteristics of Beecher's fifteen studies that could account for the 35 percent response rate.[6] Spontaneous improvement and symptom fluctuation are part of natural history and must explain improvement in some cases. Kienle and Kiene also point out that Beecher failed to account for the deterioration in some patients that offsets improvement in others. In a treatment trial of the common cold, improvement in six days was considered a positive result, ignoring the obvious fact that most colds normally resolve themselves by then. In other studies, the placebo-treated patients received additional treatments, such as nitrates for angina pectoris, which could account for some of their improvement. In another angina pectoris trial, the protocol called for switching from placebo to active treatment if angina increased, thus removing the treatment failures from the placebo group and exaggerating the apparent placebo effect. In some of Beecher's fifteen citations, Kienle and Kiene believe there is a possibility that the subjects sought to please the investigator. They also point out other design flaws such as severity scales favoring a positive answer (e.g., "much better," "better," "a little better," "the same," "worse," offer three positive choices to one negative), and irrelevant outcomes (e.g., "Do you feel better?" after antihypertension medication). Table 4-1 summarizes the factors that Kienle and Kiene claim could exaggerate the magnitude of the placebo effect in Beecher's citations.

TABLE 4-1
Some Factors that Falsely Appear to Increase the Placebo Effect[7]

Natural history of disease
- spontaneous improvement
- fluctuation of symptoms
- regression to the mean (tendency of symptoms to improve)

Additional treatment permitted by the trial protocol

Observer bias
- conditional switching of treatment if placebo fails
- scaling bias
- poor definition of drug efficacy

Irrelevant response variables (e.g., relief of headaches in hypertension trial)

Patient bias
- polite answer to please the investigator
- conditioned answers
- neurotic or psychotic misjudgment

These criticisms are important and embrace many of the issues that complicate clinical trials and the understanding of placebo effects. The factors listed in the table must be controlled if a comparison of placebo and treatment effects is to be free of bias. Natural history and other changes over time should be acknowledged when discussing the magnitude of placebo effects. Kienle and Keine perform a service in pointing out these confounding factors, but fail to disprove the presence of an important placebo effect in successful therapeutic encounters. Data from preceding (and subsequent) chapters in this book should satisfy most people that such an effect exists—albeit less powerful than Beecher suggested.

Many claim that if only we could subtract the effect of "no treatment" from the observed placebo response, we could eliminate the effect of natural history and accurately estimate the true placebo effect. Two Danish doctors, A. Hrobjartsson and P. C. Gotzsche, performed a systematic review of clinical trials that included a group that received placebo and another that received no treatment.[8] Many of these trials were testing a treatment, but for the purposes of their review, only data from the placebo and "no treatment" groups were processed. Hrobjartsson and Gotzsche were able to find 114 clinical trials that included both placebo and no-treatment groups.[9] They further subdivided these into thirty-two with *binary* (yes/no) outcomes and eighty-two with *continuous* outcomes (compared values). Each of these were subdivided into trials with subjective outcomes and those with outcomes that were recorded by an unbiased observer. The main findings of this review are that there was no benefit of placebo over "no treatment" in the studies with binary outcomes or in those where the outcomes were objective. The placebo performed better in continuous outcome trials, especially if there were few subjects. In the seventeen trials where pain relief was the outcome measure, the placebo was significantly superior to "no treatment," but the absolute improvement was small. Hrobjartsson and Gotzsche have updated their data with forty-two more recent trials that confirmed their earlier conclusions.[10] The authors' claim that their results do not support Beecher's hypothesis frustrated some experts.

Some greeted this paper with dismay. In an editorial in the same issue of the *New England Journal of Medicine*, John Bailar says, "Some myths ought to be true."[11] He compares the findings of Hrobjartsson and Gotzsche to those of Toto, the little dog in *The Wizard of Oz* who found upon looking behind a curtain that the wizard was just an ordinary man. Bailar suggests that the Danes' conclusions are too sweeping. Despite the difficulties inherent in such a review, the authors did find some placebo effect with pain and other subjective symptoms. The lack of statistical power to examine subgroups and the great variety (heterogeneity) of the results defy interpretation. Many of the trials themselves were designed to test treatments and not the placebo response, and many were of poor quality.

In another commentary, R. L. Koretz reminds us of the powerful evidence for a placebo effect reported elsewhere, for example, the results of sham surgery in the treatment of angina (see chapter 9).[12] As Hrobjartsson and Gotszche themselves state, their data do not permit an assessment of the doctor/patient relationship in the placebo and "no treatment" groups. While they separate this relationship from the placebo effect, Koretz believes (as do I) that the interaction between healer and patient is an integral part of the effect. Both Bailar and Koretz are unconvinced by Hrobjartsson and Gotszche's conclusions, but everyone agrees there is no justification for deliberate placebo treatments outside clinical trials. They would probably also agree that Beecher overstated his case, especially in view of the scientific weaknesses in his fifteen cited trials that were pointed out by Kienle and Keine.

IN SUPPORT OF A PLACEBO EFFECT

Data presented throughout this book argue for an important placebo effect in most treatments. However, Hrobjartsson and Gotszche report that the difference between placebo and "no treatment" in clinical trials appears to be small. Perhaps this is because there *is* little difference. In the 114 trial reports, both the placebo and no-treatment groups were similarly recruited, screened, and observed during a study period. Thus, many of the components of a placebo effect, including doctor/patient relationships, were common to both. The Danish review's weakness is the absence of a true no-treatment group in which these reinforcing components are absent (an impossibility). Gotzsche himself defined a placebo effect as "the difference in outcome between a placebo treated group and an untreated group in an unbiased experiment."[13] The 114 trials they reviewed were not "unbiased." An unbiased experiment may be impossible because once a subject enters a trial, he is no longer "untreated."

One trial included in the Hrobjartsson and Gotzsche review may help clarify the issue. K. B. Thomas consecutively assessed two hundred of his general-practice patients.[14] These were randomized into two groups of one hundred; the first subjected to a positive approach and the second to a neutral one (see table 4-2). He gave the patients in the first group a firm diagnosis and told them that they would be better in a few days. He explained to the subjects in the second group, "I cannot be certain what is the matter with you." Half (fifty) of the patients in each group received a placebo pill (thiamine), indicating it would help in the first group, and without such encouragement in the second. In the first group, 64 percent of the patients were improved, and in the second "negatively" treated group, only 39 percent improved. The giving of the placebo pill made no difference in either group. Thomas concludes that the doctor himself is a powerful therapeutic agent. The treatment provider's attitude and deportment is a powerful component of the placebo effect. Neither Kienle and Keine nor Hrobjartsson and Gotzsche address this issue in their reviews.

TABLE 4-2
Positive Physician Attitude versus Pills in the Placebo Effect[15]

Two hundred consecutive general practice patients with undiagnosed complaints:

	n*	Diagnosis	Physician Attitude	Improved†
Positive	50	yes	"You will be better soon"	32/50 (64%)
Positive + Pills	50	yes	"Pills will help"	32/50 (64%)
Negative	50	no	"I don't know what you have"	18/50 (36%)
Negative + Pills	50	no	"I don't know if pills will help"	21/50 (42%)

*n=number of subjects
†"positive" vs "negative" treatment p<.005

Thomas's conclusions are supported by the work of G. N. Verne and colleagues, who induced skin and rectal pain in patients with the irritable bowel syndrome.[16] They found that rectal lidocaine (a local anesthetic) reduced both pains more than a rectal placebo. In a subsequent experiment, they added verbal encouragement to these treatments. This increased the response to treatment such that the relief of skin and rectal pain to the rectal placebo was as great as that of the rectal lidocaine. Positive attitudes greatly enhance treatments.

In an earlier review of twelve trials, E. Ernst and K. L. Resch found that placebo treatment was better than "no treatment," especially for pain.[17] They also pointed out that both groups are subject to the time effects described in chapter 13 such as natural history, regression to the mean, shifting baselines, and parallel treatments. None of these data reveal much about the "true placebo effect," which is what would remain if the various time effects were known and could be subtracted from the apparent response to placebo in a clinical trial.

What the criticisms do indicate is that the placebo effect is subtle, and its scientific study requires care. Beecher's pioneering but simplistic tallying of the improvement of clinical trial subjects on placebo is an inadequate measure. Placebo research is challenging and full of pitfalls. Nevertheless, its existence is certain and vitally important to therapeutics.

DISEASE VERSUS ILLNESS

Beecher cites evidence for objective effects due to placebos. He points to skin eruptions (Dermatitis Medicamentosa), urticaria (hives), and subjective complaints such as nausea, headache, and fatigue as evidence that placebos can produce physical effects. In their critique, Kienle and Kiene point out that many of the side effects reported by Beecher existed prior to exposure to the placebo. Anecdotes are seldom useful in identifying anatomical or physical changes resulting from placebo therapy. Some would go further and say that such changes have never been proven to be due to placebo. Here we encounter the difference between disease and illness. The former is an abnormality observable by others, the latter is the person's experience (symptoms) and how she feels. The physical attributes of disease are less prone to placebo effects than the subjective symptoms of illness.

AN EFFECT, NOT A THING

Clearly, an inert pill or "no treatment" can have no intrinsic therapeutic qualities. A patient may feel better after placebo treatment
because of the therapeutic circumstances, the personality of the caregiver, the healing atmosphere, and his own receptiveness. These attitudes, actions, and circumstances benefit the patient, not the placebo
itself. Thomas and others have demonstrated that such a placebo
effect may take place without a placebo (see table 4-2). The
healer/sufferer relationship is at the heart of the matter.

HUMAN INTERACTION

The placebo effect is the product of a successful human interaction. It
requires someone who is deemed capable and who undertakes to take
care of an ill person. Healers and patients must come to share attitudes, needs, knowledge, beliefs, and a sense of empathy that create a
healing climate. A skeptical patient or an unfeeling doctor could
cancel the placebo effect or even cause a "nocebo" effect. The effect
depends upon the expectations, experience, and trust of the patient
interacting with the competence, confidence, trustworthiness, and
personality of the healer. In earlier times and in primitive societies, a
healer might be characterized as powerful. This power is subtler in
our age of equality, but it is necessary just the same.

Elements of this healer/sufferer relationship exist in most human
relationships. A salesperson who projects confidence in the product,
who is trusted by the buyer, who promises to be there if the product
fails, and who seems to care is most likely to satisfy a customer. Like
a patient, a buyer is vulnerable and in need, while the salesperson
embodies the means to satisfy the need. Similar analogies exist in
other human transactions from politics to the confessional.

Of course, healing is more than just successful salesmanship. The
feelings of suffering, loneliness, and vulnerability that haunt illness
are unique. The authority and effectiveness of the healer depends
upon how he or she is perceived by the sufferer. While elements of
the healer's power occur in other human relationships, nowhere is it
as personal as it is in the examining room. The doctor/patient relationship is arguably the oldest and most important human transaction

apart from friendship, love, and family. It is so central to health care that doctors, administrators, and planners must promote it.

CONCLUSION

A placebo can be an activity, device, pill, or almost any plausible thing. A placebo effect is a component of all healing, and may be achieved without a placebo. Nevertheless, it is understood poorly. In a randomized clinical trial, a placebo pill, device, or procedure improves patients' symptoms through placebo effects and the natural tendency of most conditions to get better. In such a trial, the test treatment must perform better than a placebo treatment to be successful. The small difference in the improvement observed in some clinical trials between placebo and "no treatment" is beside the point. Both involve the achievement of a therapeutic relationship, a phenomenon that requires no pill, device, or procedure. We must strive for conditions that optimize this relationship, thereby maximizing the placebo effect.

CHAPTER 5

ELEMENTS OF THE PLACEBO EFFECT

The placebo effect is important to all therapy, yet we understand it poorly. It deserves serious study in its own right. Rather than considering it as the enemy, a foil for "evidence-based medicine," we should adopt the placebo effect as an important clinical tool. Here, we consider several factors that may promote placebo effects.

ALLAYING ANXIETY

We experience pain through two general mechanisms, *sensory-discriminatory* and *affective-motivational*.[1] Nerves transmit impulses from an injured organ to the brain. Strike your thumb with a hammer and you instantly feel pain through sensory nerves hardwired to the central nervous system (CNS). Relief is likely to occur with analgesics such as aspirin or narcotics. Everyone experiences this acute sensory-discriminatory pain, and everyone understands it.

Affective-motivational pain is more complex. An emotional component is characteristic of many chronic painful conditions. The central nervous system plays a significant role, and many suspect that chronic-pain awareness resides there. Anxiety is usually present as well. Affective-motivational pain is typically chronic with no evidence of injury. For examples, some abdominal pains, backaches, headaches, and muscle aches are chronic and unexplained. While sometimes bitterly complained of, these chronic-pain complaints often lack objective features such as withdrawal and tenderness when touched. A person's psychological and social reactions may prevent accurate description, and obscure the exact location and nature of the painful stimulus. Doctors are seldom able to identify a precise physical cause for such pain. Analgesics are relatively ineffective for many chronic pains, but psychoactive drugs such as antidepressants (sometimes in subantidepressant doses) or tranquilizers may help.

Every pain includes some measure of both sensory and emotional awareness. Some are sensed predominantly through the peripheral nervous system (e.g., nerves to the limbs) while others are felt mainly through the CNS. Both mechanisms demand attention. A small boy bruises his knee. Through nerve transmission from the knee to the brain, he instantly feels pain (sensory-discriminatory). However, no specific treatment of the knee arrests his cry, but rather his mother's comforting embrace (affective-motivational).

Many chronic pains are unresponsive to painkilling drugs, causing many affected people to become disillusioned with conventional medicine. Alternative therapies delivered in a manner that allays anxiety or salves emotional hurts can therefore achieve positive results—at least for a time. The enthusiastic administration of a "promising" treatment could lessen the anxiety component of a symptom and may be salutary. A healer who relieves anxiety enhances her treatment, whatever that treatment may be.

CONDITIONED OR PAVLOVIAN RESPONSE

Pavlov's dog demonstrated the *conditioned response*. Normally an animal salivates when the smell or sight of food anticipates a meal. Pavlov arranged to have a ringing bell accompany the sights and smells of his dog's meal. After a conditioning period, the dog began to salivate whenever he heard the bell even in the absence of the sight and smell of food. The dog had become "conditioned." Psychologists believe that people also can be conditioned to respond emotionally or physiologically to a seemingly irrelevant stimulus. Fifty years ago, Gliedman and associates speculated that a person might be conditioned so that his expectations of a therapeutic encounter may be realized.[2] They suggested that a doctor produces a "central excitatory state" that makes patients amenable to her expectations.

Many people associate relief of their symptoms with past treatments so that repetition of a treatment may engender a conditioned response. Subtle favorable experiences with doctors, medicines, or other healing encounters could have a similar effect. Subjects who as children received treats, comforting, or were excused from school along with their treatments may become conditioned to expect them and even use illness to achieve special treatment.[3] Experimentally, administration of analgesics (painkillers) appears to augment the pain-relieving effect of a subsequently administered placebo. The subject is conditioned to respond to treatment even when the pharmacologically active component is removed.

There are other such experiments. N. J. Voudouris and colleagues told two groups of ten subjects that they were to receive an analgesic which was in fact a placebo.[4] During the conditioning, the authors surreptitiously paired placebo administration with an increase in the painful stimulus for the first group of subjects and with a decrease for the second. Subjects' placebo responses were tested pre- and postconditioning to a second type of experimental pain. Those who originally had decreased pain with placebo experienced less pain again with placebo after the second experimental pain stimulus. Once reduced pain is paired with a placebo (conditioned stimulus), relief occurs when the placebo is taken again (conditioned response). Thus, analgesic placebo responses can be "conditioned."

Physiological conditioning is also possible.[5] Recall the effect of saccharine in the immune suppression of rats previously conditioned with saccharine and cyclophosphamide. In another experiment, asthmatic children were exposed to a vanilla aroma whenever they inhaled bronchodilators to relieve the spasm of the small breathing tubes that caused their asthma. Once "conditioned," their bronchi dilated when exposed to the aroma alone—a conditioned response.

Therapeutic trials sometimes include a two-week placebo run-in period in a vain attempt to eliminate placebo responders. In some other trials, subjects are "crossed-over" from a treatment period to a placebo period or vice versa so that each subject was exposed sequentially to the treatment and the placebo control. However, such maneuvers can be counterproductive. In a crossover trial, the placebo response was greater if it was given *after* the active drug.[6] Conversely, the effect of a drug was less if it was given *after* a placebo. Patients who were switched from an active analgesic to placebo have pain relief longer than if treatment was abruptly stopped.[7] After treatment with the drug atenolol, blood pressure remained lower on placebo than if no pills were substituted.[8] Through conditioning, crossover trials or placebo run-in periods may obscure the benefit of the treatment under study. Voudouris believes that when eliciting placebo effects, conditioning is more important than telling a subject what to expect.[9] That is, it is more powerful than expectancy.

EXPECTATION

Patients are more likely to improve on a treatment if they expect and desire it to help them.[10] Improvement can be reinforced if the doctor accompanies the treatment with encouragement and if the patient has a positive attitude. In performance studies after the administration of alcohol or caffeine, the results are in accordance with what the subjects expect.[11] If you expect caffeine to improve your performance, it likely will.[12] Injections create a greater expectancy of benefit than pills, and the color of pills can influence the patient's expectations of their effect. Placebos even have side effects. In a clinical trial, investigators must warn all blinded participants about expected side effects from the test treatment. Since those receiving the placebo also are warned, they may experience side effects similar to those who actually take the treatment. Expectations may change during randomized clinical trials,[13] posing special challenges to designers of such trials. Trial doctors and nurses, friends, fear of being a "placebo responder," the need to be off medications, and other trial conditions may influence a subject's changing expectations of benefit.

Sometimes it is difficult to separate conditioning from expectancy. One experiment set out to determine the value of the brand name of a medication for the treatment of headaches.[14] The investigators compared branded and unbranded analgesics in a clinical trial of women who were either users or nonusers of the drug. The active drug was more effective when labeled with the brand, but the placebo was also more effective when taken from a branded rather than from a plain package. Thus:

> branded analgesic > unbranded analgesic >
> branded placebo > unbranded placebo.

Both the branded drug and the branded placebo were more effective in those who regularly used the brand previously. Were the women who had previously used the drug conditioned to get pain relief when taking a branded placebo, or did the sight of the brand name on the package cause them to expect relief?

Perhaps no treatment creates such expectations as surgery (see chapter 9). The preoperative rituals and commitments involved in having an operation can powerfully reinforce a person's expectation that the result will be positive. A. G. Johnson provocatively suggested that if patients are involved in the decision to operate and the choice of operation, there is a strong incentive for them to feel better.[15] Otherwise, they must admit to themselves, relatives, and others that they made the wrong choice. Johnson speculates that the expectation of postoperative improvement is even greater if a patient has paid for the surgery. Great expectations must also accentuate the disillusionment if the operation turns out badly—a nocebo effect.

F. Bennedetti and his colleagues demonstrated how specific expectation of pain relief can be.[16] In volunteers, subcutaneous (skin) injection of the irritant capsaicin induced a painful local reaction in all four limbs. Application of an inert cream relieved the pain only in the limbs to which it was applied. In addition, injecting the narcotic antagonist naloxone prevented the pain-relieving effect of the cream. The expectation that the placebo cream would relieve the pain made it happen. Bennedetti concludes that a local opioid mechanism accounts for this placebo effect. Relief appears to be mediated locally by the body's natural narcotics (*endorphins*) that could be blocked by naloxone. Whether or not endorphins explain the phenomenon, the subjects expected pain relief to occur only in the treated limbs.

Doctors can encourage expectations of benefit when they talk to patients. There is evidence that early attention to the patients' symptoms, fears, and concerns has a positive long-term outcome. One study retrospectively reviewed the case notes of 112 patients diagnosed by their doctors to have the irritable bowel syndrome thirty-two years earlier.[17] The investigators catalogued features of each doctor's record that gauge the strength of the doctor/patient relationship (presence of social history, reassurance, explanation of symptoms, discussion of test results, etc). The greater the number of these features recorded, the less likely were the patients to return to the doctor for their symptoms over the subsequent thirty-two years.

Time initially spent addressing a patient's concerns and fears may have long-term benefits.

Early enthusiasm by the promoters of a new surgical procedure maximizes the expectation of benefit and conversely reduces the perceived value of existing treatment. The so-called Hawthorne effect, where improvement results from "being studied," may also augment the expectation of improvement. If we expect something to make us feel better, it is more likely to do so.

CIRCUMSTANCES

Responses to treatment are subject to circumstances. For example, some athletes continue playing a match after sustaining a normally disabling injury. After an attack, wounded soldiers require less analgesia than civilians do with similar injuries. Adrenaline or the body's natural pain relievers might explain this, but perhaps the anticipation of athletic glory or honorable discharge also play a role. These examples illustrate the need to control for the circumstances when testing analgesics in a clinical trial. In medical practice, treatments promise to heal when the circumstances and surroundings are optimal. House calls, office visits, and hospital admissions can create potential healing environments.

CULTURE (PLACEBO AND NOCEBO)

In the world of anthropology, every tribe, culture, or society has medicine men or women who enjoy great authority among their fellows despite the incredulity of outsiders. "Medicine men" wielded power for good (and for evil), and were essential providers of treatments throughout the long history of healing. Deeply rooted in cultural traditions, these powerful individuals were widely *believed* to heal. Conversely, such important people sometimes could do deliberate harm through hexes and voodoo—a "nocebo" effect. Medicine men (and women) are so prevalent in all cultures that they must satisfy a primitive need to make sense of the human condition. No doubt, the power of religions to heal (or to harm) arises partly through this need and it may explain many of the world's great "isms" and cults. Traditional medicine also has its potentially comforting symbols and rituals, from the diploma on the wall to the taking of the pulse. Perceptive modern physicians recognize the role of culture, tradition, and ritual in the success of their own treatments.

THE DOCTOR

Among the many definitions of the placebo effect, Howard Brody suggests "a change in a patient's illness attributable to the symbolic import of a treatment rather than a specific pharmacological or physiological property."[18] This acknowledges that no pill is necessary. Healers have the power to make patients feel better irrespective of treatment. The symbolic giving of treatment by a comforting figure is crucial. The doctor *is* the placebo!

In Western cultures, the doctor became a powerful healing authority. In his 1911 play, *The Doctor's Dilemma*,[19] George Bernard Shaw depicts a doctor named Sir Ralph Bloomfield Bonington as "cheering, reassuring, healing by the mere incompatibility of disease or anxiety with his welcome presence." Shaw disliked doctors. Sir Ralph is a parody, but his character reveals something of public attitudes toward the healing powers of physicians before medicine's great therapeutic advances. (We shall get to know Bonington better in chapter 9.) Usually, placebos delivered by a doctor achieve the greatest benefit. This power incorporates a doctor's reputation; his figure, manner, and personality; the authority and confidence with which he delivers his treatment; and even the office, instruments, white coat, and disinfectant aromas that symbolize the healing profession.

A physician's attitude is important. A positive approach to her patient can be therapeutic whether or not any treatment is given.[20] A doctor can convey compassion and a positive sense of encouragement in several ways. Feeling the pulse, listening to a patient's concerns, and physical examination are examples. Surgeons notice their patients' relief when they examine an acutely painful abdomen, impressing their students with the healing potential of the "laying on of hands." Images linger of doctors braving inclement weather to attend the sick, comforting the parents of a sick child, or waiting patiently at the bedside for a fever to dissipate. (See figure 5-1.) What contemporary doctor (or nurse) can afford time for such "nonessentials"? It is a sorry comment on modern, technologically triumphant

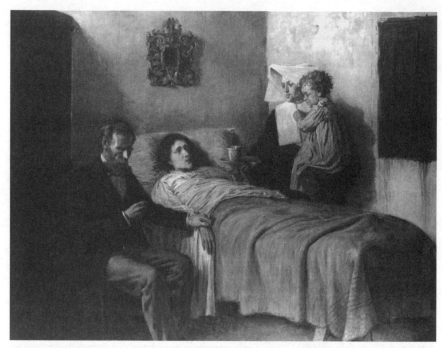

Figure 5-1: *Science and Charity* by Pablo Picasso (1897). Museo Picasso, Barcelona. (© Picasso Estate / SODRAC [Montreal] 2004.) Before 1900, medical care often occurred in the patient's home. Picasso's idealized image of the caring doctor portrays a past medical arcadia. Notice there is no white coat, although the nurse has a white bib and cap. While the doctor here could use his training in science to diagnose the patient's problem, likely pneumonia, he had little effective treatment to offer, only empathy. Compare this scene to your last visit to a public hospital. Despite the nostalgia, neither doctors nor patients would happily return to those times. Nevertheless, both sense that something has been lost.

medicine that the "art" is threatened. Physicians, patients, and society should understand what is at risk.

DIAGNOSIS AND MEANING

Brody said that diagnosis provides an understandable and satisfying explanation for an illness.[21] He means that by making a diagnosis and explaining the nature of the complaint, the physician provides something tangible to which the patient can cling during his discomfort and which explains the ailment to friends and family. A skillfully orchestrated diagnostic test can have therapeutic as well as diagnostic benefits. H. C. Sox and his colleagues demonstrated this phenomenon in 176 patients with *noncardiac* chest pain.[22] (See figure 5-2.) Two groups of patients were treated equally, except that the first group underwent testing with an electrocardiogram and a blood *creatinine phosphokinase*. These tests have little diagnostic value in this situation, yet in all respects, the tested patients fared better than the untested patients. They had less pain, less disability, and were more content with their care.

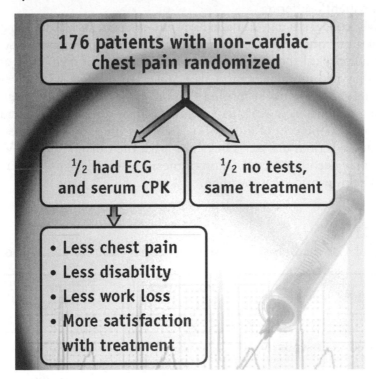

176 patients with non-cardiac chest pain randomized

½ had ECG and serum CPK

½ no tests, same treatment

- Less chest pain
- Less disability
- Less work loss
- More satisfaction with treatment

Figure 5-2: Investigators divided 176 patients, who had chronic chest pain not due to heart disease, into two groups. Both were treated identically, but in the first group, the patients were tested with an electrocardiagram and a blood level of creatinine phospho-kinase. These tests are usually abnormal immediately after a heart attack but have little diagnostic value for the chronic chest pain studied here. Nevertheless, those patients who had these tests (all negative) subsequently experienced less chest pain, less disability, less work loss, and were more satisfied with their care. These tests, of no practical medical value, increased the patients' confidence in their negative cardiac diagnoses and improved their outcomes (see text).[23]

Diagnosis helps demonstrate the healer's care and concern for his patient's suffering, confers meaning to the symptoms, and symbolically promises some control over symptoms. In providing a meaningful diagnosis, the doctor helps evoke a placebo effect. D. E. Moerman suggests that we cease speaking of placebo effects and use the term "meaning response."[24] This conveys a positive message and avoids some of the ethical dilemmas surrounding placebos. No longer is deception an issue. Is it not ethical for a doctor to provide meaning for a patient's suffering?

My colleagues and I studied seventy-six patients consulting their general practitioner for irritable bowel syndrome (a nonfatal disorder with no physical abnormality), and found that half of them were afraid that they had intestinal cancer (see table 5-1).[25] Most were given no diagnosis so it was not surprising that only 29 percent of these cancer-fearing patients were reassured following their doctor visit. Paradoxically, only 27 percent of those who had an organic diagnosis were worried about serious disease. They *knew* what their diagnosis was. When ill, people need some explanation or meaning for their suffering. Diagnosis helps provide that meaning.

TABLE 5-1
Fear of Cancer Before and After a Primary Care Consultation[26]

	Patients with Irritable Bowel Syndrome	Patients with "Organic" Disease
Worried their symptoms meant cancer	n* = 76 45%	n* = 100 27% (p<.02)
Reassured by doctor that they did not have cancer	29%	all

*n = number of patients

CONCLUSION

Whatever a placebo may be, it can itself have no therapeutic effect. It is the circumstances and manner of the giving of placebos that exert such effects. Placebo effects can enhance any treatment. Relief of anxiety, conditioned responses, expectation, culture, and the effect of the doctor's presence and personality confer benefits. Patients feel better if they can attach some meaning to their suffering. Hence, a diagnosis and explanation for symptoms is important. Doctors instinctively bring these features to bear when treating fearful, anxious patients. Neither voodoo-science nor sleight of hand, they are vital and natural components of the healing art.

CHAPTER 6

THE NOCEBO EFFECT

"Primum non nocere." (First, do no harm.)

HIPPOCRATES (460–377 BCE)*

A treatment gone awry may do physical harm. Treatment errors are understandable and alarmingly frequent[1]—the results regrettably obvious. Less obvious, however, is that an unsuccessful healer/patient interaction may nullify a treatment's benefit or even make an ill person feel worse. The personality and conviction of the healer, the hopefulness and expectant attitude of the ill person, and a positive therapeutic relationship together generate placebo effects. Conversely, their absence, or their antitheses, may have negative or *nocebo* effects.[2] A doctor with a negative attitude toward a treatment or a patient may compromise her treatment's success. An ill person who is distrustful of his healer not only is denied placebo benefits, but also may feel worse from his encounter with her. A rushed consultation in a noisy office interrupted by the phone can disturb any client, but can devastate the worried and the ill. Those very attributes that augment the placebo effect can, if misapplied, have nocebo effects. Thus, we can rewrite the therapeutic equation:

Treatment benefit = Therapeutic gain + Natural history of
illness - Nocebo effect

Note that if the nocebo effect is greater than the therapeutic gain and the natural history effects together, the treatment will make the patient worse.

---

*BCE stands for "before the common era," known to most Western cultures as BC or "before Christ."

71

PRIMITIVE NOCEBOS

Just as primitive witch doctors and medicine men have mystical healing powers to rid the body of harmful spirits, they also have the power to instill the body with evil spirits, and to cause disease or death. For example, the Cherokees believed that death resulted from disease inflicted by witches and conjurers who were connected to an evil spirit.[3] Witchcraft or magic might activate such evil spirits at the instigation of a malevolent individual. In some societies, the "evil eye" is a jealous and harmful glance. Therefore, individuals avoid situations in which they might be envied. A malevolent tradition exists in Ethiopia where landowners fear the envious evil eye from lower-class artisans.[4] Particularly vulnerable to the evil eye are enviable people who are handsome, wealthy, and have beautiful children. Sometimes, malevolent spirits can be unleashed accidentally, as in the Middle East, where too intent a gaze may be mistaken for the evil eye.

J. L. Maddox and B. A. Lex describe the infliction of disease and death through sorcery or witchcraft.[5] The medicine man seeks the assistance of spirits or divinities to accomplish his evil purpose, which may be revenge or punishment. Walter Cannon described the notion of voodoo death as the fatal power of the imagination working through unmitigated terror.[6] Such were the beliefs of aboriginal societies in Australia, New Zealand, and Polynesia, and among transported Africans in Haiti that a powerful medicine man might cause death through fear. (So much for the "stress of modern living"!) Voodoo death is also called "magical death" or "sociocultural" death.

Western observers suspiciously seek pathophysiological explanations such as dehydration or malnourishment due to the victim's fearful failure to drink or eat. Cannon believed that voodoo death resulted from an overreaction of the sympathetic-adrenal system to fear—an extreme example of the fight-or-flight phenomenon. Others have attributed it to the parasympathetic system, or an autonomic failure.[7] Modern scientists have localized the emotional component of fear to a part of the brain called the amygdala.[8] A terrifying suggestion, by creating great fear, appears to stimulate an eventual mortal reaction through cardiovascular collapse or arrhythmia. Whatever the explanation, culturally induced societal fears such as those of the evil eye and voodoo are nocebos. Whether they induce pathology or death is debatable, but they can make some people ill or worsen their existing illness.

This phenomenon has modern counterparts. Some cases of sudden death are blamed on the presence of a severely stressful situation in which there appears to be no means of control or escape.[9] The contempt, anger, or mental cruelty of others makes sensitive people ill. Such a reaction of an ill person to a healer, whether or not it is deliberately provoked, can impair or destroy the therapeutic relationship.

SIDE EFFECTS OF PLACEBOS

Beecher described the frequent occurrence of "toxic and other subjective side effects" in subjects receiving placebos.[10] Dry mouth, nausea, headache, fatigue, and sleeplessness occurred in up to half of the subjects on placebo in his review of fifteen clinical trials. Other authors point out that many people, especially women and the elderly, have such symptoms in everyday life and their occurrence in trials cannot all be attributed to placebo.[11] In support of this, M. M. Reidenberg and D. T. Lowenthal asked 414 students and hospital workers who had no illnesses or medications if they had suffered any of the twenty-five symptoms that are commonly reported as side effects in clinical trials (including loss of appetite, constipation, dry mouth, sore muscles, and bruising).[12] Eighty-one percent had experienced at least one of these symptoms during the previous seventy-two hours. Thirty of the subjects had at least six of these symptoms. This observation may partially explain the long lists of side effects in the information sheets that accompany prescription drugs.

Frequently, the side effects reported by those receiving placebos in clinical trials are similar to those receiving the test drug.[13] There are many reasons for this. Drug regulatory authorities and the principles of trial methodology demand careful surveillance for untoward effects due to the drug being tested. Investigators and nurses are blinded as to treatment, but are alert to potential side effects, seeking them out in all subjects, including those on placebo. Also, when entering a trial, all patients must be warned of possible drug effects even though they may be destined to receive the placebo after randomization. In the conduct of a clinical trial, background conversations by investigators and nurses may mention side effects, unconsciously provoking them in susceptible persons.

It is evident that many symptoms are common yet ignored in

everyday life. In a clinical trial, subjects become more aware of them. These symptoms may not be caused by the placebo itself, but are enhanced by the actions of the investigators, the circumstances of the trial, and the suggestibility and increased vigilance of the subjects. Therefore, like all other aspects of treatment testing, trial investigators must control the tabulation of side effects through double-blinding. Robert Hahn characterized reports of untoward symptoms in trial patients taking placebos as "placebo side effects," not nocebo effects.[14] Nevertheless, the labeling of a treatment with an unnecessarily long list of adverse effects itself may induce nocebo effects.

NEGATIVE ASPECTS OF THE USE OF PLACEBOS

While most acknowledge that placebo effects accompanying an effective treatment are a good thing, few would advocate the deliberate use of inert treatments. Indeed, most feel the deceitful use of sugar pills is unethical, although doctors in practice commonly deploy active or impure placebos. Moreover, the use of placebos may harm. If thoughtlessly applied, they may divert the attention of healer and sick person from important considerations that include a proper diagnosis and its promise of more appropriate treatment. Diet and lifestyle advice may be sacrificed for the mistaken belief that there is a "pill for every ill." The continuing use of a treatment, especially a useless one, serves as a constant reminder of illness, surely another nocebo effect. The deception itself may compromise the doctor/patient relationship in subtle ways. Thus, placebo effects can justly be encouraged when administering effective treatment, but a healer deliberately misleading her patient can be counterproductive.

CONDITIONS FAVORING A NOCEBO EFFECT

Hahn suggests that, like tobacco, a nocebo increases the likelihood that illness will occur but does not guarantee it.[15] He stresses the roles of expectation and emotional state in the nocebo phenomenon. In early societies, the fearful expectation that the shaman had the power to harm often made it so. Just as a modern healer can relieve symptoms through a positive attitude and a trustworthy relationship, so she can do harm through a negative attitude and lack of empathy.

Mood may negatively influence health outcomes. In a large sample of Americans, depressed people were 1.6 times more likely to have nonfatal ischemic heart disease, and 1.5 times more likely to die than those without depression.[16] It is impossible to determine whether the increase was because of health-damaging behavior due to the depression, or a direct effect of the depression itself. Cynicism, suspicion, and a pessimistic expectation that disease will occur can generate negative expectations. The doctor may be able to overcome a patient's pessimism with a positive attitude (see table 4-1) or aggravate it by being negative.

Self-scrutiny is another source of negative expectations. Physicians are familiar with *medical students' disease*, many having experienced it themselves. When studying a specific disease, it is common for students to recognize some of its symptoms in themselves. This is more than mere suggestibility. Medical students encounter the concept of illness and mortality at an earlier age than do most other people. Hence, fear may accompany the study of a disease. The reassurance of others usually resolves these anxieties, but a few students experience lingering hypochondria.

Cardiac neurosis is a common example of externally induced negative expectations. The media carry harrowing statistics about the dangers of heart disease, and doctors and associations produce sometimes-arduous lifestyle rules to prevent it. While intended to encourage a healthy lifestyle, such publicity may harm depressed and pessimistic people with already fearful expectations. Heart disease in a friend or relative, guilt that one has not measured up to the lifestyle rules, incessant publicity, and conflicting advice contrive to convince the pessimist of his vulnerability. While heart disease is inevitable for many of us, and prevention is desirable, premature incapacity due to fear of the disease is counterproductive. Cardiac neurosis is a nocebo effect.

Just as diagnosis is treatment and has a placebo effect, so failure to diagnose may have a nocebo effect. We have seen that ill people seek some meaning for their illness. Evil spirits may have satisfied the curiosity of less-educated societies, but we moderns want the facts. We worship on the altar of causality, and seek explanation, meaning, and recognition for our suffering. Few things more dissatisfy an ill person than to leave a consultation with the notion that his doctor believes that his complaint is "all in the head" or is "nothing." Diagnosis demonstrates to the patient that his complaint is taken seriously, that he has a legitimate affliction, and that his suffering is recognized as genuine.

Brody claims that diagnosis provides an understandable and satisfying explanation for an illness.[17] He means that by making a diagnosis and explaining the nature of the complaint, the physician provides something tangible to which the patient can cling during his discomfort. A skillfully orchestrated negative endoscopic examination of the stomach and duodenum can have therapeutic as well as diagnostic benefits to someone suffering dyspepsia and who is fearful of a possible ulcer or cancer. However, failure to explain the objective of the procedure and dismissive treatment of the symptoms can have nocebo effects. Recall the experiment of Sox et al.,[18] who demonstrated this phenomenon in 176 patients with noncardiac chest pain (see figure 5-1). Patients not undergoing heart tests suffered more disability, were less satisfied with their care, and were off work longer than were their tested peers, even though the tests themselves were unreliable. Recall also that among seventy-six irritable-bowel-syndrome patients who saw their general practitioner, half were afraid they had cancer and most were given no diagnosis (see table 5-1).[19] Unsurprisingly, 71 percent of these were not reassured after the doctor visit. Illness demands some explanation or *meaning*, as Brody puts it, and its absence lessens one's sense of well-being. A physician's failure to make a meaningful diagnosis and address her patient's fears and concerns may have nocebo effects.

Another phenomenon with nocebo effects is the so-called *labeling of deviance*, where a society creates labels to denote people deemed abnormal. This applies to mental disorders where strange behavior is given a psychiatric diagnosis. In the case of depression or schizophrenia, this is useful, because once categorized, those affected can be effectively treated. In other instances, however, the deviance is less clear-cut, and labeling may denote illness where none exists. A diagnosis of *post-traumatic stress disorder* to describe a person's normal response to tragedy may achieve compensation in some cases, but the putative therapy may be no better than the consolation of a good friend. Moreover, what to most people is a normal grief response becomes an illness, with the negative connotations that having an illness implies. Extreme and malignant examples of wrongful labeling occur in dictatorships, where declaring dissidents insane is a convenient excuse for incarceration.

Those who classify diseases may label people with a disorder of which they never complain. For example, there are many gut complaints with no recognized pathology known as the *functional gut disorders*. My colleagues and I developed a classification of these disorders that include *dyspepsia* and *irritable bowel syndrome*.[20] Population surveys using this classification and its definitions consistently indicate that irritable bowel syndrome occurs in 15 to 20 percent of adults. For those seeking medical attention, such labeling provides a diagnosis and informs tests and treatment. However, most people with these disorders do not seek medical attention, and the symptoms often disappear in time. Are these individuals ill just because they report symptoms in a survey? Pharmaceutical companies would certainly be glad to have them as customers. Is labeling apparently healthy and nonsuffering people with a (for them) meaningless diagnosis and thereby exposing them to unnecessary, often ineffective and expensive tests and treatments a nocebo? Hahn claims that such labeling increases peoples' "sickness repertoire" and encourages some to adopt a sick role.[21] The proclivity for diagnostic labels is skillfully parodied in the article "The Last Well Person" by Clifton Meador.[22] He cites a future report of a fifty-three-year-old man (from somewhere near Kansas) in whom scores of physicians, psychologists, and screening procedures have failed to find a single disease. Tongue in cheek, Meador chronicles the seven hours and thirteen minutes this sole remaining healthy patient devotes daily to staying healthy: following the latest diet precepts, exercise programs, or psychological fads, all with an ear to the media for the latest health revelation, simultaneously recording three major television channels for later viewing. Meador ends by speculating that his imaginary patient may live longer by doing all these boring activities, but it will also seem longer.

A subtler labeling phenomenon is a by-product of specialization. Patients with many unexplained symptoms attributed to several organs are said to have a *functional somatic disorder*.[23] However, their diagnosis is often dependent upon the specialist to whom they are referred. In the same patient, a gastroenterologist may diagnose an *irritable bowel*, a rheumatologist *fibromyalgia*, and a gynecologist *chronic pelvic pain*. Tests and therapies flow from each specialist's interpretation, and few are equipped to address the patient's fundamental psychological problems. Instead of a patient being managed by a family doctor who knows him well, he drifts from specialist to specialist, each of whose worldview may be confined to one organ. Once tests of that organ are exhausted, such a patient moves on disappointed, but undaunted in his quest to understand the meaning of his varied symptoms.

Sociologic illness, also known as *mass hysteria* or *assembly line hysteria*, is another phenomenon with nocebo implications. This describes sickness or symptoms that occur upon learning of sickness or symptoms in other people. Fear of AIDS may be almost as incapacitating as diagnosis of the real thing. Symptoms are often respiratory, triggered by a strange odor or other changes in the environment of schools or workplaces. *Sick building syndrome* may be an example. Similarly, a dramatic suicide or car accident is often followed by a larger than expected number of such incidents in the community. In the week following Marilyn Monroe's suicide there was a 12 percent increase in the usual incidence of such deaths in the United States.[24] Identification with another victim's plight may intensify one's own.

SYMBOLISM AND THE NOCEBO EFFECT

As with placebos, symbolism is an important vehicle for the nocebo response. The robes, instruments, and social position of a medicine man can instill his people with fear as well as hope. Some are fearful of hospitals, a doctor's visit, a needle, or unpleasant medicine. Individuals with normal blood pressure often become transiently hypertensive at the sight of a doctor's white coat. The symbols of modern medicine are meant to reassure and comfort. If, paradoxically, they engender anxiety, fear, even hostility, they have the potential to harm a therapeutic relationship. The doctor's manner may be frightening. The evil eye may not be deliberate, but if fearfully interpreted it can harm one all the same.

MALPRACTICE LITIGATION—
A FAILURE OF COMMUNICATION

Nothing chills a doctor/patient relationship like the threat of malpractice litigation.[25] Its occurrence causes great anxiety for patient and doctor, and makes subsequent doctor/patient relationships difficult for both. Of course, if a medical accident provokes the action, it must be resolved. However, some litigation is the result of bad communication and might be prevented if the doctor/patient relationship were optimal. W. Levinson found that primary care physicians having two or more malpractice claims, regardless of outcome, had poorer relationships with their patients than physicians without claims.[26] Using videotapes to record doctors interviewing patients, the investigators found that those without claims tended to spend more time with their patients, explain the process of the visit (interview, examination, question time), encourage their patients to talk or give opinions, and use humor (an indication of a warm relationship). The authors conclude that what a doctor says may be less important than how he says it. The process and tone of the visit have significance.

A review of obstetrical records discovered similar technical management by obstetricians who were sued and those who were not.[27] Could poor doctor/patient communication account for the suits? It seems so. Mothers of stillborn babies were interviewed about their satisfaction with their obstetrical care.[28] Those with frequently sued obstetricians were more likely to have had unsatisfactory physician/patient communications. An Australian study concludes, "The majority of formal complaints or legal actions initiated against medical practitioners in the absence of medical mismanagement are preventable."[29] Among other things, these authors suggest open and timely sharing of information. Norman Cousins, a journalist and cancer survivor who was invited to join a medical faculty, states that "proper communication is one of the most difficult undertakings on earth," and its failure is the source of much human calamity.[30]

Failure of communication takes many forms. The information may be correct, but the doctor seems arrogant or uncaring. The doctor may not be available at a critical moment, or seem to obfuscate or ignore the patient's concerns. A healer may think she is communicating, but the patient may misinterpret her or be suspicious. Some unconscious look or gesture may give offense. If perceived to be unconscious or uncaring, communication may be nocebo rather than placebo. Remember the evil eye!

Litigation experience changes behavior in unconstructive ways. Not only has the patient become aggrieved, but also the doctor usually suffers mightily.[31] He may avoid difficult cases, become wary and cold with patients, and defensively order excessive diagnostic tests.[32] Some become bitter and experience depression, marital difficulties, and substance abuse. Early retirement and even suicide are blamed on litigation. Likewise, aggrieved patients may become bitter and mistrustful, and other physicians may be reluctant to accept them as patients. A breakdown in the doctor/patient relationship, leading a patient to complain, can produce nocebo effects with far-reaching consequences.

ORGANIZATIONAL NOCEBO EFFECTS

Technology has produced great advances in diagnosis. New techniques in public health, in infections, in cardiovascular disease, and even in cancer have saved lives and improved well-being. However, better management of some problems creates new ones, and survival of acute illness expands the need for chronic care. Persons saved from one disease must ultimately succumb to another. Twenty to 30 percent of primary and outpatient care is concerned with nonfatal but chronic, functional somatic syndromes that require time, not technology.[33] Increasing costs, longer lives, and increasing demand create pressures for even more expenditure.

In chapter 17 we shall see how developed nations respond to these challenges. All must satisfy their increasingly aging populations, while creating efficiencies and management structures that contain steadily increasing costs. Managers proliferate, designing rules to govern the behavior of the doctors, nurses, and others who actually provide the care. Introducing a 1975 conference entitled *Humanizing Health Care*, David Mechanic noted that "as the terms of reference shift to efficiency and management, there has been more than a noticeable lack of concern with medicine as a humane institution and with the motivations and ethics that govern its endeavors."[34] His words resonate thirty years later. Medicine's undeniably brilliant technical successes are achieved at the cost of less time for doctors and nurses to talk to patients.

These developments have created new or altered organizations to serve health-care professionals. Health-care organizations increasingly control professional incomes and working conditions. Professional organizations are now less concerned with advances in medical care than with protecting their members' rights and financial position.

Most specialists owe allegiance to specialty organizations that ignore problems which transcend specialty boundaries. They produce endless guidelines that one family doctor protested could paper the walls of his clinic. Licensing authorities are increasingly concerned with discipline and, in response to the despicable behavior of the very few, impose rules on the many. The popular press and rising malpractice actions add conflicting and very public pressures to the daily lives of doctors and nurses. Interest groups and patient advocates add to the cacophony. No individual can work comfortably amid all these strangers in the examining room (see chapter 15).

We should contemplate how these pressures impair doctor/patient relationships. We have already explored how the interaction of a sick person with a caring healer can encourage placebo effects. Those planning and managing health-care programs should consider how their initiatives might have nocebo effects. After all, unsatisfactory patient encounters with health care ultimately cost more than successful ones. In the name of efficiency, some organizations pressure their participating doctors to see more patients and spend less time with each of them. Medicine is a business,[35] and time is money. Such an organization, be it government, an insurance company, or a health maintenance organization risks false economies. Excessive cost saving and regulation curtails doctor/patient interaction, leading to unsatisfied patients, doctor shopping, repeated testing, and litigation—nocebo effects indeed!

THE STUDY OF NOCEBOS

Nocebo effects are difficult to study. In humans, one cannot deliberately test a potentially noxious treatment that lacks therapeutic potential. Moreover, blinding a subject to a nocebo treatment runs contrary to informed consent. There are also methodological difficulties. How does one control for a nocebo? How can an experiment allow for subjects' existing positive, negative, or absent expectations? These difficulties resemble those of placebo research.

Nevertheless, some experiments have been done—some of them through protocols that might fail a modern ethical review. These tested the effects of negative expectations on subjects' subsequent experience. For example, asthmatics can be conditioned to have increased airway resistance to exhalation (bronchospasm) by inhaling a normally harmless aerosolized salt solution.[36] One subject, allergic to roses, suffered asthmatic symptoms at the sight of plastic roses.

Thus the nocebo concept is important. We need to understand why some healing encounters go wrong. They may be due to medical errors, of course. However, many failures are due to an unsatisfactory healing relationship, a failure to deal with an ill person's fears, or his unrealistic and negative expectations. The study of nocebos, and placebos, could have wide-reaching benefits.

CONCLUSION

The nocebo effect, like the placebo effect, is rooted in prehistory, where powerful persons could "magically" exert malevolent as well as benevolent effects in people. In the healing professions (as in all personal relationships), a breakdown in healer/patient communication can have far-reaching untoward effects. These are distinct from malpractice or the "side effects of placebos." Whether deliberately or unconsciously activated, these effects may be truly harmful. At best, they impair effective treatment—at worst, they aggravate fear and destroy the healing relationship. We must learn more about the causes of nocebo effects in medical care. Doctors should strive for better doctor/patient relationships: a positive and caring attitude, a meaningful diagnosis, open discussion of even the most sensitive topics, frank admission of the limitations of treatment, and realistic appraisal of what the future may bring. The many organizations that affect doctor/patient interactions should facilitate rather than constrain. Better doctor/ patient interactions prevent nocebo effects, increase patient satisfaction, reduce complaints and litigation, and improve the cost-effectiveness of medical care.

PART 2

PLACEBO EFFECT, MEDICAL EVIDENCE, AND THE DOCTOR/PATIENT RELATIONSHIP

I n part 1, we saw that a treatment benefit was the sum of the therapeutic gain, the natural course of the disease, and the placebo effect. Since the latter two can compensate for an absence of treatment effect or even a harmful treatment effect, many useless and even dangerous treatments have prospered in the history of healing. The most outrageous example in our culture was bloodletting, which must have killed many before it fell out of use. Because enthusiasm for a treatment can elicit placebo effects, and many illnesses naturally improve, we cannot know a treatment's intrinsic beneficial effects without randomized clinical trials. Part 2 begins with the principles of clinical trials and their contribution to *evidence-based medicine*. For most trials, a placebo control is essential. However, for trials of surgical procedures, psychotherapy, and complementary and alternative medicine, clinical trial design is especially difficult, and placebo control may be impossible (see chapters 9–11).

The other application of the placebo effect occurs in the doctor/patient relationship discussed in chapters 12 and 13. So important is the placebo effect to practical therapeutics that its omission can disappoint patients and increase health-care costs. Contemporary physicians cannot deceive their patients by surreptitiously offering them a sugar pill as therapy. Nevertheless, through positive attitudes and compassion, doctors can enhance the therapeutic benefits of an effective treatment. Then, the doctor is the placebo. Not everyone responds positively to placebo treatment, so we need to understand why some people do so, some of the time. Since improper use of placebos can deceive or do harm, we consider the ethics of their use at the end of part 2.

CHAPTER 7

RANDOMIZED CLINICAL TRIALS

U ntil the mid-twentieth century, all therapy was empirical. That is to say, observation and precedent guided treatment, rather than scientific proof that it was effective. Relying upon their experience, healers sought to select the best remedy for an ill person's complaint. Even today, the choice of treatment often depends upon the healer's experience or beliefs. Physicians, almost unique among healers, have sought a scientific basis for their treatments, and their most powerful tool is the *randomized clinical trial*.

A clinical trial comparing two treatments seems straightforward, but look closer and it becomes very complicated to undertake. So many circumstances, emotions, natural changes, expectations, and other influences surround any treatment that one person's response cannot be duplicated reliably in another. Even one individual who experiences a successful treatment on one occasion cannot be guaranteed it on the next. Moreover, the art and science of treatment testing concerns many disciplines (see table 7-1). Each brings its expertise and bias to the subject, and no human can master them all. Nevertheless, healers must take responsibility for the validity of their treatments. Doctors and patients must be able to interpret the available evidence when choosing therapy. Here we discuss the principles and pitfalls of clinical trials, and the importance of placebo control. First, let us briefly review the history of randomized clinical trials.

TABLE 7-1
Some Disciplines and Institutions Concerned with Clinical Trials and Placebos[1]

Advocates
Alternative Medicine
Clinical Medicine
Consumer
Epidemiology
Ethics
Formularies
Fund Managers
Health Economics
Hospitals
Law
Marketing
Pharmaceutics
Pharmacology
Pharmacy
Philosophy
Politics
Regulatory Authorities
Social Science
Statistics

THE HISTORY OF CLINICAL TRIALS[2]

Some attribute the earliest clinical trial to Nebuchadnezzar II, who, according to the book of Daniel, gave royal youths a rigid diet of meat and wine for three years. Daniel persuaded the eunuch who monitored the trial to permit himself and three others a ten-day diet of peas and beans with water. As a result of this intervention, these four were recorded to be fairer in countenance and fatter in body than the others.[3] Daniel notwithstanding, few treatments were submitted to scientific scrutiny before the Enlightenment (the seventeenth and eighteenth centuries). Throughout the Middle Ages, medicine stagnated in the rigid traditions of Hippocrates and Galen. The contents of medieval pharmacopeias were called *galenicals*, which only slowly disappeared from modern formularies. While Galen and his followers never tested their treatments, he appeared to recognize placebo effects. Even during the Enlightenment, medical science lagged behind physics, chemistry, and astronomy. There were some glimmers of progress, however. In the sixteenth century, Ambrose Paré conducted a series of controlled experiments in burn victims. The side of a patient's burned face that was treated with onions fared better than the other side treated conventionally with materials that damaged tissue. In 1547 Paré also treated wounds with a "digestive concoction" consisting of eggs, oil, and turpentine. He observed that healing was better with this concoction than the usual cautery with boiling oil. Such early examples of controlled experiments showing old treatments to be harmful were rare before the twentieth century.

The first controlled clinical trial is often attributed to James Lind of the Royal Navy.[4] During long sea voyages, many contemporary sailors suffered or died of scurvy, a potentially fatal disease characterized by internal bleeding. In 1600, four East India Company ships, only one of which had lemon juice on board, sailed from England. Scurvy was minimal on the lemon ship, but on the others with no lemons, many sailors became incapacitated. We now know that scurvy is due to the dietary lack of fruits and vegetables containing vitamin C. In 1747 Lind, a naval surgeon on board HMS *Salisbury*, undertook to test citrus fruit against the established treatments of the day. To discredit these treatments and convince naval authorities of the value of fruit, Lind entered twelve shipboard sailors "in the scurvy" into a trial where each of six pairs received a test treatment. Diet and surroundings (the bilge) were similar for all. He gave one pair two oranges and one lemon daily, while he treated the other pairs with contemporary remedies such as seawater, vinegar, and "elixir vitriol." Recovery occurred only in those receiving oranges and lemons.

However, science-based medicine was a tough sell in the eighteenth century. It took another fifty years before the British Navy acted upon Lind's convincing discovery! Some challenged Lind's own conviction.[5] Note that the trial subjects had similar disease, surroundings, and diet, so that only the treatment varied among the six pairs. There was no placebo control or blinding. Nevertheless, Lind's work led eventually to the eradication of scurvy at sea. Henceforth British sailors were referred to as "limeys" because of their daily citrus ration. With several refinements, controlled clinical trials are now commonplace in all fields of medicine. It is sobering that future generations will regard many of today's unproven treatments with the same amazement that we behold seawater, boiling oil, and vinegar.

Once infected with smallpox, a person is immune to reinfection. Therefore, deliberate infection with smallpox was seen as a way to prevent the disease. There are reports of this in tenth-century China.[6] In 1722, after observing the "inoculation" in Turkey, an aristocratic couple deliberately infected six convicts with material from smallpox lesions. The convicts survived, and one subsequently exposed to smallpox proved to be immune.

Edward Jenner is widely acclaimed as the originator of vaccination. However, before Jenner, many had observed that milkmaids infected with cowpox seemed to be immune to the far more serious smallpox, and were known for their uniquely unblemished faces. In 1774 a Dorset farmer named Benjamin Jesty used a knitting needle to inoculate himself, his wife, and two children with cowpox.[7] When the children were later inoculated with smallpox, they were unaffected. When he proceeded to vaccinate his milkmaids, neighbors recoiled at such "bestial" treatment. A nonphysician with no connections to a medical audience, Jesty's accomplishment was only recently recognized. Nevertheless, he was the first "vaccinator." It was not until 1796 that Jenner transferred cowpox material from "the hand of Sarah Nelmes to the arm of James Phelps."

In 1798 Jenner published *An Inquiry into the Causes and Effects of the Variolate Vaccine*. The paper describes twenty-three persons with cowpox who were resistant to smallpox inoculation. The study was uncontrolled in the sense that some would have acquired natural immunity to smallpox, and the control group was historical (previously observed unvaccinated subjects). Nevertheless, the disease was very infectious and his observation that it was preventable is remarkable. Pearson, a contemporary country doctor, observed that three subjects with cowpox were immune to smallpox inoculation, and two without it acquired the more serious disease. In 1800 an American, Benjamin Waterhouse, inoculated fourteen boys with smallpox, twelve of whom had been vaccinated previously. Only the two unvaccinated boys acquired smallpox. Despite the ethically unacceptable practice of deliberately inducing smallpox (even in convicts), these early clinical scientists founded the discipline of immunology and made major contributions to public health.

While vaccination eradicated smallpox only in 1980, it has saved millions of lives in the two hundred years since Jenner's observations. Acceptance of their findings was slow, but Lind and Jenner established scientific bases for the prevention of scurvy and smallpox. Indeed, they justifiably might be acclaimed among the founders of evidence-based medicine.

The above experiments were controlled in that the outcomes of the treated persons were compared to those of similar persons with unproven or no treatment. No placebos were employed. Perhaps the first placebo control was in 1801, when John Haygarth of Bath compared the "electromagnetism" of metal rods known as "Perkins tractors" with wooden "placebo tractors" in relieving rheumatic symptoms. He demonstrated no difference in outcome.

In a nineteenth-century French trial, Pierre Louis discovered that bloodletting (or venesection, the deliberate, supposedly therapeutic removal of blood) made no difference to the outcome of seventy-eight patients with pneumonia. Despite this, physicians continued to employ this potentially harmful treatment well into the twentieth century. Venesection could benefit patients only through a placebo response and the propensity of most diseases to improve.

In 1847 the Hungarian Ignaz Semmelweis noted that maternal deaths at childbirth were more numerous in women whose babies were delivered by physicians and medical students than by student midwives. Reasoning (before knowledge of microbes) that the former had more contact with cadavers, he introduced thorough hand washing. This resulted in a 50 percent drop in maternal mortality. In 1870 Joseph Lister, the pioneer of antisepsis, compared the outcome of a small number of amputation cases treated with an antiseptic to that of similar patients in the past. While his new cases did better, the use of historical controls delayed acceptance of his conclusions—a pity.

In 1881 the great French scientist Louis Pasteur conducted a randomized controlled trial of an antianthrax vaccine in sheep threatened with anthrax infection. He compared the fates of twenty-five sheep inoculated with the vaccine with twenty-five others. When they subsequently were infected with the bacteria, all of the unprotected sheep died, and all those protected by the antitoxin survived.

In 1898 J. Febiger, a German scientist compared antitoxin made from horse serum with plain horse serum (a blood product from which cells and clotting proteins have been removed, now known to contain antibodies) in the treatment of diphtheria patients. While the horse serum was not called a placebo, that was its function. He demonstrated no difference in the patients' outcomes between the two treatments. Another early twentieth-century double-blind technique compared the effects of alcohol to an inert, but similar, material that functioned as a placebo control. By the 1930s, trials comparing different treatments for angina pectoris were commonplace.

According to A. K. and E. Shapiro,[8] the concept of double-blinding is attributable to Harry Gold.[9] In 1932 Gold began a *single-blind* comparison of the cardiovascular drug aminophylline to an inert lactose pill (which has no pharmacologic effect) for the treatment of angina pectoris. He called it the "blind test" since the subjects did not know whether they received aminophylline or lactose. Early in the trial, Gold became aware that the investigators biased the results by their attitudes and leading questions. He belatedly introduced the concept of *double-blinding*, where neither patient nor physician knew who received active drug or lactose. Publication of this negative study in 1937 ended the use of aminophylline for cardiac pain. Another innovation was the realization that test substances and placebos should resemble one another so that recognition would not be possible. In their paper, Gold and his colleagues listed many factors that could influence the response of an individual to a treatment and explained why these made double-blinding and placebo control necessary. These confounding factors include, spontaneous changes (we would call this "natural history"), changes in weather, eating habits, doctors, work, domestic affairs, and so on. The double-blind principle developed slowly over the 1940s, as Gold and his colleagues struggled with its complexities. Apparently, the first use of the word *placebo* to describe inert controls was in a 1938 therapeutic trial of cold vaccines, but Gold quickly embraced the idea. Many credit Gold for the beginnings of double-blind placebo-controlled trials that are, or should be, the standard today.

The randomized trial that finally changed the way new therapies were tested was a 1948 comparison of streptomycin and no treatment for pulmonary tuberculosis.[10] Streptomycin was a newly available antibiotic, but it was in very short supply. It was urgently necessary to determine whether it worked. Sponsored by the British Medical Research Council (MRC) and designed by H. Bradford-Hill, this trial for the first time proved the efficacy of an important new therapy.

Curiously, this trial was neither double-blinded nor placebo controlled, but the randomization protocol was innovative. Less well known is a 1944 MRC trial of patulin (a penicillin abstract) for the treatment of the common cold.[11] Patulin was heralded by the press ("More valuable than penicillin?"), and promised to help the troops fight better. A trial was organized among civilians, not an easy task in wartime Britain. Subjects received the active drug or placebo through concealed allocation. The drug proved to be no better than a placebo, saving the armed forces an expensive diversion from the war effort. Significantly, it was double-blinded and placebo controlled. These two trials set standards for the investigators who followed.

Since World War II, placebo-controlled (or comparator-controlled) trials have become the preferred method of validating therapies. No pharmaceutical firm can dream of marketing a new prescription drug without scientific proof of its efficacy and safety that satisfies regulatory authorities. However, in our passion to understand the therapeutic effects of new treatments, we have neglected to examine why so many people improve on placebos.

WHY ARE CLINICAL TRIALS NEEDED?

Sometimes, new treatments produce such a dramatic change from the inevitable mortality that preceded them that they require no clinical trial. Such was the case with insulin for diabetes and penicillin for pneumococcal pneumonia, although trials were later necessary to establish these drugs' value in certain situations. The advantages of lancing a boil or setting a fracture are manifest. However, the efficacy of most therapeutic innovations is less obvious. After most treatments, some people improve, some do not, and some worsen. One patient's or one doctor's favorable therapeutic experience is "anecdotal evidence," insufficient to convince us that it is useful for others. We need to know from collective experience whether most of the time a treatment will benefit most patients who have similar characteristics.

Even some treatments that seem self-evident and make common sense may be subject to bias. The healer administering a treatment believes it will make the treated person better and in turn convinces the patient. If the outcome is good, everyone is content. Unfortunately, it is possible that "everyone" has been deceived! Even if a medicine has known pharmacological effects, a single happy result is insufficient to prove that it is truly effective. Most patients recover naturally. Improvement occurring after a treatment reinforces its reputation. A cold runs its course in a week, so any remedy can "cure" it.

Some would argue that if a person feels better after a treatment, there is no reason to question it. Apart from the personal and public deception countenanced by such an attitude, there are practical reasons to be skeptical. Drugs are costly, and almost all have untoward effects that offend Hippocrates' ancient admonishment, "Do no harm." A drug that harms even one patient is justified only if the disease is serious, and many others can expect some good. Unproven treatments may raise false hopes and distract from better ones. Thus, drugs—indeed, all treatments—require evaluation.

Since improvement of a single patient is unconvincing, practitioners may cite a *series* of patients. A surgeon may claim that a specific operation cures most of those with a particular disease. Physicians may become enthusiasts when a drug is apparently successful in several patients. Both are subject to bias. Moreover, early success of a treatment through happenstance reinforces doctors' confidence in it, and they spread the word to colleagues. This process enhances the placebo effect and may perpetuate many useless treatments. Little may be lost if the treatments are inexpensive, harmless, and for minor illnesses, but consider the potential harm of greatly publicized but ultimately worthless cancer cures (as discussed in chapter 16)!

Randomized, controlled clinical trials are designed to avoid bias. They have revolutionized how physicians think and practice, and have greatly augmented their effectiveness in curing disease and relieving suffering. Regulatory authorities such as the US Food and Drug Administration and the European Agency for the Evaluation of Medicinal Products must approve new drugs before physicians may prescribe them. The approval process requires randomized clinical trials and is long, arduous, and expensive. The failure of new products to be released in a timely manner frustrates many, but the alternative is to permit uncontrolled use of costly, useless, and potentially harmful drugs.

BIAS

Colloquially, "bias" means to influence, sway, or favor an argument. In research, it describes any factor or process that deviates the results or conclusions of an experiment away from the truth. Anecdotes are very liable to bias. A treatment and a successful outcome may be connected by coincidence only, yet because they occur together, cause and effect may be wrongly assumed. When another patient appears with a similar problem, the healer relies on her experience and employs the same treatment. However, coincidence does not imply cause. Most illnesses improve with time, and the healer's enthusiasm and the patient's expectations can have beneficial effects. How else can one explain the centuries-long use of leeches, ritual purging, and many other noxious therapies?

A series of cases can repeat an anecdote and merely compound the bias. Only with suitable and contemporaneous controls can we begin to evaluate a treatment's usefulness. Historical controls, where previous patient outcomes are compared with those after a new treatment, can introduce bias if the circumstances change. For example, the enthusiasm of the doctor and the hopeful expectations of the patients for the new treatment are absent in a historical control period. The randomized, controlled trial seeks to avoid such biases, yet bias may still occur at any stage of the trial from patient selection to analysis. Buyer beware! Readers of a clinical trial report should understand its biases before buying its conclusions.

J. Kleijnen[12] and his colleagues suggest subtle methodological errors that may bias a trial. Using a *balanced placebo design* investigators can, in parallel, conduct two placebo-controlled randomized trials of a single treatment. If one has a different trial condition, they can determine the effect of that condition on the outcome. For example, the effect of the test drug appears to be lessened when there is informed consent in one of the parallel trials, or if the patient knows he is likely to receive a placebo. In longer trials, if the subject experiences an improvement on the drug, he may realize he is not on placebo and upwardly adjust his expectation of improvement. Put another way, when a study is unintentionally unblinded and the subject realizes he is on the test drug, its actions and the placebo effect become synergistic. Similarly, an investigator can influence outcome if she knows that one group is less likely to get a placebo than another is. Bias lurks everywhere in testing treatments.

ELEMENTS OF A CLINICAL TRIAL

A. Bradford-Hill, the designer of the streptomycin study, defined a clinical trial as "a carefully and ethically designed experiment with the aim of answering some precisely framed question."[13] Christopher Bulpitt modified this to define a controlled clinical trial as "a carefully and ethically designed experiment which includes the provision of adequate and appropriate controls by a process of randomization, so that precisely framed questions can be answered."[14] However, no definition can embrace the many and detailed elements that constitute the modern randomized, double-blind, placebo-controlled clinical trial. Since bias may appear in many subtle ways, it is countered by sophisticated methodology, the elements of which follow (see table 7-2).

TABLE 7-2
Elements of a Randomized Clinical Trial

Hypothesis: a clinically relevant research question (precisely framed)

Subject selection and generalizability: a representative population

Random selection of study groups using concealed allocation

Double-blinding

Control group (usually placebo) identical to treatment group but without the test treatment

Predetermined endpoint

Predetermined primary outcome measure

Compliance

Intention-to-treat analysis

Appropriate, transparent **statistical evaluation** of data

Publication of results even if negative

Responsible discussion of conclusions

Hypothesis

All research should begin with a carefully stated hypothesis that conveys what investigators expect the experiment to prove. A hypothesis for a randomized clinical trial may be stated: "Will the symptoms of patients receiving a drug be more improved [at a certain endpoint with a precise outcome measure] than those of other patients with similar disease and circumstances receiving an externally identical placebo?" A trial should have only one primary objective, since multiple outcomes statistically weaken the conclusions. Secondary objectives may help create hypotheses for future studies, or even support the primary objective. However, their successes or failures do not affect the success or failure of the study, which must be determined solely by the outcome of the primary objective. In the main, investigators should focus a clinical trial to answer a single, precisely framed research question.

Subject Selection and Generalizability

To test a treatment for a population of patients with a certain disease, investigators may conduct a randomized, controlled clinical trial. If the results of the trial are to be applied to this population, the trial's subjects must be representative. That is, the selected patients must resemble the larger population in age, sex distribution, stage or severity of disease, other treatments, and environmental factors that might influence the course of the disease. Such a representative sample is often difficult to achieve. In a serious or terminal disease such as cancer, recruitment is relatively easy since regional cancer centers often handle all the cases in their area. However, ambulatory patients with relatively benign illnesses attend doctors in many places, and there are reasons why many of them might be unwilling or unable to participate in a time-consuming trial. These include the need to work or look after their children, lack of confidence in the proposed treatment, insufficient symptom severity, unwillingness to take a placebo, and *exclusion criteria* such as other disease or medication that render them ineligible.

For some complaints such as headache, backache, fibromyalgia, or irritable bowel syndrome, only a few subjects with the symptoms seek medical care, and even fewer are referred to the university centers where clinical trials are usually conducted. Irritable bowel syndrome (IBS) patients in such centers constitute less than 10 percent of all those with IBS symptoms and are more likely to have coincidental depression and other diseases than the remainder in primary care or those who do not consult doctors.[15] Thus, the results of a clinical trial conducted among these few referred patients may not be *generalizable* to primary care IBS patients, let alone the majority who seek no medical care at all. Similar selection bias occurs in trials testing treatments for headache, dysmenorrhea, and backache. When interpreting the results of a clinical trial, careful scrutiny of the selection process is essential in order to determine to whom the results apply.

Randomization

Investigators next must randomize the selected subjects into the two or more arms of the clinical trial. In a trial comparing a medication to placebo, the subjects receiving each treatment should be randomly allocated to remove the possibility of bias and ensure the comparison groups are as similar as possible. Randomization is achieved in many ways from the tossing of a coin to random allocation by computer. Techniques do not concern us here, but a successful randomization should result in comparable subjects in each treatment group. To avoid bias, someone other than the investigator should do the randomizing, and throughout the trial, investigators should have no opportunity to learn to which group the patient is assigned. This process is termed *concealed allocation.*[16] Bias could occur if the investigator selects which group a patient enters or if he knows a subject's allocation.

The reader of a clinical trial report can judge the effectiveness of randomization by comparing the characteristics of the treatment and control subjects. The first table in a trial report commonly presents such a comparison by listing relevant demographic features such as age, gender, use of other treatments, and duration of illness (see table 7-3). Generally, the larger the trial, the more likely will concealed allocation produce demographically similar groups. Such data should also include factors that might, if not evenly distributed between treatment groups, bias the results. For example, any study of respiratory disease should have similar rates of tobacco use in each treatment group.

TABLE 7-3
Hypothetical Demographic Characteristics of Two Groups Entered in a Randomized Clinical Trial

	Treatment Group N=80	Placebo Group N=82	Difference
Age (mean years)	39 (range 28–49)	40 (range 24–55)	NS
Sex (% Female)	76	78	NS
Race (% white)	93	90	NS
Symptom Duration (months)	13 (range 9–15)	18 (range 11–14)	NS
Other Drugs	4	3	NS
Dropouts	13	2	P<.05

This hypothetical "Table 1" in a clinical trial report shows sundry information in the two groups. When compared statistically, there are no differences between the groups in age, sex, race, symptom duration, or the use of other drugs, suggesting that random (and concealed) allocation to the groups was successful. However, the greater number of dropouts in the treatment group during the trial suggests a bias, possibly due to side effects of the drug being tested. Whatever the outcome data, it is important to use an "intention-to-treat analysis" where the dropouts are considered as "treatment failures."

Blinding

If, upon entering a trial, a patient knows that he is receiving a drug rather than a placebo, his outcome might be influenced in several ways. If the treatment is new and promising and the outcome is subjective, he may be biased toward a positive outcome. Sometimes, a patient may respond to questions about outcomes in ways designed to please the investigator. His responses may also influence the way the investigator records the results. Attitudes may even change during a trial.[17] For these reasons, subjects in clinical trials are blinded, that is, they do not know which treatment they received until the outcomes are determined at the end of the trial.

As Gold discovered during the 1930s, the investigators and those judging outcomes may also introduce bias in overt and subtle ways. During allocation of subjects to treatment groups, investigators could influence the chosen treatment allocation, subtly indicate a preference for one treatment, or influence a patient's compliance with the study protocol. Even the most inscrutable investigator cannot control the beliefs of his coworkers and the enthusiasm that often attends a new treatment. Individuals charged with gathering study data may also be influenced by their beliefs about the treatment and interpret the data accordingly.

Where only the subjects are blinded in a randomized controlled trial, it is said to be *single-blind*. When both subjects and investigators are blinded, the trial is *double-blind*. If a third person is also blinded and independently assesses the trial process and results, the trial becomes *triple-blind*.[18] Ad absurdum, if the statisticians or data analysts are different persons again and also are blinded, the trial is *quadruple-blind*. In practice these latter two terms are seldom used, but the principles are nevertheless important.

Endpoint

The endpoint is the time when the outcome is determined, usually, but not always, at the end of the trial. For example, the endpoint of the study of a chronic painful disorder, illustrated in figure 1-1, is during the last of twelve weeks. The success or failure of the trial is judged by an improvement in the outcome measure during that week compared to the beginning of the trial (baseline). There are several possible endpoints: the last day of the trial, the average of several periods within the trial, or even the occurrence of an event that the tested treatment is designed to prevent, such as a heart attack. Like other features of good trial design, the endpoint must be determined in advance.

Outcome Measures

In some trials, the outcome is clear-cut and easily measured. Examples might be weight gained due to a nutritional supplement or lost through a weight-losing diet, the occurrence of an event such as a stroke or admission to a hospital, or the shrinking of a tumor as measured by an imaging technique. However, in many cases the outcome determination relies on the patient's opinion about how he feels at the endpoint compared to the baseline. Such a subjective outcome measure requires seamless double-blinding to prevent bias.

Subjective outcomes may be determined in numerous ways. A simple method is to request a simple "yes" or "no" to a question such as, "Compared to before the treatment, is your symptom improved?" This two-choice outcome is called *binary*. Alternately, a five-point *ordinal scale* might be used as in the following example:

Compared to before the treatment, is your "symptom":
        "much better,"
        "better,"
        "the same,"
        "worse," or
        "much worse"?

Note that this scale balances so the number of "better" and "worse" choices is equal. There are sometimes seven or nine choices. These replies are difficult to compare statistically because the intervals between them are unequal. For this reason, investigators may choose a measurable *visual analogue scale* (VAS):

much worse	worse	same	better	much better

0   10

In this example, the subject is shown a line usually with 0 at one end, 10 at the other, and a legend with the ordinals indicated above. The line under "same" is the midpoint indicating five out of ten. The subject then indicates with a mark on the line where the severity of his symptom fits. In a trial, investigators may measure how much the patient's assessment of his symptom severity changes between the baseline and the endpoint on an ordinal or VA scale. Ordinal and VA scales must be balanced with the neutral point in the middle to avoid a *scaling bias*.

Sometimes investigators need to consider more than one disease manifestation in an outcome measure. One way is to declare the primary outcome measure to be the most important symptom or sign, relegating other outcomes as secondary. Some diseases or "syndromes" manifest several subjective symptoms and/or objective signs. Investigators have tried to overcome this difficulty by designing severity indexes or symptom scores. One example is the Crohn's disease activity index (CDAI).[19] Table 7-4 illustrates several features of Crohn's disease (a chronic intestinal inflammatory disease) that are combined to provide a single measurable index. Note that symptoms (diarrhea), medication use (antidiarrheals), physical observations (abdominal mass), and laboratory tests (hematocrit) are incorporated into a single score. Each item is weighted according to its importance. Investigators can compare this index at the endpoint to its value at the baseline. The CDAI has been indispensable to the development and testing of new treatments for Crohn's disease.

Other times, a combination of symptoms describe a *syndrome*, such as irritable bowel syndrome. Unlike Crohn's disease, there are no objective findings, but abdominal pain, altered bowel habit, and well-being are considered meaningful. Improvement in the pain alone is deemed insufficient to describe improvement in the syndrome. To circumvent this difficulty, a *global outcome measure* is employed.[20] For example, in testing a new drug for the constipated phase of the irritable bowel, the subjects are asked, "Please consider how you felt this last week in regard to your irritable bowel syndrome, in particular your overall well-being, and symptoms of abdominal discomfort, pain, and altered bowel habit. Compared to how you felt before entering the study, how would you rate your relief of symptoms during the past week?" A risk of this composite endpoint is that "general well-being," can measure mood (e.g., anxiety or depression)

TABLE 7-4
Crohn's Disease Activity Index (CDAI)[22]

These 8 criteria comprise the CDAI. Each item's weight is in brackets. For definitions of terms, consult the glossary.

[x2] 1. Number of liquid or very soft stools in one week.

[x5] 2. Sum of 7 daily pain ratings: 0=none; 1=mild; 2=moderate; 3=severe.

[x7] 3. Sum of daily ratings of general well-being: 0=generally well; 1=slightly below par; 2=poor; 3=very poor.

[x20] 4. Symptoms or findings presumed related to Crohn's disease:

   a. arthritis/arthralgia

   b. skin/mouth lesions, pyoderma gangrenosa/erythema nodosum

   c. iritis/uveitis.

   d. anal fissure, fistula, or perirectal abscess.

   e. other bowel-related fistula, e.g., enterovesicle, etc.

   f. fever over 37.8°C, or 100°F.

[x30] 5. Use of diphenoxylate, loperamide, or other opiate for diarrhea: 0=no, 1=yes.

[x10] 6. Abdominal mass: 0=absent; 0.4=questionable; 1=present.

[x6] 7. 47 − hematocrit (males); 42 − hematocrit (females).

[x1] 8. $\dfrac{100\text{x ([standard weight]} - \text{[actual body weight])}}{\text{standard weight}}$

rather than IBS. In addition, one of the several combined factors might drive the outcome.[21] For example, improvement in constipation may produce a positive outcome even when pain and well-being are unaffected. Thus, a new drug might seem to be effective against IBS when the benefit could be due solely to its laxative effect.

There is a difference between *within-patient* and *within-group* comparisons of trial outcomes. In the former, each patient's outcome is recorded according to predetermined criteria, and the number of improved patients (*responders*) compared between the groups. Here the outcome is *binary*. An outcome of death is binary in that there are only two possibilities, death or not. The statistician need only compare the number of deaths in each treatment group, the difference being the therapeutic gain. Binary outcomes are also possible in a trial where outcome success is defined prior to commencement, such as a diastolic blood pressure below 80, or a weight gain above five kilograms.

For within-group comparisons, the outcomes of the subjects in each group are averaged so that the outcome is *continuous*. In continuous outcomes, the outcome measure is a value, and at the endpoint, the mean values are compared among the various treatment groups. For example, a mean 60 percent improvement in a symptom in the treatment group and a mean 40 percent improvement in the placebo group indicate a therapeutic gain of twenty.

Compliance (Adherence)

In any trial, some subjects will drop out after they are randomized and before the endpoint is reached. Reasons to drop out include intervening disease, other commitments, dramatic worsening of the condition, disillusionment in the trial, belief the treatment is a placebo, side effects, and failure to follow the trial protocol. To ensure the subject is getting the treatment, investigators may phone them periodically or count the pills remaining at the endpoint.

Dropouts can destroy the trial if too few remain to allow statistical evaluation. Analysis of the outcome data, using only those who have stayed in to the end, is called a *per protocol analysis*. If 13 percent of subjects fail to finish the study in the treatment group compared to 2 percent in the controls, they can bias the results (see table 7-3). To counter this bias, researchers should employ *intention-to-treat analysis*. Here, dropouts are considered to be treatment failures and included as such in the interpretation of the study. Sometimes, if subjects are in the study long enough, the time of their last recorded data becomes the endpoint. If the dropouts are equally balanced among the treatment groups, the intention-to-treat analysis may produce results similar to the per protocol analysis. If however, the dropouts are all in one group, they may indicate some dissatisfaction with the treatment, and must be deemed treatment failures. If they drop out because they feel better on their treatment, yet are considered treatment failures, another bias is introduced.

Analysis

For analysis of the results of a clinical trial, we must rely upon the arcane world of statistics. The average person need not be a statistician to interpret clinical trial data, but a few terms and concepts are useful to know. The *therapeutic gain* or *absolute benefit increase* is the actual increase in good outcomes between treatment group patients over control patients. Some call this the "delta." For binary data, it is expressed as the percent of treatment group patients with good outcomes minus the percent of placebo group patients with good outcomes. In figure 1-1, the weekly therapeutic gain is the difference between the dots representing the percent of patients improved by the treatment and the percent improved by placebo. The *number needed to treat* (NNT) is the therapeutic gain (percent) divided into one. Thus, the NNT is the number of patients that must be treated for one additional good outcome to occur. If the number is small, say four, the improvement of the test treatment over a placebo might be "clinically significant." If the NNT is high, say eighteen, the treatment may not be worth using. The therapeutic gain and NNT may help the non-statistician interpret a trial report, but they do not obviate the need for investigators to perform statistical analyses.

The statistical terms found in many trials include the *p-value* and *confidence intervals*. They are the investigator's holy grail, and are the products of statistical calculations of comparison data derived from an experiment, in this case a clinical trial. Normally, a statistically significant conclusion accepts a 5 percent minimum chance of error. As pollsters often say, their data are correct "nineteen times out of twenty." A statistically significant difference that has a 5 percent chance of error between the outcomes of two arms in a randomized clinical trial is usually reported as "p<.05." A value "p<.01" is highly significant, while "p<.06" is insignificant. This convention provides a convenient threshold to distinguish two values from one another, but whether the statistically significant result is *clinically significant* is another matter. The therapeutic gain, the NNT, the gravity of the illness being treated, and the cost and adverse effects need all be considered when treating a patient. It is essential to remember that "p<.05" means that there is a 5 percent chance the differences between the two groups occurred by random chance rather than because of the effect of the treatment. Thus, one trial in twenty could show a statistically significant difference when no real treatment effect exists. This is a *type I error*. A more stringent p-value, say "p<.01" reduces the risk of a type I error. However, the study may now fail to show a difference when one exists, a so-called *type II error*. Either way, 100 percent certainty is a statistical impossibility.

Many prefer the *confidence intervals of the mean* as a statistical tool. This interval is a range of values with upper and lower limits for a population. If sufficient population samples of similar size are tested, 95 percent of the intervals will contain the true mean value. The narrower the range, the more confident we can be that the data are accurate. Where confidence intervals are compared between two populations, a difference is demonstrated by the failure of the confidence intervals to overlap.

There are several caveats when interpreting statistics. Too few subjects in the trial will result in insufficient *power* to show a difference between two sets of data (type II error). Taking into account the expected difference and the required p-value, the investigators should estimate the number of subjects necessary for the trial results to show a difference, and they should record this figure in the methods section of the trial report.

Another caution is that statistical testing in an experiment should focus on the primary outcome measure. In a clinical trial, this might be pain or some other clinical phenomenon. If this is declared the primary outcome before the study, then "p<.05" means that the pain is relieved by the tested treatment with 95 percent confidence. Secondary outcomes may be tested as well, but only to support the primary outcome and suggest items that may be explored in other trials. If there must be two primary outcomes, a statistical maneuver is necessary to compensate for the increased chance of a positive result in one of them. Ad absurdum, the more outcomes analyzed, the more likely a chance positive result will occur.

Statistical tests such as the T-test or regression analysis are beyond the range of this volume. As David Sackett explains, few investigators understand more than the rudiments themselves, and must collaborate with statisticians.[23] For further explanation, the reader should refer to one of the texts that appear in the notes. Investigators have a responsibility to report their findings in as clear a manner as possible, so the unsophisticated reader can use the information. If the statistics are convoluted, it is likely that the results are of marginal clinical significance. Finally, statistics are only as reliable as the data to which they are applied. A clinical trial may be flawed through defects in any of the elements described above. Statistical redemption of flawed data is a mirage.

Placebos in Clinical Trials

Placebo controls are not always necessary. If there is another drug of proven efficacy for the treatment of the subjects in the study, then it can serve as a comparator. However, it is statistically difficult to demonstrate no difference between two treatment outcomes because of a possible type II error. If the established drug is proved to be very effective, then its use as a comparator is sound. However, a new drug that is "equivalent" to a marginally effective one actually could be no better than a placebo. If the new drug is completely safe, one can argue for a placebo control if withholding an alternate treatment for the duration of the trial will not harm the subjects.

As explained in the first section in this book, the use of the word *placebo* to describe the control device for a clinical trial forever changed its meaning. Doctors no longer give placebos to please a patient. A new treatment is compared to a placebo to ensure that it is more effective. As such, the placebo must resemble the treatment in every possible way including color, size, and taste. In the case of medication, disguising the placebo and active pills or capsules is relatively straightforward. Difficulty arises only when the test drug has effects, other than the primary outcome, that the patient easily recognizes. For example, anticholinergic drugs used to treat bowel pains cause a dry mouth. Once the patient (or investigator) realizes that he is on the test drug, the trial is no longer double-blind.

In trials of dietary, psychological, or surgical treatments, placebos are less easy to disguise. Devices are controlled in many ways. One example is Haygarth's two-hundred-year-old trial where wooden rods controlled for the electromagnetic metal "tractors" in the treatment of arthritis. In the case of a machine, investigators accomplish placebo control by switching it off. Whatever the proposed treatment, the control group must receive a placebo or alternative treatment that neither subjects nor investigators can distinguish from the treatment being tested.

DESIGN OF RANDOMIZED, CONTROLLED TREATMENT TRIALS

How can the above elements be consolidated into a randomized clinical trial? There are many trial designs and I shall briefly describe only a few. Figure 1-1 illustrates a design for validating a medication for a chronic painful condition. Here the subjects are randomly selected patients submitted by concealed allocation to drug treatment and placebo treatment groups. Prior to commencing treatment, a two-week run-in period permits the investigators to make baseline observations. Then the subjects are randomly allocated the test drug or an outwardly identical placebo pill. Subsequently, they are assessed weekly (for twelve weeks) with a previously agreed-upon primary outcome measure. The endpoint could be the last week of the study, or an average of twelve weekly measurements. In figure 1-1, a four-week follow-up period demonstrates what happens when the treatments cease.

There are many variations of this model. There may be no run-in, and the baseline is estimated at time zero. The treatment period may be shorter or longer. There may be several treatment arms to the study with each group of subjects receiving different doses of the drug. Some studies test survival or the prevention of an event over a long period. Others address treatments for an infection say, over a week or less.

A *crossover trial* features two successive treatment periods between which the groups switch treatments. In crossover designs, each subject serves as his own control. Comparison of symptoms on drug and placebo is now possible for each patient. This provides a statistical advantage but creates new problems. For many disorders with shifting baseline values, consecutive treatment periods may not be comparable. More seriously, an effective drug's benefit may spill over into a subsequent placebo period. As mentioned in an earlier chapter, if a potent pain-relieving drug is given first, the subsequent placebo effect is heightened, whereas if the placebo is given first, the efficacy of the drug is lessened. In the second period, there may be a residual pharmacological effect from the first. Some trial designs attempt to minimize sequential effects by inserting a short *washout* period at crossover. In every type of trial, the principles are similar and essential if we are to credit the results.

Not only drugs can be tested by a randomized, double-blind, placebo-controlled clinical trial. Many believe that a firm mattress is beneficial for lower back pain. Researchers in the Mediterranean island of Mallorca challenged this belief with a randomized trial comparing firm with medium-firm mattresses provided by the investigators, blindly installed, and randomly allocated to 313 patients with uncomplicated lower back pain.[24] Using VAS scores, there were three primary outcomes (allowed for statistically) at the ninety-day endpoint: improvement in pain while lying in bed, pain on rising, and disability. The medium mattresses resulted in better outcomes in intention-to-treat analyses at the endpoint and throughout the ninety days. In addition, those sleeping on the medium mattresses were more likely to favor the desirable fetal position, possibly because there was less pressure on the hips and shoulders. This result is especially compelling because so many believed that hard mattresses were better.[25]

WHO PARTICIPATES IN CLINICAL TRIALS?

Subjects in randomized, double-blind, placebo-controlled clinical trials are people like you and me. Without them new drug testing could not occur. Whether or not participants derive any benefit from participation, they perform a valuable public service. Nevertheless, those invited to participate in a controlled trial should consider several issues.

Will Being in the Trial Help Me?

This depends on many things. Obviously, if a participant receives the active drug and the drug proves effective in the trial, he may benefit.

However, it is possible that the drug will prove ineffective, or that he will receive the placebo, or even be one of a few in whom an effective drug fails. There are less tangible benefits. A trial offers the opportunity for patients to learn about their disease. They may interact with experts and learn of research efforts. Close observation by doctors and nurses managing the trial can have health benefits unavailable to those not in a trial. Occasionally, a trial may provide an early opportunity to receive a truly advanced treatment.

Who Is Doing the Trial?

One is reassured if a university hospital or family-practice establishment supports the trial. Nevertheless, the study need not be at a university, as the mattress study shows. Often, a pharmaceutical company funds the research, and some contract research establishments will conduct their trials in community practices. Institutional ethics committees must approve all proposed trials and also evaluate their value and safety. The principal investigator at the study site should be a physician who is knowledgeable about the treatment and disease under study. No trial can proceed without a competent study nurse who monitors patients' progress, collects data, and oversees the trial's conduct. Study coordinators and statisticians manage the collected information.

Will I Be Harmed by the Trial?

It is impossible to guarantee complete safety. Nevertheless, pharmaceutical houses test drugs extensively before they offer them to humans, and most randomized clinical trials are safe. Pharmaceutical firms, licensing authorities, and ethics committees are unlikely to approve a drug for trial if they have any safety concerns, especially if the disease is not life threatening. For cardiac disease or cancer, however, some degree of risk is acceptable, provided the possible benefits are sufficient. In the end, potential subjects must make their own judgment. Nobody should enter a trial without giving *informed consent*, and participants should feel free to seek advice or withdraw at any time. The principal investigator should describe the test treatment, including how it might improve the patient's condition. She should explain all known and theoretical risks as well as the probability that one might receive the placebo. The Declaration of Helsinki outlines the elements of informed consent and the ethics of human experimentation (see chapter 14).

Should I Participate in This Trial?

A prospective participant should be satisfied that the conditions described above are in place and that the results of the study will be published whatever the outcome. He should also accept the disruption of his life by trial routine and prohibition of certain drugs, foods, or pregnancy (if female). If, in addition, he is comfortable with the study personnel, he should consider it. Participants must feel that treatments for their disease are presently unsatisfactory and be committed to help find better ones.

CONCLUSIONS

Randomized, placebo-controlled, double-blind clinical trials are the cornerstone of modern scientific medicine. Trials evolved over two centuries but became serviceable only after World War II. They seek to replace the anecdote, the series, and "experience" as the basis of medical decision making. To be credible, a randomized, controlled trial must be designed to answer a single, precisely framed clinical question, such as, "Is treatment X better than placebo for patients who suffer a disease where the stage of the disease and the social and physical environments are similar?" Researchers address the question by randomizing a typical or representative group of patients through concealed allocation to receive either the test treatment or an apparently identical control treatment. In double-blind fashion, the two groups' outcomes are compared without bias at the endpoint. Like the perfect poem, the perfect clinical trial is likely unattainable. Even the statisticians permit a 5 percent error. Nevertheless, randomized controlled clinical trials are the essential building blocks for evidence-based medicine—the subject of the next chapter.

CHAPTER 8

EVIDENCE-BASED MEDICINE

"[T]he placebo effect is the only single action which all
drugs have in common and in some instances it is the only
useful action that the medication can exert."

STEWART WOLF (1959)[1]

Before 1700, mysticism, anecdote, belief, tradition, and experience were more prevalent than science in the healing arts.
During the Enlightenment, there were major advances in our understanding of human anatomy, physiology, bacteriology, and biochem-
istry. Slowly, those practicing therapeutics and surgery began to base
their treatments on the new knowledge, and the practice of medicine
became rational and science based. However, proof that most therapies, even if science based, were effective was not forthcoming until
the mid-twentieth century. Only with the development of the randomized, double-blind, placebo-controlled clinical trial did physicians have a tool to evaluate treatments, and separate their benefits
from those of the placebo effect and the course of nature.

Since randomized, controlled clinical trials for new treatments
have become the norm, it does not mean that all that went before is
fallacious, nor does it mean that all that physicians now do is evidence
based. Lack of proof of efficacy does not prove lack of efficacy. What
trial evidence does mean is that for most patients for many diseases,
there is scientific evidence that favors certain treatments. These treatments are by no means the only measures that healers should use, nor
do all patients resemble the subjects of a given clinical trial. Nevertheless, we can begin to feel confident that therapeutics has entered a
new age, where increasing randomized clinical trial data support a
greater proportion of the treatments that doctors can prescribe for

111

patients. The therapeutic questions science has yet to answer seem limitless, and the validation of treatments will never be complete, but the beginning has been impressive.

Now, we shall consider how the evidence from randomized clinical trials can help doctors make their treatments science based. So far, the terms "doctor," "physician," "healer," and "health-care professional" have appeared interchangeably. Here, "doctor" or "physician" seems most appropriate, since medicine has led the search for a scientific basis to treat patients. Dentistry and nursing are based largely on clinical research, too, but practitioners of psychotherapy and complementary and alternative medicine have much catching up to do. Yet, as we examine the expanding science of medical therapeutics, we must not forget the art of healing. The placebo effect indicates that more than science is required to make most ill people feel better.

DEFINITION OF EVIDENCE-BASED MEDICINE

We can define *evidence-based medicine* as the "conscientious, explicit and judicious use of the current best evidence from clinical care research in making decisions about the care of individual patients."[2] Thus, physicians must conscientiously follow the literature to discover new data that might help them treat their patients. This is a tall order, as there are hundreds of medical journals of varying quality, and most of their reports are complicated and difficult for doctors or nondoctors to read. To discover the best treatment, physicians need to consult the current medical literature and study the methods section of each relevant report to ascertain if the research adheres to the principles of randomized trials such as generalizability, randomization, blinding, predetermined outcome measures and endpoints, and intention-to-treat analysis.[3] "Judicious use" infers that the physician must judge whether her patient fits the description of the subjects on whom the treatment was tested. Then, after considering the patient's preferences, the side effects, and the cost, both can decide whether to use it.

THE NEED FOR CLINICAL TRIALS: NATURE AND THE PLACEBO EFFECT

In the physical sciences, experiments answer questions with precision, so controls are often unnecessary. Before a known weight dropped from a known height hits the ground, it will attain a velocity that can be precisely calculated. It is even possible to accurately allow for variables such as wind, altitude, and atmospheric density. Provided the calculations are correct, the experiment will produce identical results on subsequent occasions. In biology, experiment is less precise. Not only are many of the biological inputs in an experiment unknown, but animals' behaviors are unpredictable. To measure the energy expended by a rat negotiating a maze, scientists must control for variations in the participating animals' motivation, hunger, fear, and conditions in the maze during each experiment. In a clinical experiment, investigators must not only control for biological variables, they also must account for a vast range of environments, emotions, behaviors, and psychologies that enrich and complicate people's lives. Since these human attributes may influence the course of a disease during a clinical trial, trial subjects must be randomized so that the treatment and control groups can be reasonably expected to be similar. Meanwhile, "lurking in the shadows"[4] between science and emotion is the placebo effect, reminding us that double-blinding is needed as well.

HOW USEFUL ARE RANDOMIZED, CONTROLLED TRIALS?

Clinical trials cannot be perfect. Given the human imperfections of the investigators, the trial subjects, and the physicians that must use the data, much can go wrong between a hypothesis and the consulting room. While the randomized, controlled trial is the best tool we have for evaluating treatments, we should briefly consider its advantages and limitations.

Advantages

The above arguments summarize the need for randomized, controlled trials to prove that medications are effective. However, there are other advantages. If the drug is distributed to pharmacies without clinical trials, then harmful effects may not be noticed or reported. The randomized trial permits a close examination of the drug in action. Harmless side effects like headache may be tolerable if the drug is useful, but kidney damage or untoward interaction with another drug is another matter. Clinical trial evidence often causes the eventual removal of some useless or even harmful treatments from medicine's repertoire. Historical examples include Lind's discrediting of seawater or vinegar to treat scurvy, Louis's demonstration that venesection made no difference to the outcome of pneumonia, and Haygarth's exposure of the uselessness of electromagnetic tractors. Chapter 9 describes common surgical procedures that randomized controlled trials demonstrated to be no better than sham surgery.

Removal of expensive, useless, and costly treatments from the repertoire not only protects patients but also saves money. The process of discarding old tests and treatments is more difficult than it should be. In 1939 E. F. Du Bois declared, "[A]ny young neophyte can introduce a new drug. It requires a man of large experience and considerable reputation to destroy an old one" (quoted by Stewart Wolf).[5] The judicious use of randomized, controlled trials should make the task easier.

By scientifically scrutinizing disease, patients, and treatments, investigators gain new knowledge. One subject's side effect may be another's salvation. Clinical trials first tested a drug now known as Viagra for the treatment of hypertension but failed to demonstrate any benefit over current treatment. When after the trial the investigators sought to collect unused pills from the subjects of the trial, they discovered that some men were reluctant to part with them. Investigation revealed that the pills improved their erectile function. Rather than fall into the dustbin of pharmaceutical history, Viagra proved successful in new trials and is now a useful and best-selling drug for a purpose its developers would never have discovered without the original carefully monitored clinical trial. Like Alexander Fleming's fortuitous contamination of a bacterial culture with penicillin mold, some of the greatest therapeutic discoveries are accidental. Such accidents require opportunities for prepared minds to observe.

Clinical trials improve the confidence in and the reputation of medical care. Subjects gain the opportunity to learn about their illness and get exemplary treatment. Clinical trials provide the scientific basis of medicine and therefore they are here to stay.

Limitations

Even a carefully conducted randomized clinical trial may produce falsely negative results. An insufficient number of subjects may result in a type II error. A flaw in the entry criteria, too many dropouts, or a poorly chosen outcome measure may also weaken a trial's applicability. Failure may be due to something mundane such as choosing an inadequate formulation or dose of the test drug. Randomized trials lack precision to detect small benefits. More disturbing is the possibility of a false positive result, thus legitimizing a useless therapy (type I error). Remember, no statistics can be 100 percent accurate. The danger of false negative and false positive trials is that their conclusions become set in stone. As far as we know, such instances are rare, but unless we subject falsely categorized treatments to retrial, or careful postmarketing follow-up, we may never know the truth about them.

The protocols of trials permit little opportunity to optimize the dose of a drug for individual subjects. In real life, the dose is adjusted according to the patient's age, size, and possibly physiologic measures such as pulse and blood pressure. These adjustments would compromise blinding in a trial, which is why some dosing questions remain unaddressed. Some claim that placebos are unnecessary if the outcome measure is objective as in death or stroke.[6] However, placebos control for more than the outcome itself. Changes in the attitudes, incentives, and behaviors of a person entering a clinical trial can themselves alter the outcome.

Some complain that randomized clinical trials delay the availability of valuable new treatments. From the preceding discussion, it is obvious that this is an untenable position. If the treatment were known to be useful, there would be no need for a trial. Using ineffective treatments wastes money and risks harm. Where the disease is fatal, pressure to approve a new drug prematurely can be irresistible. Patient-advocacy groups often chafe at the delays in their members' access to new drugs, but science should not be rushed. Some will remember the approval of the sedative drug thalidomide. Only when it was given to pregnant women after its release did the world learn of its horrific damage to the fetus. Others claim that assignment to a control group in a clinical trial can delay a person's use of the test treatment. Here again, the argument is two sided: those on the treatment may fare no better, or even worse, than those on no treatment or on a placebo. Furthermore, participation in a trial may be itself beneficial.

Randomized clinical trials are very expensive. The pharmaceutical industry estimates that the cost of bringing a drug from conception to regulatory approval is $800 million[7] or more,[8] and clinical trials are the most costly component. Such trials are required not only for regulatory approval for a drug but also to persuade patients or insuring authorities to pay for it. The requirement for expensive clinical trials may inhibit the development of some new drugs, especially if the potential for sales is small.

Evidence-based medicine has a pharmaceutical bias toward new drugs. Other or older treatments are often neglected. Only if it can foresee a profit from drug sales will a firm take on the required expense for research and development. Thus, the needs of patients with common diseases such as ischemic heart disease, cerebral vascular disease, and the common cancers are served best. An uncommon disease implies uncommonly low returns and commands less pharmacological interest. Most treatments are untested, and many are not even drugs. Who will sponsor the necessary clinical trials? Occasionally, a treatment generates controversy, spurring governments or private granting agencies to initiate or support clinical trials. Some individual investigators undertake small, valuable trials at little cost. However, many patients with rare diseases or in poor economies are ill served, and some older treatments remain at large without ever having their efficacy and safety established.

USE OF RANDOMIZED CLINICAL TRIAL RESULTS

Regulatory authorities such as the Food and Drug Administration (FDA) depend upon evidence from clinical trials to approve or disapprove new drugs submitted by the pharmaceutical industry. Such trials also help health-care administrators decide which treatments to pay for. Academics participate in clinical trials and teach evidence-based medicine. At the heart of this effort is the physician who must herself interpret the results of myriad studies of unequal quality. The patient needs to know the evidence as well, and his most reliable source is the physician who also knows his personal medical history.

When applying the results of a clinical trial to her practice, a physician must determine if her patient is demographically similar to the trial participants, and if his complaint fits that examined by the trial (generalizability). Exact fits are elusive, so a doctor must judge many factors when choosing a treatment. Controlled trials can provide solid information to guide decision making. Unfortunately, the careful assessment of a clinical trial reported in a medical journal is difficult and time consuming. The reports are often flawed, of doubtful relevance, or simply obscure. Many sources of information are available, such as reviews written or presented by academics, data provided by drug company representatives and patient advocates, and stories presented by the media.

Academic Reviews

Academic physicians are the principal independent source of a doctor's information. Reviews published in the medical literature are of three types: the review article, the systematic review, and meta-analysis. Their quality is variable and prone to the writer's personal bias. Academics also participate in lectures, symposia, consensus conferences, and refresher courses.

Review Article

The traditional way to summarize information for physicians is the review article. Textbooks are generally more comprehensive than review articles, but share many of their characteristics. Customarily, a medical-school professor writes the article. She has usually made a career studying the disease or treatments in question, so the editor considers her well suited for the task. Often, the article deals with a broad subject such as a disease. It is usual to cite a large number of references throughout a narrative description of the disease's prevalence in the community, clinical symptoms, pathophysiology, diagnosis, and treatment. If skillfully written and published in a peer-reviewed journal, such reviews are helpful and useful updates for busy doctors and other researchers.

Nevertheless, there are criticisms. Many reviews are too exhaustive for busy doctors. A review naturally reflects the writer's opinions. Despite an extensive reference list, the reader cannot be assured that all the relevant literature was covered. Unpublished or foreign language material may not be included. The reviewer may be a biased consultant for a firm or advocacy group. Doubtful data may be uncritically accepted or conflicting evidence unresolved. P. C. Gotsche found that forty-four of seventy-seven reports of randomized trials cited a disproportionate number of articles favorable to the drug that was being tested.[9] In response to critics, editors have begun to insist that reviewers describe their selection of citations and declare any pharmaceutical consultancies or other potential conflicts. Better journals require a blind vetting of reviews by two peers. Since a broad review often declares opinions or facts with few supporting details, readers should examine the cited references.

Systematic Review

A systematic review has a narrow focus; that is, it addresses a specific clinical question. Unlike the review article, it must abide by certain rules.[10] Reviewers must decide in advance which scientific articles, usually randomized controlled trials, they must include in the review. The search for qualified reports must be comprehensive, requiring the use of databases such as those of Medline, Pub Med, or the Cochrane library. Finding unpublished material that meets the inclusion criteria may require an inquiry of drug manufacturers or a survey of peers. To insure that the material is valid, each included report should be examined according to the characteristics of a good randomized trial as outlined in table 7-2. To ensure that that a systematic review's interpretation will be reproducible, two or more experts should independently read all the included reports and work out any differences in evaluating the data before proceeding.

Meta-analysis

A step beyond the systematic review, the meta-analysis was defined in 1976 as "the statistical analysis of a large collection of analysis results from individual studies for the purpose of integrating the findings." This process seeks to increase the accuracy of clinical evidence in the following ways.[11] Where several studies are too small to show a significant difference between treatment groups, their combination will increase the power of their data. When the reports disagree, combining them may resolve uncertainty. Combined trials may contain data that answer questions not addressed in the initial trials. Meta-analysis is not simple vote counting but rather a combining of data from like trials. Trial data may be weighted according to quality and number of subjects. Meta-analysis demands hard conditions. All the included trials must fulfill the features described in chapter 7. The various study populations should be comparable, and the conditions of the trial, the endpoints, and the outcome measures should be as similar as possible. Sadly, too often these conditions are unmet. H. S. Sachs and his colleagues reviewing this "new type of research," found that 72 percent of eighty-six meta-analyses failed in at least one of six major areas of study design.[12] Furthermore, unless, the trials to be meta-analyzed are well executed and similar to one another, no amount of statistical manipulation can redeem them. "Garbage in—garbage out!"

To be sure, there have been important and successful meta-analyses. Consider the problem of respiratory distress associated with infant prematurity.[13] Several small studies addressed the use of an inexpensive short course of corticosteroid medication to women expected to deliver premature babies. None had the power to demonstrate a benefit, but a meta-analysis of the data from these studies did show a treatment advantage and convinced doctors to adopt it. Nonetheless, it is worth noting that this effort had rare advantages. The populations in the several trials were identical: pregnant women at risk of premature delivery. All were treated with corticosteroids, and mortality and infant respiratory distress were finite outcome measures. Compare these features with those in the example trial of a chronic painful disorder illustrated in figure 1-1. To meta-analyze several studies of this sort, reviewers would have to satisfy themselves that each trial recruited similar subjects, that the features of their disorders were identical, that each fulfilled the conditions for randomized trials (outlined in the previous chapter), and that they all used the same predetermined endpoint and outcome measure to determine success or failure.

These conditions are unmet in many systematic reviews. An example is a meta-analysis of clinical trials testing the efficacy of "antispasmodics" in the treatment of IBS.[14] In the rest of this paragraph, square brackets indicate features of a good systematic review listed by A. D. Oxman that are absent from this meta-analysis.[15] The review included disparate drugs deemed to relieve colon spasm, yet spasm is unproven as a cause of irritable bowel [unclear focus, misguided hypothesis]. Abstracts and unpublished reports were not sought [probable publication bias]. Entry criteria were seldom stated and the reviewers permitted inclusion of articles that could include up to 49 percent of subjects who did not have IBS [inappropriate entry criteria]. The included trials had one or more of five different outcome measures [unassessed validity, incomparable outcomes].

Dissimilar drugs, variable endpoints, dissimilar outcome measures, and faulty or nonexistent entry criteria are not considered in the data analysis [faulty data analysis]. These and other drawbacks do not support the authors' conclusion that the disparate "antispasmodic" drugs are useful in treating irritable bowel syndrome.[16] Regulatory bodies and physicians apparently agree, since few of these are approved for IBS treatment in more than a handful of countries, and "antispasmodics" are gradually falling out of use. Relegation may take a while, but prescribers eventually vote with their prescription pads.

Meta-analysis has become a medical fad. Notwithstanding some notable successes, few trial data are suitable. A futile quest to make flawed trials into gold is alchemy. It not only wastes researchers' time, but it also befuddles the literature. We need more and better clinical trials, not rehashed faulty data.

Consensus Conferences

Because most clinical questions are not, or cannot be, answered by randomized, controlled trial or systematic review, experts may tackle issues at "consensus conferences." Using available data and focused debate, doctors can arrive at "best practice" or state-of-the-art recommendations. While such exercises are an opportunity to capitalize on the expertise and wisdom of the participants, they often make determinations on inadequate or inappropriate evidence.[17] Their frequent reliance on pharmaceutical sponsorship invites bias. Nevertheless, consensus reports can be useful in advising the busy doctor. To ensure that the guidelines are relevant, users, for example, family doctors, should be represented on guideline committees. Importantly, intense discussion by peers of therapeutic dilemmas should stimulate the quest for better evidence.

Industry Representatives and Advertisements

Drug detail personnel are trained to sell drugs, which is their principal responsibility. While they have become better educated as to the use of their companies' products, their view of the patient and his problem is narrow. Their usefulness is in their accessibility to the busy doctor who may see them in her office. A good drug salesperson will describe the approved indications and dosing of the drug, how it is believed to work, and what untoward effects are likely. After all, he has an interest in the success of the product, and its incorrect use is counterproductive. Nevertheless, his advice is biased and needs to be examined critically. Patient advocates provide useful information to patients, but they are not a source of scientific evidence for physicians.

For obvious reasons, drug advertisements in medical journals are biased. Too often, they are strategically juxtaposed with a relevant article in the journal. Less obvious is their inaccurate use of citations. A Spanish study found 287 separate advertisements for antihypertensive and lipid-lowering medication in major medical journals.[18] Of 125 citations for claims made in the advertisements, only 102 could be retrieved, and 18 percent of them were not randomized trials. In nearly half the others, the citation did not support the advertisement's claim, usually because it recommended the drug for patients to whom the study results did not apply. Another study found that 92 percent of advertisements were not in compliance with the FDA criteria for advertising, and half would lead to improper prescribing if they were the doctor's only source of information.[19] Angry at this report, pharmaceutical companies withdrew many advertisements from the journal that published it.[20]

The Media

Regrettably, the popular media are sometimes sources of misinformation. While the press can publicize health problems and warnings, it seems unable to deal adequately with clinical dilemmas. The journalist's zeal to dramatize and his inclination to focus on cures or disasters are at odds with the incremental nature of medical research. Today's breakthrough may be tomorrow's bust; we hear about the former, but seldom the latter. Moreover, the dramatic and oversimplified exposition of the results of complicated clinical trials may confuse rather than enlighten. For example, excited expositions of the latest dietary data tug the eating public back and forth among evil calories and essential elements, inviting cynicism or despair. Since most alleged dietary flaws or virtues would exert their damage or benefits over long periods, even lifetimes, and since no study has lasted that long, common sense and a wait-and-see attitude seem appropriate.

Some investigators have difficulty explaining their results to health reporters. Even medical journals sometimes permit authors to present data in the most arresting manner—and it is then reproduced in the press. The data on hormone replacement therapy are of great public interest but difficult to understand. Table 8-1 illustrates two ways to display the data. The percentage increases suggest a dramatic difference and a good headline.[21] These figures seem formidable and are liable to confuse and frighten rather than enlighten women who must make a decision whether to continue the drug. The absolute data that were published in the original report indicate a truer picture and provide a basis for patients to decide what is best for them.[22] Neither method addresses the cosmetic benefits and symptom relief for which many started the drug in the first place. Few press reports distinguished estrogen/progesterone combinations from estrogen alone where the risk was shown later to be negligible. Such sensationalism is a nocebo.

TABLE 8-1
Two Ways to Present the Risks and Benefits of Estrogen plus Progesterone in Postmenopausal Women

Outcome	Relative Risk (excess or reduction)	Absolute Risk in 10,000 Person Years*
Increase in Heart Attacks	29%	+7 Cases
Increase in Strokes	41%	+8 cases
Increase in Breast Cancer	26%	+8 cases
Reduction in Colon Cancer	−37%	-6 cases
Reduction in Hip Fractures	−33%	-5 cases

* total number of all subjects' years of exposure to the drug

In a large population where the risk of an adverse event is uncommon, the relative risk may seem large as it does in this case. In fact, the increases and decreases shown here do not represent many cases, yet they make great headlines. An estimate of absolute risk (also shown here) permits a more sober assessment. Not factored in these data are the improved quality of life and other benefits that led to the treatment in the first place.

The Web provides information on some subjects, but it is difficult for nonexperts to distinguish legitimate sites from those with an angle.

PUBLICATION BIAS

It is a fact of scientific life that trials that fail to show superiority of a test treatment over a control are less likely to be published than positive trials.[23] This means that any literature review in the topic will suffer publication bias; that is, the review will be biased away from the truth toward a verdict that the drug is effective. The fault lies at many levels. Editors are often blamed, since negative trials are seen as less newsworthy. Citations are a mark of success for journals and few editors want unquotable articles cluttering their valuable pages. Only a minority of trials registered with the FDA are ever published and these are not normally retrieved in systematic reviews.[24] I suspect, though, that the problem is usually elsewhere. Investigators are human, and failure to prove a hypothesis can be discouraging. Laziness, lack of time, new interests, or an unwillingness to face a publication setback all work against the very difficult task of preparing the data for the peer-review process. Some trials are buried because their flawed designs or incompetent executions are an embarrassment to all. Sponsors of trials may see no advantage in the publication of contrary data. Indeed, some pharmaceutical firms are suspected of suppressing information that they believe might comfort the competition.[25] Worse, there seems to be little relationship between the diseases for which there are published randomized, controlled trials and the global burden of disease.[26]

Publication of all randomized trials is a public responsibility.[27] Not only does publication bias distort the truth, but also suppressing a failed trial precludes an opportunity to help future investigators learn from its mistakes. Moreover, stifling the results of a randomized trial is a betrayal of the participants who investigators persuaded to enter the trial by lofty claims of research and better medical treatment for others. They (and the public) need to know the outcome of their efforts. Evidence-based medicine depends on *all* the evidence. Reviewers must seek it out.

The solution is not straightforward. Journal pages are finite and cannot accommodate all randomized trials. Tongue in cheek, some propose a *Journal of Negative Results*. But who would sponsor, let alone buy, such a journal. For their reviews, the members of the Cochrane Collaboration collect all the relevant published trial material as well as any data that can be unearthed from elsewhere. Their registry contains more than four hundred thousand records, mainly published articles from developed countries.[28] Keeping the Cochrane Web site current requires the dedication of hundreds of volunteer Cochrane collaborators. The Cochrane library is at http://www.cochrane.org/cochrane/revabstr/mainindex.htm. While Cochrane rightly resists pharmaceutical funding, it seems it will eventually need independent support to maintain its momentum. There are also some national registries.

An international global registry has been proposed. The World Health Organization employs unique trial identification numbers for trials approved by its ethics review board. The ideal would be an international registry where all trials would be available when approved. Not only would this help avoid publication bias, but it would also help prevent duplication or repetition of faulty methodology. In a worthy initiative, the editors of several of the world's leading medical journals are insisting that clinical trials be publicly registered at the outset, or they will not be considered for publication.[29] This is only a partial solution as it will be neither comprehensive nor mandatory, and authors would be free to publish elsewhere.

CAN EVIDENCE-BASED MEDICINE BE RELIABLY DISSEMINATED AND INTERPRETED?

Academics affiliated with medical schools conduct most randomized controlled clinical trials and reviews and publish their work in the medical literature. While specialists within their own discipline can absorb the results, the material is so vast and of such variable quality, that it must overwhelm most primary-care physicians, to say nothing of the public. Where, then, can one acquire and manage this data? As noted, one source is the Cochrane database. This is the most complete collection of data on a multitude of clinical questions. Some family-practice journals helpfully provide brief Cochrane updates for their subscribers.[30] Regrettably, many of the reviews conclude a treatment *may* be effective (in other words, it has not been proven ineffective), deplore the inadequate data, and merely call for randomized, controlled trials. This leaves doctors and patients with inadequate advice. Should they use the treatment?

The quality of a clinical review might be judged by the quality of the journal that publishes it. Is it peer reviewed? Is the journal widely read? Is it independent with paid subscribers or sent free to all members of an organization? How dependent does it seem to be on pharmaceutical advertising; is there a surfeit of advertisements among the articles? Do some of these relate to subject matter in the same issue of the journal? How prone is a journal to enhance its exposure through quotes in the media? The reputation and accomplishments of the author are important, as is the institution from which she hails. Careful attention to subsequent letters to the editor, reviews, or commentary in other journals may help one judge an author's opinions. Readers should regard an enthusiastic report with skepticism. If it sounds too good to be true, it likely is.

Scientific publishing seems likely to get much more complicated.[31] Since the portal that brings the best research to light is the prestigious journal that then owns the copyright, some see scientific publishers as monopolies that present financial barriers to scientific knowledge. Moreover, since public institutions such as the National Institutes of Health support much scientific research, the resulting data should be freely available. One solution is to make all scientific papers available on the Internet within six months of publication. A worrisome development is the notion that the Internet should replace journals entirely. The resulting erosion of peer review, editorial control, and other barriers to bad science may do more harm than good. Incorrect information or too much irrelevant information is more dangerous than no information.

SUMMARY AND CONCLUSIONS

If there were no placebo effect, and the natural course of a disease were predictable, there would be no need for randomized, controlled trials. The anecdote would reign supreme in medical decision making. What happened once, in the same circumstances, would happen again. However, this is seldom the case, and the principle of evidence-based medicine that controls for placebo and natural effects is here to stay. In order to cope with the results of so many controlled trials, physicians require independent assembly and evaluation of the available data. Reviews, systematic reviews, and some meta-analyses are the best sources of medical information, but they have limitations. Biased or sensationalized information from the pharmaceutical industry or the media is counterproductive. Much treatment remains to be validated by clinical testing, and much of what is proven is not readily available to busy doctors, a subject we address again in part 3. The next three chapters address randomized trials in therapeutic disciplines where controls are especially difficult: surgery, psychological treatments, and complementary and alternative medicine.

CHAPTER 9

CAN SURGERY BE A PLACEBO?

"Cheering, reassuring, healing by the mere incompatibility of disease or anxiety with his welcome presence. Even broken bones, it is said, have been known to unite at the sound of his voice."

SIR RALPH BLOOMFIELD BONINGTON IN
THE DOCTOR'S DILEMMA, BY GEORGE BERNARD SHAW[1]

Surely, surgery has no placebo effect! After all, the patient is asleep while something mechanical is done to fix the patient's condition. An incision is painful, a nocebo if anything, and unlikely to make a patient better unless whatever is wrong is rectified. Yet, incredible as it seems, surgery can exert powerful placebo effects. Recognition of this widely ignored phenomenon has important implications for the practice of surgery and for the rational administration of health care. This is because a confident surgeon, performing a seemingly logical procedure backed by anecdotal recounts of success, can produce a happy result even when the procedure itself is later realized to be useless. Conceivably, such a surgeon could even overcome a bad operation. Surgeons, like Shaw's Bonington, and like other health professionals, instinctively learn the value of a positive attitude to maximize the benefits of their operations.

HISTORICAL NOTES

From earlier civilizations, a number of surgical procedures of undeniable benefit have emerged. Often the results are instantaneous, gratifying, and lasting. An excellent example is the draining of an abscess. Presumably, this began with the use of a sharp stick to lance boils that are visible as hot, red, painful swellings in the flesh coming to a white head just under the skin. Release of the pus from such a lesion instantly relieves pain, permits the area to heal, and allows the fever to subside. The incision may even be lifesaving. No one has ever questioned the virtues of such a procedure, although experts may argue about the timing of the intervention, the type of incision, and whether or not to use antibiotics. Now with well-timed operations, surgeons drain abscesses in the abdomen, chest, brain, teeth, and elsewhere. Other procedures with rightfully unquestioned benefits include the alignment and immobilization of broken limbs; caesarian section; and surgical relief of obstructions of the intestines, the bile ducts, or the ureters. These operations never can be submitted to randomized clinical trials, other than to compare techniques. Doing nothing would be an unacceptable control.

In contrast, medical history is littered with operations that are not so obviously useful and that fall by the wayside when later generations of doctors realize their futility or even their harmfulness. Bloodletting is a classic example of a treatment, now known to be harmful, that was widely accepted as a treatment for everything from infections to anemia to malaise. Bloodletting likely began serendipitously as a treatment for *dropsy* or swollen legs where one of several causes is heart failure. Before the days of diuretics, removal of some blood could temporarily reduce the load on a failing heart. Perhaps encouraged by the benefit in such cases, and ignorant of the cardiovascular effects of the procedure, our forebears resorted to bloodletting for many ailments. George Washington died in 1799 of inflammatory obstruction of the larynx.[2] Despite his enfeeblement, his doctors bled him four times, removing over five pints of blood. According to Dr. James Craik, the youngest of the attending physicians, Dr. Elisha Cullen Dick, "was averse to bleeding the General . . . if we had acted accordingly to his suggestion . . . and taken no more blood from him, our good friend might have been alive now. But we were governed by the best light we had; we thought we were right, and so we were justified."[3] What Washington needed was a tracheotomy!

In 1794 Benjamin Rush (another signatory of the Declaration of Independence) expressed enthusiasm for venesection and gushed, "Thank God, of the one hundred patients who I have visited, or prescribed for [venesection for yellow fever], this day, I have lost none, . . . Never before did I experience such sublime joy, as I now felt in contemplating the success of my remedies."[4] Rush's prestige popularized the treatment, to Washington's detriment. Louis's debunking report a generation later only slowly gained attention, and venesection continued into the twentieth century. We need not return to the prescientific age to find similar examples. A century ago, a British surgeon named Arbuthnot Lane attributed many symptoms to *chronic intestinal stasis*.[5] He believed that absorption of toxins from the colon led to such disparate conditions as depression, premature senility, rheumatoid arthritis, changes of vision, and hair loss. The science of bacteriology developed in the late 1800s. Many writers noted the colon's rich bacterial population, and blamed many illnesses on colon stasis where thriving bacteria caused *autointoxication*.

To prevent this imagined self-poisoning, Lane led a campaign to remove colons. Lane's views had considerable influence and reinforced the ritual purging that lingers to this day. Nineteenth-century European writers believed that the colon was a useless and dangerous "encumbrance." One declared that "every child should have its large intestine surgically removed when 2 or 3 years of age."[6] This is a cautionary tale. Lane's implausible hypothesis never was submitted to scientific inquiry—it only died at the hands of skeptics. The line between truth and humbug often can seem obscure.

Examples of futile surgical procedures within living memory include the opening of the abdomen "to let in a little light and air" for intestinal tuberculosis, and the fixation of a supposedly "floating" kidney.[7] Surgeons operating on the abdomen for other reasons often removed the appendix to prevent appendicitis and performed tonsillectomies to prevent tonsillitis. These operations had a flawed rationale and lacked a valid scientific underpinning. They disappeared as time demonstrated their futility and even harmfulness. The unquestioned adoption of such procedures could do nothing for patients, so their persistence for decades can only be explained by what occurred in the minds of both doctors and patients. The placebo effect can overcome the shortcomings of even harmful interventions.

ENTHUSIASTS AND SKEPTICS

In 1961 H. K. Beecher described the sequential roles of enthusiasts and skeptics in the evolution of new surgical techniques.[8] In the 1950s, for example, enthusiasts hailed internal mammary artery ligation as an effective treatment for angina pectoris. Beecher summarized the results of three uncontrolled trials on 213 patients under-going this operation. Thirty-eight percent of subjects achieved complete relief of their symptoms. Later, other surgeons, who were skeptics, achieved complete relief of symptoms in only 6 percent of similar patients with the same procedure. Lincoln's aphorism comes to mind, "You can fool some of the people some of the time, but not all of the people all of the time," except that here there was no intention to deceive. Enthusiastic surgeons believed that the operation was successful. Only when science proved the procedure worthless was it finally abandoned (see below).

As with any treatment, a new operation begins with an idea. Whether tenable or not, the enthusiast adopts and promotes the idea, convincing his patients of its therapeutic possibilities. Early apparent success is all the confirmation that is required. The medical and lay press uncritically report the "breakthrough" and other surgeons and patients clamor for information. The originator becomes an advocate, his or her career often benefiting from the discovery. The attendant publicity raises expectations and hope overcomes reality to install the procedure in the surgical repertoire. A century ago, William Osler had this phenomenon in mind when he facetiously urged doctors to use a new treatment while it still had the power to heal.[9]

Then, untoward effects appear, the human and financial costs become evident, and skeptics question the operation's benefit. Subsequent successes appear less remarkable than the original and the originator fades from public view. Gradually the procedure falls out of use, or it is proven to be useless and possibly harmful. Osler notwithstanding, a conservative attitude to surgical breakthroughs is usually wise.

> "Be not the first by whom the new are tried,
> Nor yet the last to lay the old aside."[10]

Thus, colectomy for apoplexy, mechanical antiesophageal reflux devices, removal of the lower half of the body for cancer (hemicorporectomy), small intestinal bypass for obesity, and fixation of fallen kidneys each had its day before being relegated to the dustbin of medical history.

CONTROLLING SURGICAL TRIALS

A Surgical Placebo?

Compliance to the principles of evidence-based medicine is necessary for the approval of new prescription drugs. In industrialized countries, a new drug must pass efficacy and safety hurdles set up by regulating authorities such as the Food and Drug Administration. Then, the sponsoring pharmaceutical firm must convince doctors and those who must pay for the drug that it is useful. No such process applies to surgery. New operations or new indications for old ones are introduced with little more than local hospital scrutiny. Surgery is a fix-it specialty, where something anatomically abnormal can be repaired to restore health.

There is no sinister intent here. Belief in surgery is widespread. Surgeons are uniquely positioned to maximize the placebo effect. They receive deference from the support staff, and are often "a last resort" for colleagues. The preoperative ritual prepares the patient to enter the operating cathedral, where he is put quietly to sleep while others toil to relieve his pain and suffering. Surgeons are by nature positive, enthusiastic, and confident. Who would want a surgeon who was otherwise? Patient attitudes are important as well. While "lumpectomy" is sometimes as effective as removal of the breast for cancer, many women choose the latter to be rid of it.[11] Moreover, the patient has invested much in the decision to undergo an operation. Amid the hope, the expectation, and the need to be better, few would be glad to admit their decision was a bad one.

Sham Surgery

When the outcome measure is subjective, for example, feeling better rather than relieving obstruction, the results of surgery cannot be compared fairly with the results of doing nothing. How, then, can we evaluate a surgical procedure scientifically, and prove its benefits for certain patients? One technique is to use sham surgery. In order to provide a control group to evaluate a surgical procedure, researchers randomly divide prospective subjects into two groups. The first group undergoes the operation under study. The second group has sham incisions with no operation. The group allocation is unknown to the subjects themselves or to the investigators who must monitor the outcome.

Though these maneuvers embody the elements of a randomized, controlled trial, they provoke unique ethical challenges. Briefly, these challenges center upon the withholding of possibly effective treatment during the trial, the complications of the incision or anesthetic, and the difficulty in achieving truly informed consent. In a drug trial, an inert placebo pill serves as a harmless control. In contrast, a surgical sham incision is painful and potentially harmful. This poses yet another ethical dilemma. While sham surgery in a trial creates risks for the few, continuing to use a procedure without proving its utility risks harm for the many. You may ask, "If many or most patients improve after a surgical procedure, what's the harm?" The answer is that the cost is too high, there is risk, and the placebo effect is illusory and transient. If the benefit is simply a placebo effect, surely it is unethical to continue doing the procedure. Yet, other than the natural waning of enthusiasm described above, there seems no easy way to identify and discredit useless operations scientifically. Despite these issues, trials controlled by sham surgery have occasionally produced remarkable and revealing results.

EXAMPLES OF RANDOMIZED CONTROLLED SURGICAL TRIALS

Understandably, few surgical trials measure up to today's exacting scientific and ethical standards. The following examples illustrate how such trials can be useful and expose their drawbacks.

Internal Mammary Artery Ligation

Angina pectoris is exercise-related chest pain due to increased oxygen demand by the heart muscle (myocardium) that results from diseased or occluded coronary arteries. Relief occurs if the circulation through these arteries to the heart can be improved. The internal mammary arteries originate from the great arteries in the neck and descend either side of the breastbone. Based on some experimental evidence (since repudiated) it was thought that ligation of these arteries might divert blood through the great vessels above the heart into the coronary circulation, thus improving the heart's circulation and myocardial oxygen supply.[12]

The operation was simple: small bilateral neck incisions, identification of the arteries, and the placement of ligatures. The procedure required no entry into body cavities and there were few complications. The notion was appealing, and surgeons adopted the operation with enthusiasm. Early reports showed improvement in the angina in up to 91 percent of cases and complete relief in up to 64 percent. There was even objective evidence of improvement, including electrocardiograms that were more normal, improved exercise tolerance, and less need for antiangina medication. Such results contrast with previous estimates that spontaneous remissions of angina occurred in only 14 percent of men and 19 percent of women.[13] One surgeon enthused, "with surprising regularity the human subjects have been relieved of pain almost immediately, long before new coronary blood vessels could have grown in."[14] Thus, many thousands of patients with severe angina were treated by internal mammary ligation in the 1950s. I remember observing such an operation as a medical student.

But, as Beecher predicted, skepticism soon surfaced.[15] Many surgeons doubted the theory underlying the procedure. Demonstration of postoperative improvement in coronary blood flow was not forthcoming, and improved angina did not correlate with improved coronary blood flow. After the initial trials, the percent of people improved by the procedure began to decline. In 1958 one skeptical surgeon placed a ligature around the internal mammary arteries of two subjects but did not tighten it.[16] These subjects experienced great subjective improvement in their angina after the incision and nonligation, yet no further improvement when the surgeon later tightened the ligatures by pulling the suture ends left protruding through the skin.

In 1958 E. G. Dimond undertook a small trial in eighteen patients, of which five had a sham operation.[17] Improvement occurred in ten of the thirteen ligated patients and in all of the sham-ligated patients. Three ligated and two nonligated subjects respectively reported complete relief. Those relieved had increased ability to exercise free of pain and a reduced need for drugs. A year later, L. A. Cobb studied seventeen patients whose activity was seriously limited by angina.[18] The surgeon made skin incisions under local anesthesia and at that moment was shown a card that randomly indicated which patients to ligate. Occluding the mammary arteries produced no better results than the sham operation when a blinded observer assessed the outcome. Most subjects in both groups had subjective improvement and many had improvements in exercise tolerance and drug requirements.

These small trials are of very great importance. They signaled the abandonment of internal mammary ligation as a treatment of angina pectoris. They illustrated the potentially powerful placebo effect of surgery. They demonstrated that a properly blinded and randomized controlled surgical trial could produce useful knowledge and exposed the need for more careful evaluation of the utility of surgical procedures. Yet they failed to signal a new age of controlled surgical trials. They stood alone for years, and only recently have surgeons reintroduced sham operations as research tools.

The Cobb study illustrates why sham surgery failed to prosper. Statistical experts claim the small number of patients provided insufficient power to prove no difference between the two groups. Moreover, it appears that the patients were not told that they might receive sham surgery, only that a new technique was being evaluated. Such an explanation would be unacceptable by modern interpretations of "informed consent." Ruth Macklin notes that truly informed consent is impossible in the highly charged atmosphere surrounding an impending surgery, and declares that sham surgery is "ethically unacceptable."[19]

A skin incision to expose a superficial artery is one thing, but the notion of exposing a sham-operated patient to the risks of an incision in the abdomen or burr holes in the skull escalates concern. Furthermore, *no* incision or anesthetic is 100 percent safe. Hence, there is a dilemma! The need to protect the individual from harm now trumps the future common good, which is to identify and discard costly, risky, and harmful surgery. It must be so! We need alternative methods to evaluate surgery, arguably the most costly and risky of all medical acts.

Arthroscopic Surgery for Osteoarthritis of the Knee

Osteoarthritis is a chronic degeneration of the joints featuring destruction of the cartilage that covers the articular surfaces of bones where they meet in the joints, accompanied by some inflammation of the *synovial membrane* that encases the joint cavity. Unlike other types of arthritis, the degree of inflammation is not great and anti-inflammatory drugs are not very effective in relieving the joint pain. At least 12 percent of people over age sixty-five have frequent knee pain due to osteoarthritis, and disability is common. *Arthroscopy* is the inspection of the joint cavity through an instrument sequentially inserted into the knee via three small skin incisions. Theoretically, *lavage* (washing) of an osteoarthritic joint at the time of arthroscopy removes harmful debris that has accumulated from the degenerative process. *Debridement* consists of smoothing out the rough edges of the joint surfaces to permit better function.

Randomized, controlled trials of these procedures compared to no treatment (no sham incision) suggested that this operation improved knee pain. These studies were not blinded, and whether or not a subject had surgery would be painfully obvious to him and those who evaluated the outcome. Meanwhile, in the United States in 2002, more than 650,000 such procedures were performed, each at a cost of $5,000 (over $3 billion total).[20] Clearly, there are many enthusiasts. However, there are skeptics. To determine if these procedures truly relieve knee joint pain and improve function, J. B. Moseley and his colleagues conducted a randomized, double-blind, controlled trial of knee lavage and debridement versus sham surgery.[21]

One hundred eighty patients participated, sixty having three small incisions in the knee (sham surgery or placebo group), sixty-one having arthroscopy and lavage through the incisions, and fifty-nine having arthroscopy and debridement. These numbers were predetermined to be sufficient to detect differences in outcome among the groups. A research assistant revealed the treatment allocation to the surgeon only after the patient was draped in the operating room. The surgeon manipulated the surgical instruments in a similar manner before each patient. The allocation to surgery or sham incision was concealed from the patients and the observers, but not, of course, the surgeon and anesthetist. The sham-operated patients received light sedation, which produced amnesia and simulated the operated subjects' general anesthesia.

Informed consent included the written statement, "On entering this study, I realize that I may receive only placebo therapy. I further realize that this means that I will not have surgery on my knee joint. This placebo therapy will not benefit my knee arthritis." Forty-four of the patients decided not to play a part in the trial, but once in, only 16 of the 180 subjects withdrew. The study was conducted in a veterans' hospital, and a single surgeon performed all the procedures.

Over 90 percent of the subjects were male, and the groups were demographically similar.

The main outcome measure was pain severity twenty-four months after the procedure recorded on a twelve-item self-reported ordinal scale. Data were collected at two and six weeks, and six, twelve, eighteen, and twenty-four months. Secondary measures of pain and knee function were recorded as well. The patients in all three groups had about 50 percent improvement as measured by the pain scale, and there was no significant difference in any outcome measure between the three groups. The authors deftly conclude, "If the efficacy of placebo lavage or debridement in patients with osteoarthritis of the knee is no better than that of placebo surgery, the billions of dollars spent on such procedures annually might be put to better use."[22]

Appearing forty-three years after the internal mammary artery ligation trial, this research had to overcome rigorous ethical hurdles. Informed consent is demonstrably present. The possible harm of the sham surgery is minimized through superficial incisions and the use of sedation rather than general anesthesia. Follow-up in all groups was beyond the normal clinical standard. Neither of the groups undergoing lavage or debridement fared any better than the placebo group. In fact, it seems to have been an advantage to be in the placebo group since those patients recovered slightly faster from the effects of surgery. From the data, it would seem henceforth unjustified to perform lavage or debridement in osteoarthritic knees that have the characteristics of the knees of the patients entered in this trial.

There are criticisms, to be sure,[23] but they seem minor in the face of the evidence. The subjects were mostly men (whereas osteoarthritis is more common in women), and the refusals and dropouts may have skewed the study toward subjects with greater expectations. Maybe the surgeon was insufficiently skilled. These caveats are unlikely to have affected the results or the conclusions. The onus is now on remaining enthusiasts to disprove this study's conclusions.

It is too early to say if this report will result in the termination of knee lavage and debridement, but the authors have done a great service to health care by casting serious doubt on expensive and invasive procedures. They have also demonstrated that in some cases, scientific study of the efficacy of surgical procedures is possible. Moreover, they have again demonstrated the placebo effect of surgery itself.

We should strive to discover better ways to duplicate the impressive improvement seen in these "sham-operated" patients.

Parkinson's Disease: Treatment by Implantation of Fetal Cells in the Brain

Parkinson's disease is a chronic, progressive disease of the brain resulting in tremors, muscular rigidity, and physical incapacitation. The cause is the loss of neurons from centers in the base of the brain that produce a chemical transmitter of nerve impulses called *dopamine*. One treatment is the oral administration of levodopa. This drug provides imperfect replacement therapy for dopamine and commonly causes adverse reactions. One hypothesis is that the injection of human embryo neurons into the base of the brain might provide a living source of dopamine. Experimentally, such transplanted tissue "takes" in animals. Such is the enthusiasm of some surgeons that many centers have set up programs to treat severe Parkinson's disease in this way. Champions of the operation publicized their results in the news media in many countries.

Many features of Parkinson's disease make it liable to a placebo effect. The disease fluctuates in severity. It is worse when the sufferer is anxious or stressed, and better when he is content or at rest. The response to medication is itself variable, and in clinical trials the patients in placebo control groups show substantial functional improvement. Skeptics began to doubt the favorable reports. Then, a multicenter randomized, controlled trial of bilateral fetal nigral transplantation in patients with Parkinson's disease produced disappointing results. The authors concluded, "Fetal nigral transplantation currently cannot be recommended as a therapy for [Parkinson's disease]."[24] Of more importance to us, a companion study compared the quality of life in the patients before and after surgery according to whether they believed that they had the active transplant or the sham procedure.[25] Those who believed they had received the transplant said they had greater improvement in physical functioning than those who believed their surgery was a sham. The authors attribute this perceived improvement, without objective improvement, to the placebo effect.

Surgical implantation of embryonic cells in the brain is very different in complexity to internal mammary artery ligation and knee lavage. Not only are Parkinson's patients debilitated, but the fetal tissue must be implanted via "burr holes" drilled through the skull. Although the technology is sophisticated, burr holes are more threatening to patients than skin incisions. While some question the performance of this unproven treatment on patients with Parkinson's disease, the proposal to test its efficacy with a surgical trial using sham burr holes encountered great criticism.[26] Here is another ethical paradox. It is apparently permissible to perform untested, very invasive, and potentially harmful surgery on many people without knowing if it is effective, yet to some it is unethical to subject a few people to sham surgery to establish whether an operation is beneficial or not. Randomized, controlled trials such as the one described above can save many from harm, inconvenience, and great costs.

Here, as in law, the rights of the few properly outweigh the welfare of the many. Resolution of this dilemma should be a priority. We need to find alternative means of evaluating surgery and to resist bandwagon acceptance of dangerous procedures based on enthusiastic anecdotes.

COMMENT

What accounts for the large placebo response to surgery? A first requirement is an ill person. Next, we need an operation believed by many (patients, doctors, relatives, journalists, and others) to be just the thing for that illness. The surgeon himself must project confidence, and the nurses, orderlies, interns, and other members of the team should reinforce his healing power. The person hopes and expects to get well. The emotional capital he invests in the procedure may be amplified if a fee is invested as well. Minimizing the importance of a disappointing result is preferable to an admission that he made a mistake.[27] Add to these the admission to a hospital, the signing of consent, the preoperative medication, the surgical gowns, and the entry into the operating cathedral where green angels of care tend to basic needs while the anesthetist prepares the patient for temporary oblivion. These positive circumstances are ideal for a placebo effect. The surgery itself is usually beneficial, often restorative, and sometimes lifesaving in its own right. Yet no one should underestimate the effects of kindness, encouraging words, and positive circumstances to make the ill person feel better still. For each procedure, we need to be sure that these are not the only reasons patients feel better.

OTHER EVALUATIONS

Comparisons of Two Surgical Procedures

Other methods to evaluate the efficacy of surgical treatments or devices require no sham surgery, blinding, or deception. Timely removal of an acutely inflamed appendix is a long-accepted practice, substantiated by the bad outcomes if the inflammation is allowed to become a generalized infection. Normally, a small incision ("laparotomy") in the right lower abdomen permits the surgeon to remove the diseased appendix. Recently developed laparoscopes can penetrate even smaller incisions in the abdominal wall, permitting appendectomy through instruments controlled outside the abdomen. A Hong Kong study randomly assigned seventy patients with acute appendicitis to each of two demographically similar groups.[28] One group had laparoscopic appendectomy and the other had the traditional incision. Pain scores, analgesic use, reintroduction of food, and length of hospital stay were the same in both. However, laparoscopic surgery took 75 percent longer than traditional surgery, and, in fourteen patients, a full incision proved necessary because laprascopic surgery was technically impossible. This has implications for other operations. In the case of a diseased gallbladder, the benefits of laparoscopic removal seem so obvious that nobody contemplates a controlled trial to test the procedure. Yet without such testing, some may doubt its advantages in the light of the Hong Kong appendectomy experience.

Gallstones obstructing the exit from the gallbladder may cause pain and severe complications if not treated. Their removal with the gallbladder (cholecystectomy) after attacks of pain due to obstructing gallstones is accepted surgical practice. However, a process called *lithotripsy* is a newer alternative. Machine-generated shock waves shatter the gallstones into fragments that pass "harmlessly" through the biliary system. In 1992 a British Department of Health–sponsored study compared cholecystectomy with lithotripsy and found similar benefits but greater cost for lithotripsy.[29] Surprisingly, the response to lithotripsy was the same whether or not the stones were cleared from the gallbladder, and the benefit appeared to last for several years. Since there was no sham lithotripsy control, we cannot be sure how much of the benefit was due to the procedure itself, the natural history of gallstone disease, or the placebo effect. Possibly, the introduction of a new treatment for gallstones that does not require general anesthesia or abdominal incision increased patients' expectations and exaggerated the placebo effect. The lack of blinding prompts doubt that lithotripsy is as effective as cholecystectomy.

Evaluation of Therapeutic Devices

History is replete with healing inventions of boundless imagination. In 1801 Haygarth compared the "electromagnetism" of metal rods with wooden placebo rods in relieving the symptoms of five patients.[30] Healing was believed to be due to an electromagnetic effect of the metal. Four of the five were relieved of their symptoms with this device, and the same results occurred with wooden imitations the next day. The experiment "clearly proved what wonderful effects the passions of faith and hope can produce on disease." Haygarth concluded, "An important lesson in physic is here to be learnt, the wonderful and powerful influence of the passions of the mind upon the state and disorder of the body. This is too often overlooked in the cure of disease"—a wise and prescient exposition of human susceptibility to the placebo effect.

However, old notions die hard, and the therapeutic benefits of physical forces in many conditions were believed until the middle of the eighteenth century and beyond. In 1849 Alexander Cumming extolled the virtues of electrogalvinism.[31] A modern variant is the practice of *pulsed magnetic field therapy* for failure of fractures of the tibia (shinbone) to unite after one year. Prior to 1984, there were reports of success with this therapy in healing broken bones that previously failed to heal (nonunion). A British research team randomly allocated patients into two groups.[32] The first received pulsed magnetic field therapy, while the second, a control group, underwent the same procedure with the magnetic field turned off. Five of the nine patients treated with the machines plugged in had their tibias united within twenty-four weeks. However, five of the seven patients treated with the apparatus *unplugged* healed in the same period. (Is that Shaw's Sir Ralph Bloomfield Bonington's voice we hear in the background?)

It seems electromagnetism might produce nocebo as well as placebo effects. Some people living near power transmission lines have been concerned that their electromagnetic emissions cause cancer.[33] A poorly executed study found several leukemia patients were from homes near transmission towers. In a classic example of confusing coincidence with causality, this information led to an industry of lawsuits, microwave measurers, periodicals (*Microwave News*), books, hundreds of studies, and a huge stake in the concept. It took two decades and several scientific commissions to debunk an idea that should never have been credited in the first place.

CONCLUSIONS

Many surgical procedures produce benefits of dramatic and undoubted benefit. Lancing an abscess or removing an acutely inflamed appendix are examples. However, some surgery is done to relieve subjective symptoms, especially pain. The emotionally charged accoutrements of surgery—the confidence of the surgeon, the expectations and hopes of the patient, the masks and gowns, the rituals of consent, preoperative preparation, scrubbing, and anesthesia—predispose us to placebo effects. Surgical trials that employed sham operations have dramatically demonstrated placebo effects in surgery and the futility of a few procedures. Comparison trials and careful postoperative follow-ups are useful in evaluating an operation's efficacy but are much less rigorous tests of an operation's utility. Double-blind testing of all new surgical procedures would be desirable were it not for ethical concerns. No common good that might result from validating a surgical procedure can overcome the possibility that some subjects undergoing sham incision might be harmed. Nevertheless, such trials are possible for some procedures. We need new methods of evaluation for most. In the light of the internal mammary artery experience, how much current coronary artery surgery can claim to be evidence based?

There are lessons to be drawn from the data presented here. Trials of surgical procedures that employ sham-operated controls demonstrate that surgery conveys a substantial placebo effect. Moreover, it leads us to suspect that some operations, especially those with subjective outcome evaluations, would prove themselves useless if submitted to properly designed trials. Like any other treatment, an operation has outcomes that cannot reliably be predicted by its rationale. Designing methods for the scientific evaluation of surgical procedures should be a health-care priority. Meanwhile, surgeons should continue to conduct themselves in a manner that maximizes beneficial placebo effects in their patients.

CHAPTER 10

PLACEBO EFFECT
AND PSYCHOTHERAPY

"Psychotherapy: Effective treatment or effective placebo?"[1]

Humans have always been perplexed by madness.[2] Some primitive societies attributed special powers to the insane who
became medicine men or priests. Shamans even feigned madness
during their healing rituals. Most civilizations stored the insane where
they could not be seen, such as in the eighteenth- and nineteenth-century asylums and madhouses of Europe, and later, in state and provincial hospitals in North America. Originally designed for therapy and
study, they gradually filled with the incurable. Therefore, there was
little progress in therapy, and the welfare of the mentally ill was often
neglected. The discipline of psychiatry was born amid controversy
over the causes of insanity. A little over a century ago charismatic figures like Freud and Jung began to change the way the mentally ill
were regarded, and developed means of treatment based on personal
anecdotes that later critics "castigated as tales from the Vienna
Woods."[3] Nevertheless, by 1900, largely through the efforts of Freud
and others, some mentally ill people had a human face at last, and
those with financial resources had somewhere to turn for help. The
next major development was the use of drugs to manage emotional
and mental disorders. Psychopharmacology revolutionized management of the severely mentally disabled and by 1960 became a routine
method of treatment. The ability to discharge most of the inhabitants
of mental hospitals confirms the value of medication, mitigated some-
what by finding too many of them sleeping on our streets.

PSYCHOPHARMACOLOGY

The efficacy of a psychoactive drug in the treatment of depression or other mental disorder may be tested by a randomized, double-blind, placebo-controlled trial (as outlined in chapter 7). The entry criteria are usually derived from the definitions of the disorders found in the *Diagnostic and Statistical Manual of Mental Disorders*, 4th ed. (DSM–IV),[4] and outcome measures can be designed to show symptom improvement. As in other drug trials, an inert pill designed to resemble the treatment pill serves as the placebo. (I shall not discuss psychoactive drug trials further in this chapter.)

PSYCHOTHERAPY

Psychotherapy is any purely psychological method of treatment for mental or emotional disorders. B. J. Cohen explains it as "a form of treatment in which an individual who is suffering some distress comes to a socially sanctioned healer, who in turn attempts to relieve this distress by using personal influence to mobilize change in the sufferer."[5] An incomplete list of psychotherapeutic techniques appears in table 10-1. Psychiatrists and psychologists, trained in certain techniques, practice formal psychotherapy. However, consciously or otherwise, other healers practice psychotherapy with no special training. Doctors, alternative care practitioners, and clergymen practice informal psychotherapy as part of their healing encounters. No doubt, the ministrations of the ancient medicine man were often a type of psychotherapy. Talking to a good friend might be psychotherapeutic, too.

TABLE 10-1
Some Types of Psychotherapy

Analytical (psychoanalysis)
Behavioral
Biofeedback
Cognitive
Cognitive Behavioral
Existential
Family
Group
Hypnotism
Interpersonal
Marital
Relaxation
Supportive

CONTROLLED TRIALS FOR PSYCHOTHERAPY

Until the advent of psychopharmacology, psychotherapy in some form was the mainstay of psychiatric treatment, and it remains an important component today. Here, we need to consider the special problems encountered when conducting randomized controlled trials to establish the efficacy of psychotherapy. For psychotherapy research, what is the placebo control? What can serve as the inert treatment control analogous to the lactose pill and sham procedures used in other therapy research? Our purpose here is not to criticize the use of time-honored psychiatric techniques. Rather it is to point out the scientific difficulties of proving their efficacy. Psychotherapy in any of its forms requires evaluation that takes into account the placebo effect and the natural history of mental illness. In the era of evidence-based medicine, tradition, charisma, anecdote, and experience no longer suffice.

The many psychotherapy techniques and schools do not concern us here except as examples (see table 10-1). What does interest us is how we might prove that these techniques are efficacious and how psychotherapy relates to the placebo effect. Some techniques are very expensive, requiring long periods of training by the therapist and many lengthy sessions with the patient. How do we know that this effort is justified? Freud and others championed their techniques through force of character and skillful use of anecdote. This is not good enough in our era of collectively funded medical care. It begs the question, What is a suitable control treatment for randomized trials of psychotherapy? As the editor of the *Lancet* asks, is "psychotherapy effective treatment or expensive placebo?"[6]

According to Cohen, all types of psychotherapy have elements in common. These include:

- an emotionally charged, confiding relationship with a helping person;
- a healing setting (the doctor's office);
- a rationale, conceptual theme, or myth that provides a plausible explanation for the patient's symptoms and prescribes a ritual or procedure for resolving them; and
- a ritual or procedure that requires the active participation of both patient and therapist and that is believed by both to be the means of restoring the patient's health.[7]

A visit to a doctor can have similar characteristics. So, is Cohen in reality describing some elements of the placebo effect in family practice?

Until recently, acceptance of psychotherapy was unquestioned. It had what epidemiologists call *face validity*; that is, it made sense to manage a freshly bereaved patient's depression by "talk[ing] out ills rather than forking out pills." Crude attempts to evaluate psychotherapy began in the 1950s.[8] One study found that patients' improvement on psychotherapy was no better than that of non-patients with similar symptoms.

A 1980 meta-analysis of five hundred clinical trials showed that psychotherapies were superior to untreated controls.[9] This meta-analysis had many of the flaws discussed in chapter 8 and included so many different types of psychotherapies, subjects, diagnoses, and outcomes, that it must be interpreted with skepticism. The control subjects in most randomized controlled trials believe they might receive an active therapy and therefore expect to get better, but that is not the case with the "untreated controls" in this review. Once an individual with mental illness enters a trial as a "no treatment" control, he knows he will have no treatment and so is not blinded. If not entered in a trial, but simply and unobtrusively observed, the subject does not experience the trial's conditions and therefore is not a true control. Therefore, untreated patients are unsatisfactory controls. Oddly, the authors of this review considered placebo treatment a form of psychotherapy. When reanalyzed, the same data showed no difference in outcome between psychotherapy and placebo treatment.[10]

It is easier to criticize such studies than devise better ones. The question remains: Does a trained therapist using any psychotherapeutic technique provide a better outcome for a mental disorder than the best efforts of a caring physician or any other caring person? Since many psychotherapy techniques are very time-consuming and expensive, the question is of great interest.

PLACEBO CONTROLS FOR PSYCHOTHERAPY TRIALS

Randomized, controlled trials for psychoactive drugs can employ placebo controls in a similar manner to other randomized clinical drug trials. However, placebo controls in psychotherapy trials are problematic. Even if we decide that placebo therapy is not a form of psychotherapy, the problem of devising suitable sham treatments remains. Investigators can attempt to provide the control group with all the caring and therapeutic arrangements of the treatment group except the specific intervention under study, and blind the participants and investigators as best they can. Another strategy is to compare an unproven psychotherapy to an already proven one, but some critics might argue there are no proven psychotherapies. Both could theoretically be the same or worse than no treatment.

In 1989 I. Elkin and colleagues published the results of a randomized controlled trial of the treatment of depression.[11] This collaborative study sponsored by the US National Institute of Mental Health compared cognitive psychotherapy, interpersonal psychotherapy, an antidepressant plus case management, and placebo and case management. (The placebo resembled the antidepressant pill, and "case management" meant continued standard treatment that would be given outside the study.) All treatments were accompanied by significant improvement in symptoms and functioning compared to the baseline. There was a trend for the severe cases of depression to improve more in the antidepressant group, while the placebo treatment was least effective. The psychotherapy groups lay somewhere in between.

However, among all four groups there was no difference in the improvement of subjects with mild depression, which is a very common condition. Thus, this study does not settle the issue.[12] How good a control was "case management?" It is still possible that certain types of psychotherapy may be better for certain patients, but Elkin's trial could not prove that. Moreover, all four groups had some form of psychotherapy, including the two groups with case management, and all the patients were examined, diagnosed, and monitored. These manipulations are powerful forces for improvement. The study lacked a true control group that was treated the same way as the treated groups without placebo or psychotherapy. Is such a control possible?

A recent randomized clinical trial of treatments for "moderate to severe functional bowel disorders" illustrates the difficulty.[13] One group in the trial received *cognitive behavioral therapy* by a trained therapist. In twelve weekly hour-long sessions, the therapist and patient "focused on the influence of attention, personal appraisal, sex-related cognitive schemas and illness attributions as related to the gastrointestinal symptoms as a means of developing more effective coping strategies." To control for this elaborate treatment, a second group received "twelve weekly modified-attention control sessions . . . where the participants reviewed their symptom diaries, read educational materials mainly taken from a book on functional gastrointestinal disorders, and then discussed the information with the therapist."

The same therapist provided both the cognitive and control (placebo) treatments. As a result, the two treatments superficially resembled each other but the study was single-blinded. In such a long trial with many sessions, is it possible for a therapist trained in cognitive behavioral psychotherapy to approach these two sets of patients with the same degree of enthusiasm and impartiality? Most clinical trial experts would say no, because they believe that with psychotherapy, more so than with drugs, the therapist's enthusiasm, expectations, persuasiveness, and conviction are part of the therapy. How can that be maintained equally for treatment and control patients? Is it not possible that one day the therapist might enthuse, "Oh, good, a cognitive-behavioral candidate, I can use my skills," and another day sigh resignedly, "Here comes a control patient, I need a coffee break"? There are verbal and nonverbal cues that transmit such attitudes. Also, is it not possible that "modified attention control" is good therapy after all? Paradoxically, it would be difficult to disprove the hypothesis that identical subjects left with a caring family doctor might do as well or better at less cost than subjects getting either cognitive behavioral therapy or its putative control. This otherwise exceptionally well-planned study is haunted by these conundrums.

PLACEBO RESPONSE IN RANDOMIZED PSYCHOTHERAPY TRIALS

Joan-Ramon Laporte and Albert Figueras summarize the placebo responses in randomized clinical trials of psychotherapy or drugs in the treatment of anxiety, depression, schizophrenia, or dementia.[14] They chose the three most commonly cited trials of each. The placebo responses in these trials ranged from 21 to 70 percent, although the diversity of the trial designs makes comparison difficult. It would be very valuable to understand the factors that account for this substantial placebo response and its apparent variability. Psychotherapy or not, we can all agree that maximizing the placebo effect is a good thing for a healer to do.

THE PLACEBO EFFECT IS THERAPY

Disappointed at the small therapeutic gain achieved by the treated group compared to controls in a randomized trial, investigators often lament that the placebo response is too high. One pharmaceutical representative once asked me incredulously, "If even placebo would give [*sic*] therapeutic effects . . . would this have a negative impression on [his company's] drug therapy?" Another glance at figure 1-1 reveals the reason for such worries. While the test drug improved more than half of those taking it, the placebo treatment improved over 40 percent. It is tempting for some to believe that if only the placebo response were less, than the "real" drug would show to better advantage.

Such sentiments expose a lack of understanding of placebo responses in clinical trials and in the real world. As stressed in part 1, improvement in the treated individual is the sum of the tested treatment's effect, the placebo effect, and the effect of the treated condition's natural history. While it is impossible to determine the relative roles of drug, placebo effect, and nature in any individual, collectively in the example, the drug can take independent credit for only about 10 percent of the improvement in the treated subjects. This difference is significant, to be sure, but without the help of nature and placebo effect, the drug's benefits would be far less impressive. The message here is what many healers know instinctively: for most illnesses, time is an ally, and a positive approach enhances treatment. In this sense, placebo therapy is a form of psychotherapy, and one we should recruit and encourage.

THE FALL OF AN ICON

In his book *Fall of an Icon*,[15] Joel Paris critically appraises psychoanalysis in historical and contemporary terms. In the 1950s and 1960s, the chairs of psychiatry of most North American medical schools were held by psychoanalysts whose hegemony owed everything to the writings of Freud and his disciples. The escape to New York and Boston of many European analysts before and during World War II accounts for its greater popularity in the new world than in Europe. When Paris was training in Montreal, American and Canadian psychiatry trainees aspired to be analysts, and to be analyzed oneself was part of the training—a rite not unlike that seen in some primitive societies.

Classical Freudian analysis split into many variants,[16] each with its champion, yet none tested the efficacy of their treatments. By the 1960s, medicine had a tradition of evidence-based practice, but psychiatry had none. The skepticism of others forced many analysts to leave academia and join institutes where analysis reigned supreme.[17] It was becoming clear that such treatment was ineffective for psychosis, and analysis came to serve anxiety, depression, and other conditions formerly known as neuroses. The advent of psychoactive medication changed all that. Younger psychiatrists began evaluating the new drugs for psychoses, and later for all psychiatric conditions. Strikingly successful results were demonstrated in randomized clinical trials, and pharmacotherapy permitted many psychotic patients to function in society. Psychoanalysis could demonstrate no such benefit for any of the disorders it addressed, and mainstream psychiatry moved toward evidence-based drug therapy and away from the myriad analytic techniques. While not yet extinct, classical, long-term analysis is relegated to treatment of drug-resistant cases where its efficacy still begs examination.

Attempts to compare one type of analytic technique with another often result in no verdict.[18] If they are all similarly effective, what is their common feature? Paris states that such therapy is a relationship, not the application of a theory. Novices, and even sympathetic university professors, achieved as good results as experienced therapists, suggesting that technique and training made little difference. While it seems impossible to design a placebo treatment to compare to analysis, many features of analytic-therapy results resemble the placebo effect. "Technique plays a lesser role than the doctor/patient relationship,"[19] says Paris, and later, "Time is the healer, but the analyst gets the credit."[20] Thus, the placebo effect and natural history of illness could account for analytic success, which could likely be achieved by other, less costly means.

Fifty years ago, Freud was a twentieth-century icon. Now it seems he will be scarcely remembered in the twenty-first century. Nevertheless, Paris credits him with introducing humanity to psychiatry along with the concept that human beings are more irrational than rational. Perhaps this theme is a suitable text for the next chapter.

CONCLUSIONS

Defenders of formal psychotherapy point to the improvements they see in their patients, whose improved social and work functioning is measurable. Such a defense is increasingly untenable. We have seen the futility of relying on anecdote and uncontrolled trials, and have become aware of the improvement wrought by time and the placebo effect. The large choice of psychotherapy treatments could be interpreted as indirect evidence that no treatment has an advantage. We need to consider the possibilities that psychotherapy success is a placebo effect, or that inducing a placebo effect is psychotherapy. What elements do psychotherapy and placebo effect share? If we understood these, we would be better equipped to manage all illnesses. Does it boil down to a committed, caring, and respected caregiver combining evidence-based techniques where they exist with an exemplary healer/patient relationship? Are there patient characteristics that signal receptiveness to the putative advantages of psychotherapy and placebo therapy? We need answers to these questions if psychotherapy is to be evidence based.

CHAPTER 11

COMPLEMENTARY AND ALTERNATIVE MEDICINE

"Any mummery will cure, if the patient's faith is strong in it."

MARK TWAIN[1]

U p to 70 percent of people in Western countries use complementary and alternative medicine (CAM).[2] Annual use is 16 percent in Canada and 5 percent in the United States (table 11-1).[3] These figures exclude self-medicating users of herbals, vitamins, and other dietary products. A 1999 survey found that 73 percent of Canadians had used at least one alternative therapy at some point in their lives.[4] Chiropractic therapy was the most frequently employed at 36 percent, followed by relaxation and massage, at 23 percent, and prayer, at 21 percent. Europeans are even more likely to use CAM,[5] and Australians pay more for CAM than for prescription drugs.[6] The estimated $3.8 billion Canadians spent on these treatments was almost twice the capital expenditure for the nation's hospitals. Many seek more than one CAM treatment, and most CAM users are also under the care of a physician (see table 11-1). Most did not report their CAM treatments to their doctors, and 39 percent thought it was none of their business.[7] There was one CAM visit for every three visits to a medical doctor. Everywhere CAM is part of the therapeutic landscape.

TABLE 11-1
Use of Healing Professions in the United States and Canada*[8]

Use in Last 12 Months	United States	Canada
Physician	66%	79%
Chiropractor	4	15
Acupuncturist	1	1
Homeopath/Naturopath	.4	1
Massage Therapist	2	3
Any CAM Provider	5	16
Physician Only	63	68
CAM Provider Only	1	2
Both CAM Provider and Physician	4	14

*Self-medication with herbals or vitamins is excluded. Number of people surveyed in the
United States: 16,000; in Canada: 70,884.
  Data from: 1996 Medical Expenditure Panel Survey (United States).
              1996 Canadian National Population Health Survey.

WHAT IS CAM?

Definition is difficult because of the rich diversity of CAM treatments. Table 11-2 contains an incomplete list compiled by an ad hoc advisory panel to the Office of Alternative Medicine (OAM) at the US National Institutes of Health (NIH).[9] That the austere, evidence-based NIH should have such an office is a remarkable development in itself. In 1998 this office opened a "complementary medicine field"[10] within the Cochrane Collaboration.[11] The goal is to establish an Internet-accessible registry of controlled CAM trials, and evaluate them through systematic reviews. There are 695 journals devoted to CAM and two-thirds of the articles retrieved in this initiative are not in conventional medical databases such as Medline. With the Cochrane organization, the OAM seeks to overcome the publication bias and to capture relevant material published in other languages.

TABLE 11-2
Classification of Alternative Systems of Medical Practice

Alternative Systems of Medical Practice

Acupuncture*
Anthroposophically Extended Medicine
Ayurveda
Community-Based Health-Care Practices
Environmental Medicine
Homeopathic Medicine*
Latin American Rural Practices
Native American Practices*
Natural Products
Naturopathic Medicine
Past Life Therapy
Shamanism*
Tibetan Medicine
Traditional Oriental Medicine

Bioelectromagnetic Applications

Blue Light Treatment and Artificial Lighting
Electroacupuncture*
Electromagnetic Fields*
Electrostimulation and Neuromagnetic Stimulation Devices
Magnetoresonance Spectroscopy

Diet, Nutrition, Lifestyle Changes

Changes in Lifestyle
Diet
Gerson Therapy
Macrobiotics
Megavitamins*
Nutritional Supplements*

Herbal Medicine

Echinacea (purple coneflower)*
Ginger Rhizome
Ginkgo Biloba Extract*
Ginseng Root
Wild Chrysanthemum Flower
Witch Hazel
Yellowdock

Manual Healing

Acupressure
Alexander Technique
Biofield Therapeutics
Chiropractic Medicine*
Feldenkrais Method
Massage Therapy
Osteopathy
Reflexology
Rolfing
Therapeutic Touch
Trager Method
Zone Therapy

Mind/Body Control

Art Therapy
Biofeedback
Counseling
Dance Therapy
Guided Imagery
Humor Therapy
Hypnotherapy
Meditation
Music Therapy
Prayer Therapy*
Psychotherapy
Relaxation Techniques
Support Groups
Yoga

Pharmacological and Biological Treatments

Antioxidizing Agents
Cell Treatment
Chelation Therapy
Metabolic Therapy
Oxidizing Agents (Ozone, Hydrogen Peroxide)

---

*Discussed in text

The National Library of Medicine and the NIH National Center for Complementary and Alternative Medicine (NCCAM) propose the following definition; "[A] CAM therapy is one that is used instead of ('alternative') or in addition to ('complementary') the conventionally accepted therapy for a condition." Fortunately, the debate over CAM has become more dispassionate, abandoning pejorative terms commonly used a generation ago. "Quackery" and "charlatanism" are superseded by "unconventional," "alternative," "unorthodox," "irregular," "drugless," or "complementary." Some call orthodox medicine "regular," "mainstream," or "biomedicine." CAM practitioners prefer warm and fuzzy descriptors like "holistic," "allopathic," and "natural," while uncompromising medical doctors might choose "unscientific" or "unproven." Such judgmental terms can inflame rather than inform the discussion. Many people with chronic complaints adopt several healing practices and most include biomedicine. "Medical pluralism" demands an awareness of all healing techniques.[12]

Medical school curricula seldom include CAM. Nevertheless, nineteen surveys of mostly primary-care physicians in Western countries indicate that many refer to CAM practitioners and about 15 percent practice some form of CAM themselves.[13] In these surveys, many physicians believe some CAM is useful, especially young and female doctors. Physicians must be prepared to discuss CAM with their patients and assist them with their decisions to use or not to use it.[14] Liability is possible if essential information is omitted or incorrect.[15]

HISTORY OF CAM

The history of CAM is the history of healing itself. CAM and early medicine shared many characteristics, and were competitors even into the twentieth century. Both were innocent of the scientific method. As A. K. Shapiro and E. Shapiro asserted, "[U]ntil recently, the history of medical treatment is essentially the history of the placebo effect."[16] Babylonians four thousand years ago used *mandrake*,[12] a Mediterranean plant extract, for pain relief, and it accompanied Tutankhamen in his tomb. We now know mandrake contains the drugs *atropine* and *scopolamine*, whose excessive use must have done more harm than good. As noted earlier, despite knowledge of the blood's circulation, and the weakening effects of anemia and blood loss, some doctors and others bled patients for serious diseases. During the Enlightenment, improved knowledge of physiology and pathology caused medicine, or *biomedicine*, to stand apart from other healing traditions. Physicians, unlike CAM practitioners, began to base their treatments more on rational or plausible theories springing from the new science and less on the doctrines of antiquity. Nonetheless, the process was slow and some egregiously unscientific medical practices persisted into the twentieth century.

Medicine, no less than CAM, promoted implausible, useless, and sometimes dangerous therapies. Thus, mainstream and unconventional medicine shared more than either would have cared to mention. Many old medical treatments were harmless, but harmful bloodletting and ritual purgation took centuries to abolish. Such are the powers of nature and the placebo effect that they can conceal a treatment's harm. Medical science after 1800 led to more rational medicine and surgery. However, with few exceptions, evidence-based medicine began only after World War II, permitting medicine to define itself ever more distinctly from CAM.

Just as some conventional treatments are CAM, so some CAM can become conventional. Nitroglycerine began as a homeopathic treatment.[18] The purple foxglove provided William Withering (1741–1799) with a potent extract for treating dropsy (edema).[19] The extract contained *Digitalis purpurae*, the precursor of digoxin, a valuable and commonly used heart medication. It took decades to develop a reliable digitalis preparation and learn that the drug is effective only for swelling caused by heart failure, but not for that due to kidney or liver disease. W. K. Kellogg's promotion of healthy cereals presaged the high-fiber diet, now commonly recommended by doctors for constipation.[20]

T. J. Kaptchuk and D. N. Eisenberg remind us that medical pluralism has long existed in the United States.[21] In 1800 there were only about five hundred doctors trained in recognized medical schools to serve a population of around seven million. Sundry surgeons, barber-surgeons, botanical healers, midwives, apothecaries, cancer doctors, bonesetters, inoculators, abortionists, and sellers of nostrums cared for the sick. There were also religious and ethnic healers such as native medicine men, voodoo healers in New Orleans, and Dutch zieckentroosters (comforters of the sick) in New York. Later, Christian Science and other religions played healing roles. Lacking information of the outside world, pioneer families adopted folk medicines such as copper bracelets for arthritis and chicken soup for colds.

Intense rivalry among the various healing fraternities spawned colorful rhetoric and political gamesmanship. The founder of homeopathy, Samuel Hahnemann, claimed medical doctors practiced a "non-healing art . . . which shortened the lives of ten times the number of human beings as the most destructive wars and rendered many millions of patients more diseased and wretched than they were originally."[22] Oliver Wendell Holmes reposted that homeopathy was "a mangled mass of perverse ingenuity, of tinsel erudition, of imbecile incredulity and of artful misrepresentation."[23] Holmes was equally critical of his own profession, claiming "that if the whole material medica, as now used, could be sunk to the bottom of the sea, it would be all the better for mankind,—and all the worse for the fishes." This lively debate owed much to the placebo effect and nature—the only forces that could sustain useless or even harmful treatments.

No doubt, Hahnemann and Holmes were both correct. In the nineteenth century, many medical treatments were dangerous and much of CAM was fraud. The American Medical Association began as a buttress against medicine's rivals and through its Committee on Quackery punished members who dared to practice unorthodox medicine. Unorthodox practitioners' associations were also hostile to their members' collaboration with competing therapists. With the wisdom of hindsight, it seems that these various healing interests were equally self-serving. Except for surgery, few nineteenth-century treatments exist today. Nevertheless, CAM now thrives alongside scientific medicine, and some believe that each may have a role.

IS CAM QUACKERY?

"Quacksalver" is from an Old Dutch word meaning someone who boasts about his treatments. In seventeenth-century English, it was shortened to "quack" meaning an "ignorant pretender to medical skill; one who boasts to have knowledge of a wonderful remedie [sic]; an empiric or imposter in Medicine" (Oxford). "Mountebank" and "charlatan" have similar meanings. The nineteenth-century "snake-oil salesman" is another synonym. A Web site called *Quackwatch* informs the public against fraudulent medical claims.[24] As mentioned, these terms do not soothe the fevered CAM debate. Most CAM practitioners believe in the power of their treatments, as do most physicians in their not always science-based treatments. We cannot consider true believers to be quacks.

Unscrupulous and fraudulent practitioners know their product is valueless and yet sell it to the gullible often at outrageous prices. Perhaps "quack" is appropriate here. The distinction may be difficult. How can observers be certain if a practitioner believes or does not believe in his healing technique? As a gastroenterologist, I am incredulous that anyone can believe the claims of colonic lavage therapists. In the end, I think it best that we avoid the term "quack" altogether.

CAM AND BIOMEDICINE IN CONTEMPORARY SOCIETY

The debates concerning CAM and modern biomedicine reflect the duality of healing—the art and science of medicine. CAM in its many forms requires a worldview constructed by faith. To benefit, one has to believe in a treatment's healing power. In contrast, medicine demands proof and takes pride that it is "evidence based." Nevertheless, the frontier is more blurred than it appears. Some complementary therapies have a plausible rationale, and some even show promise in clinical trials. Conversely, much of what medical doctors do can be as rooted in belief, tradition, and theory as CAM. Alternative practitioners may treat a cold with echinacea, and family doctors may prescribe an antibiotic. Neither practice is evidence based.

Biomedicine is most successful in dealing with acute diseases with a known cause. Examples are pneumococcal pneumonia cured by penicillin, or angina pectoris (heart pain) cured by unblocking coronary arteries. It is with these *organic* or *structural* disorders that medical technology and evidence-based medicine excel. However, doctors are less successful if the condition is chronic and its cause is unknown. Examples are some backaches and headaches, chronic fatigue, and irritable bowel syndrome, sometimes called *functional disorders*. Sufferers of these as opposed to sufferers of structural disorders are more likely to seek treatment by CAM. The terms *organic* and *functional* are not very satisfactory but are widely used. Organic disorders are structural and recognizable, and their consequences apparent on examination. They belong firmly in the physical world and, like the speed of a weight dropped from a height, are subject to measurement and specific manipulation. Functional disorders are unfairly linked with psychological problems, and the thoughtless consider them unreal or of little importance. They are invisible to others, so their recognition requires the testimony of sufferers. Often considered to be in the world of the mind, cognition, or feeling, disorders of function are more difficult to understand and manage than those of structure.[25]

Separation of mind and body is usually attributed to the seventeenth-century philosopher René Descartes,[26] and succeeding generations have grappled with his *"dualism."* Modern writers such as G. L. Engel decry the separation and point out the role of the mind in even an obviously physical disease such as cancer.[27] There are two conspicuous contradictions in the distinction between functional and organic diseases. The first is that patients with organic disorders have emotional reactions to their disease. These may be fear, worry, hopelessness—in fact, the whole range of human emotion and imaginings. Wise healers recognize this and care for a patient's emotions as well as his body. The mind-body interaction is most complex in a chronic organic disorder such as rheumatoid arthritis. Chronic disability, pain, and lack of dramatic cure have devastating effects on such a patient's worldview and social functioning. Some reactions to pain and disability such as giving up and excessive dependency are destructive, while others, such as actively pursuing rehabilitation and retaining a positive social attitude, are constructive. In such a situation, perhaps both biomedicine's palliative drugs and some forms of CAM are of service. CAM, so long as it does no harm, is then complementary, offering solace where biomedicine comes up short.

The second contradiction in the organic/functional dichotomy is that functional disorders may have organic features. Indeed, reductionists (those who believe all symptoms have a simple explanation) might claim that all illness, even all human behaviors, have a physical/chemical basis. Migraine headaches have visual abnormalities and brain changes. Irritable bowel syndrome manifests itself with constipation and diarrhea. Such observable changes are not just in the mind.

A discussion of CAM must address two essential questions. Is CAM's "success" due entirely to the placebo effect and the natural evolution of the disease? Can CAM be harmful? Before addressing these questions, we should consider some of the more common CAM treatments and the difficulties in evaluating them. There can be no attempt to include all the more than three hundred such treatments in use, nor to explain the meaning of the many types of CAM listed in table 11-1.[28]

EXAMPLES OF CAM TREATMENTS

Chiropractic

Chiropractic is the most prevalent CAM treatment.[29] There are sixty thousand chiropractic school graduates practicing in the United States. One out of three people in North America and Great Britain sees a chiropractor. Spinal manipulation and the chiropractic catchword *subluxation* date from Hippocrates, but the profession's epiphany is assigned to September 18, 1895, when Daniel David Palmer reported his first spinal adjustment. Over the following century, chiropractic pursued an uneven course, and strong personalities disputed many matters. However, the resistance of organized medicine diminished in 1975 when the Supreme Court found the American Medical Association guilty of antitrust violations. Now, there are numerous chiropractic schools, licensing examinations, and recognition by all fifty states. In the United States, Medicare, more than half of the health maintenance organizations, and 75 percent of private insurers cover chiropractic. The issue of third-party funding mandates risk/benefit analyses.[30] In 2004, facing a fiscal crisis, the Ontario government withdrew (delisted) coverage for chiropractic treatment.

A charged atmosphere still characterizes the chiropractic debate.[31] Nevertheless, chiropractic has been submitted to more randomized clinical trials than other CAM treatments. Two chiropractors, W. C. Meeker and S. Haldeman, reviewed the history of chiropractic and evidence for its efficacy.[32] They indicate that the profession is at a crossroads. Many chiropractors chafe at the term CAM and wish to be regarded as legitimate health professionals. Working against them are several factors: the tenuousness of subluxation as the fundamental flaw that chiropractic strives to heal, the great variety of adjustment techniques offered, and the paucity of supporting evidence. Trial design difficulties include inadequate blinding, unsuitable controls, and unsatisfactory outcome measures.

D. C. Cherkin and colleagues compared chiropractic manipulation with an educational booklet for the treatment of low back pain.[33] However, this is not a blinded, controlled study. Chiropractic is a dramatic, personal contact procedure conducted by enthusiasts—placebo forces that cannot be matched by a booklet. Despite this advantage, chiropractic was found only marginally superior yet cost about $430 compared to $153 for the booklet (including visits). Skeptics suspect that chiropractic, without the placebo effect, might be no better than the booklet.

Meeker and Haldeman found seventy-three randomized clinical trials of spinal manipulation in the English-language medical and chiropractic literature. Forty-three were trials of manipulation for low back pain, and thirty favored manipulation. Only eleven of these were "placebo controlled," and eight were positive. According to E. Ernst, just two of these back trials were "sham manipulation controlled" and of adequate quality. Meeker and Haldemen admit that even the positive trial results are not convincing. Their overall view is modestly optimistic, while that of Ernst is mildly skeptical. The fierce views of others can be found in letters to the editor that followed these two articles.[34]

Childs et al. applied criteria to predict which patients with back pain would respond to manipulation therapy.[35] In a randomized clinical trial they found that those who met the criteria had better results with manipulation than with exercise. An editorial lauds the attempt to select patients most suitable for therapy, but criticizes the inadequacy of exercise as a control, the frequency of dropouts, the "trivial effects," and the questionable generalizability of the results.[36] Since the patients knew their treatment (exercise plus manipulation versus exercise alone), the trial could not be blinded, and bias seems likely.

Chiropractors must design a placebo treatment that can satisfy the need for trials to be double-blinded. Not to be forgotten is that chiropractic occasionally does harm. Massive stroke due to dissection of the vertebral artery is a rare complication of neck manipulation. Until better efficacy and safety data are forthcoming, it seems to me that the Scottish verdict "not proven" applies and readers must make up their own minds.

Acupuncture

Acupuncture in Chinese medicine is traced from the third century BCE.[37] Health is seen as a balance between yin and yang and the five elements: wood, fire, earth, metal, and water. *Qi* is said to be the life energy that flows through body meridians that are accessible by a skilled acupuncturist. The Chinese attribute great cures to acupuncture. A delegation of Western anesthetists visited China in 1974 to observe the use of acupuncture for general anesthesia during dental extraction and major surgery.[35] Since there were strong cultural and political reasons for acupuncture to succeed and the analgesia was not total, the visitors doubted its applicability elsewhere. Attempts to introduce it to Western operating rooms were unsuccessful. Nevertheless, acupuncturists are licensed in forty-one states[36] and about one million Americans are treated annually, primarily for pain.[37] Many hospital pain clinics include acupuncture among their therapeutic tools.

Evidence for efficacy is scant. Six of eight Cochrane reviews are for painful conditions.[41] In five, the data demonstrate no benefit of acupuncture over placebo. In two, there is insufficient data to come to any conclusion. Some data seem to support the use of acupuncture for headache, but the reviewers require more trials to be certain. A systematic review of fifty-one trials of acupuncture for chronic pain found twenty-one that were positive.[42] However, two-thirds of the studies were of low quality, and they account for the positive results. The Cochrane reviewers concluded that there was "limited evidence that acupuncture is better than no treatment for chronic pain and inconclusive evidence that acupuncture is more effective than placebo, sham acupuncture or standard care." The authors' suspicion that there is a publication bias further weakens the already weak support for acupuncture. Two single-blind, randomized clinical trials test the use of acupuncture to treat chronic mechanical neck pain and osteoarthritis of the knee.[43] The first showed statistically but not clinically significant improvement. The second reported improved function and pain relief after twenty-three true acupuncture treatments over twenty-six weeks compared to sham acupuncture, but 25 percent of subjects had dropped out by then. The fact that the therapists knew whether the patients were receiving sham, rather than real, acupuncture undermines the data. There is no suitable (placebo) control for the acupuncture needle. Several variations of acupuncture complicate the task of proving that any of them work. These include burning herbs on the needles (moxibustion) or connecting them to an electric current (electroacupuncture).

Following dental surgery, acupuncture was no better than sham treatment in achieving pain relief.[44] However, whether real or sham, patients who believed they were receiving acupuncture were more likely to improve. Dominicus So interviewed sixty-two acupuncture patients before and after their qi was restored to harmony.[45] Attaining their stated therapeutic goals was most likely if their expectations of the treatment and the acupuncturist were low. Evidently, high expectations invite disappointment. Tellingly, the author concludes that "perceived acupuncture outcomes seem not to be related to placebo effects and patient expectations, but rather to client-practitioner relationship factors." Indeed!

Acupuncture is not always harmless.[46] Pneumothorax (punctured lung), spinal lesions, and septic infection suggest a rare and careless exuberance with the needles. More common and therefore more noteworthy is that infected needles transmit Hepatitis B virus. A Japanese acupuncture clinic recorded only sixty-four minor adverse events among 55,291 treatments, sixteen of which were "forgotten needles." They claim that negligence, ignorance, or poor sterilization practices account for the serious complications reported by others.

Acupuncturists must do better research if they are to convince the public in Western countries that the benefit of acupuncture is more than a placebo effect or that medical care plans should pay for it. They also must sterilize their needles or use disposable ones.

Homeopathy

At the end of the eighteenth century, a German doctor named Samuel Christian Hahnemann proposed the three principles of homeopathy.[47] The principle of *similars* held that a treatment could be selected by how similar its toxic effects resembled a patient's symptoms. Cinchona bark produced effects similar to malaria; ergo, greatly diluted doses should treat malaria. The homeopath selects treatments by how closely its effects resemble the patient's disease. The second principle was that treatments retained their activity when *diluted* in a series of steps of 1:10 or 1:100, with each dilution shaken. Hahnemann claimed that great dilutions retained the vital nature of the drug and had clinical effects. J. P. Vandenbroucke and A. J. de Craen point out that at recommended dilutions (greater than Avagadro's number [6.023 x 10^{23}]), no drug is detectable, indeed no molecule may remain.[48] The third principle, *holism*, held that the remedies are best when before dilution, the drug's effects most closely mimic an individual patient's symptoms. Thus, a disease might have more than one treatment according to its specific manifestations in a patient.

Homeopathy became a rival for unscientific medicine, still wallowing in dangerous therapeutic ventures such as venesection and arsenic. A contemporary medical journal labeled homeopathy "a cheat" with little advantage over placebos. The antipathy grew throughout the nineteenth century, particularly as homoeopaths used statistics to show superior outcomes in their own hospitals (perhaps because in medical institutions, some therapies were dangerous, or the patients were more seriously ill). However, the American Medical Association needed the homeopaths to refer their patients to its developing medical specialties, and homeopathy adopted some conventional medicines such as diphtheria antitoxin. Thus in 1903 the AMA buried the hatchet and invited the homeopaths to join. Assimilation led to a decline in homeopathy until its recent resurgence.

W. B. Jonas and his colleagues assessed six systematic reviews of clinical trials that address the question, Is homeopathy superior to placebo?[49] Because the trial designs, treatments, and outcomes are very different, interpretation of the combined data is difficult. Many had a small sample size, which invites bias, as well as inadequate blinding. The largest trials tended to be negative, and there is likely a publication bias. Despite these substantial criticisms, four of the six systematic reviews claim that homeopathy is better than placebo. However, the authors of three of these admit that their results are not convincing because of shortcomings and inconsistencies. Vandenbroucke points out that conventional medicine is quick to dismiss these results since they are theoretically untenable.[50] The authors of one systematic review "would be ready to accept that homeopathy can be efficacious, if only the mechanism were more plausible." It is not easy for the scientifically minded to accept Hahnemann's principles or the therapeutic value of dilutions where the active principle is undetectable.

Jonas also reviewed the results of homeopathy trials for individual diseases. While some are tentatively favorable, the quality of the studies permits only equivocation. The trials tend to be small and flawed. One negative example is a randomized, double-blind, placebo-controlled trial of homeopathy for pain control after bilateral wisdom teeth were sequentially removed.[51] Homeopaths selected and diluted their medicines to 10^{30}. Their solutions and placebo (water) were randomly given to patients, beginning three hours postextraction. Pain scores remained identical after treatment, and the subjects showed no preference for the medicine. However, the homeopaths protested they were unable to individualize the dose and timing of their treatment. With so many possible homeopathic programs, a limitless number of such trials would be required to prove none of them worked. Observers must use their own judgment. If you think such treatment is ridiculous, you will reject it. If not, you may try it. In such a case, who should pay for it?

Herbal Medicine

Twelve percent of Americans spend more than $5 billion annually on herbal remedies. In North America these remedies are largely unregulated and manufacturing quality control is voluntary.[52] The European community has directed a double standard for different types of medicines.[53] In order to bring herbals under regulation, proof of their efficacy is waived, while it is still required for conventional medicines. Tellingly, after paying US$283 million in 2002 for herbal medicines, the German health authority reduced the number of those approved to four in 2004. This demonstrates growing gaps between what is expected for conventional and nonconventional therapies, and between regulatory approval and reimbursement by health-care plans. In the future, we can expect much more discussion of these gaps.

There are many herbal compounds including Chinese herbal mixtures, and study is hampered by the lack of standardization and quality control. A. G. M. De Smet lists contaminants, including digitalis, microorganisms, pesticides, toxic metals, painkillers, and arthritis drugs, that could alter an herbal's quality.[54] Several herbals, such as St. John's wort, interact with prescription drugs. Some are toxic to the heart, liver, nervous system, or kidneys. For example, kava used for anxiety[55] rarely causes liver damage that may require a liver transplant.[56] Yet herbals' principle selling point is that they are "natural" and therefore safe. (But arsenic is natural, too!) Randomized trials evaluate a "small fraction" of the thousands of available herbal medicines. We describe three examples here.

Echinacea

Echinacea was first used medicinally by native Americans,[57] who iron-ically were free of colds prior to the arrival of Europeans. Neverthe-less, it became a popular cold remedy in Europe and has a renewed popularity in North America. Several upper respiratory viruses cause the common cold, which is responsible for lost productivity and bac-terial complications such as sinusitis. A Cochrane review included "sixteen trials [eight prevention trials and eight trials on treatment of upper-respiratory-tract infections] with a total of 3,396 participants . . ." and concludes that "[t]he majority of the available studies report positive results. However there is not enough evidence to recommend . . . echinacea preparations for the treatment or prevention of common colds."[58] Ernst agrees that the evidence for echinacea in pre-venting colds is weak and reminds us of a probable publication bias.[59]

P. B. Barrett and his colleagues randomly assigned echinacea or placebo to 148 students when they "believed they were coming down with a cold."[60] They were then instructed to take four of the assigned capsules six times in the first twenty-four hours and three times daily thereafter for up to ten days. (The placebo capsules contained alfalfa and both contained peppermint to disguise the taste.) The endpoint was the last day before the subject answered "no" to the question, Do you think you are still sick today? Subjects were monitored throughout, and double-blinding was confirmed by asking subjects to identify what they had taken. The protocol accounted for possible confounders such as other medications, gender, and the duration and severity of symptoms at entry. The mean duration of the cold was 6.27 days for those taking echinacea and 5.75 days for those on placebo (no statistical difference). At endpoint, the severity of fourteen individual symptoms was similar in the two groups.

So, is this negative trial the last word on echinacea for the common cold? It is not. First, many lesser-quality trials were deemed positive. The authors admit that they might not have detected a small difference and that the healthy young participants might handle colds differently than others. Although the capsules used here were care-fully analyzed and contained 125 mg *E. augustifolia* root, 62 mg *E. purpurae* root, and 25 mg *E. purpurae* herb, they also contained thyme. These contents differed from those of other available preparations. R. B. Turner points out that neither the "active" principle of echinacea nor its mechanism of action are known.[61] Therefore, we are unable to confront fundamental issues such as dose, bioavailability, and pharmacokinetics. There are other criticisms. "Once the cold has started, it may be too late for echinacea." "The product used was not the best choice." "It should be gargled." "Alfalfa is not a placebo, but may itself ameliorate colds!"

The proportions of the three echinacea plant species differ in the many available products. Moreover, "potency" may vary according to whether the root or flower is used, how the active ingredients are extracted, and even the season of harvest. Colds get better in two to ten days (mean six), so that any treatment will be accompanied by a cure eventually. These data will not dissuade believers, but buyers beware. Even if some echinacea were effective for colds, the product you choose may not be.

St. John's Wort

An extract of this plant is promoted for the treatment of mild depression, but it is unknown which of several chemical constituents is the active agent. Like some prescription antidepressants, it appears to affect the metabolism of chemical mediators in the brain. Reviews suggest that short-term use of St. John's wort is more efficacious than placebo for the treatment of mild to moderate depression.[62] However, the trials are faulty, and there is no support for the extract's use in major depression. Recent large randomized trials fail to demonstrate antidepressant effects. De Smet cautions that some preparations may differ substantially from those tested.[63] Moreover, St. John's wort interacts with several drugs, including antidepressants. The most notable side effect is photosensitivity (excessive skin reaction to ultraviolet light). A Cochrane review concludes that the herb's efficacy compared to regular antidepressants is unknown, but at usual doses it has fewer untoward effects.[64]

Ginkgo

The Chinese used ginkgo fruits and seeds for thousands of years and claim they have a diverse pharmacology and numerous uses. In improving memory loss, Ernst judged eight studies to be of good quality and seven to show encouraging results.[65] Because of experimental evidence that the herb improves blood flow, it was tested in five "good" randomized trials for the treatment of "intermittent claudication" (leg pain on walking due to poor blood supply to the legs). The herb improved pain-free walking distance compared to controls. However, it was no better than pentoxyfylline, a prescription drug, and both were less effective than walking exercises.

The Cochrane collaborators reviewing ginkgo for cognitive impairment and dementia found that "Ginkgo biloba appears to be safe. . . . Many of the early trials used unsatisfactory methods and were small, and we cannot exclude publication bias. Overall there is promising evidence of improvement in cognition and function associated with Ginkgo. However, the three more modern trials show inconsistent results."[66] Scientists suspect that gingko's only role is that of a placebo. On the other hand, those who believe that the ancient Chinese possessed unique wisdom can apparently use ginkgo safely. Meanwhile, active principle, dose, formulation, mechanism of action, and long-term effects remain mysteries.

Vitamins and Infection

Some use vitamins to prevent and treat disease. The Cochrane Collaboration concluded that "[l]ongterm daily supplementation with vitamin C in large doses daily does not appear to prevent colds. There appears to be a modest benefit in reducing duration of cold symptoms from ingestion of relatively high doses of vitamin C. The relation of dose to therapeutic benefit needs further exploration."[67] The 8 to 9 percent reduction in symptom days is indeed a "modest" benefit. Given the publication bias, a clinical benefit seems unlikely.

T. A. Barringer and his colleagues address the question, Does daily multivitamin and mineral supplement prevent infection in diabetics?[68] They recruited 158 people with type II diabetes over forty-five years of age. Each participant took one tablet daily for a year: seventy-eight took the supplement and eighty took a placebo. Infections and infection-related absenteeism were greater in those receiving placebo and the differences were highly significant. In an editorial, W. Fawzi and M. J. Stumpfer pointed out that the subjects in Barringer's trial were diabetics prone to malnutrition and infections.[69] The small size of the study, the imperfect blinding, and the observation that the supplemented subjects were initially better nourished cast doubt on the results. Trials of this sort are difficult to execute and interpret. Even if it were true, prevention of infection in a small number of diabetics does not justify vitamin supplements for everyone.

Vitamins act as coenzymes that permit normal biochemical reactions to occur in the healthy body. Sufficient vitamins are provided by a normal diet. Some believe that if a small amount of a vitamin is good, huge amounts should be better. They have yet to prove their point. It seems from the above data that supplements may help malnourished diabetics resist infection.[70] There are specific indications for specific vitamins, such as vitamin D supplementation for those unexposed to the sun in winter and folic acid during pregnancy. However, vitamin supplements for healthy people on a normal diet are another matter. Mega doses of vitamins A and D can be harmful.

The vitamins A, β-carotene, and E have antioxidant activity that is believed to be capable of preventing diseases. A Cochrane review of fourteen randomized trials addressing the prevention of gastrointestinal cancer not only found that these vitamins were of no benefit, but also that overall mortality seemed greater in those taking the vitamins than in the controls.[71] Another meta-analysis showed that high-dose vitamin E increased the risk of all-cause mortality.[72] Vitamins A and D have long been known to be toxic in high doses. Clearly, excessive vitamin ingestion is too much of a good thing.

Irresponsible claims for vitamins are parodied by the wonderful story of vitamin O.[73] Newspaper advertisements claimed that vitamin O was helping thousands of people enjoy healthier lives. Testimonials claimed dramatic results, such as, "After taking vitamin O for several months, I find I have more energy and have become immune to colds and flu." Dr. Koch recommended it for astronauts to ensure they had enough oxygen to maintain their health. A two-ounce vial sold for $20.00. Fifteen to twenty drops three times a day "maximizes your nutrients, purifies your bloodstream and eliminates toxins and poisons. . . ." It is described as "stabilized oxygen molecules in a solution of distilled water and sodium chloride"—also known as salt water! Much more oxygen is available to the body from a single breath than from many liters of vitamin O, but some were persuaded that it was the perfect antidote to pollution and deforestation. Only after thousands were duped was the fraud exposed and the makers of vitamin O prosecuted. "Dr. Koch" is fictional, there is no "vitamin" O, and the deception was deliberate. The terms "quackery" or "charlatan" come to mind here. It seems the word "vitamin" conveys the notion of health and cure, and the need seems insatiable. Only a little persuasion was required to gull the gullible to pay for vitamin salt water!

Colonic Hydrotherapy

> ". . . find her disease
> And purge it to pristine health."
>
> MACBETH 5.3.53

Do you remember Arbuthnot Lane, the British surgeon who removed colons to prevent "autointoxication"? Nowadays, no hospital operating committee would permit such an abuse. Nevertheless, the belief that colon toxins cause illness persists and finds expression in colon hydrotherapy or colon lavage. Colon cleansing dates to antiquity, and Louis XIV, equipped with his royal enema chair, commanded daily enemas.[74] In hospitals, doctors order enemas or an oral laxative solution to clean the colon for diagnostic tests or surgery. Colon hydrotherapy establishments elsewhere are known irreverently as "colon laundries."

One Web site explains the rationale of such therapy:

> Our bowel—the sewer system of the body—becomes sluggish and ceases to eliminate the toxic waste that the hard working liver has dumped into it for elimination from the body. This results in a cesspool of fermenting, putrefying toxic waste, which is eventually reabsorbed by our bloodstream to again pass through and wash every cell and organ as it circulates around our body. IS IT ANY WONDER WE GET SICK! A toxic bowel if left unchecked can lead to . . . arthritis, skin problems, migraines, poor memory, lethargy, toxic overload and at worst, may lead to cancer of the bowel. Natural Colon Health and Colonic Lavage . . . may be beneficial for a multitude of health problems, including irritable bowel, Colitis, Diverticulitis, Crohn's Disease, Candida, and Chronic Fatigue Syndrome.[75]

Through PubMed or Google, I am unable to find any clinical trial reports of hydrotherapy for any disease or symptom. It certainly would be difficult to design a placebo control. The National Center for Complementary and Alternative Medicine omits hydrotherapy from its classification (see table 11-2). Nevertheless, colonics have a following. Consider this headline: "Constipation Affecting 90% of Canadians." I knew we were reserved, but 90 percent constipated! It reminds me of the musings of Mma Ramotswe, the heroine of *The Ladies No. 1 Detective Agency*, who "felt sorry for people who suffered from constipation, and she knew of many who did. There were probably enough of them to form a political party—with a chance of government perhaps —but what would such a party do if it was in power? Nothing, she imagined. It would try to pass legislation, but would fail."[76]

One hydrotherapy claim is that overweight people can lose ten to twenty-five pounds after a colon cleansing. Of course, what is lost is not fat, rather water and a small amount of feces. Hydrotherapy is not without risk. Dehydration can have serious consequences, and untrained personnel have perforated colons. The claim that hydrotherapy can diagnose cancer is false.

Distant Healing, Prayer

Eighty-two percent of Americans believe in the healing power of prayer. A review of fifty-seven admittedly poor studies found a positive effect.[77] Letters in response to these data expose the intensity of feeling on this subject. The religious implications of prayer place it outside our discussion of placebos and alternative therapy—or do they? Suppose prayer treatments were to be considered mainstream treatment. Should they then be included in health-care packages? If so, could religion itself be denied? Would any religion's prayers qualify? How would we decide?

CAN OR SHOULD CAM BE EVIDENCE BASED?

Those who espouse evidence-based medicine wish to apply its principles to CAM.[78] That would require randomized, controlled trials similar to those used to approve new drugs. They argue that a pharmaceutical company may not sell a new drug without such trials; therefore, it is illogical that similar requirements not apply to the sale of megavitamins, herbs, health foods, or homeopathic medicines. Some have been tested in placebo-controlled trials. However, for chiropractic, acupuncture, touching, colonic lavage, and spiritual or lifestyle manipulation, the challenge is to design suitable controls (as we have seen in surgery and psychotherapy).

For conventional medicine, ignoring CAM is not an option.[79] Open minds are needed if we are to determine which CAM is best to complement medical science. The difficulty is demonstrated by an uncontrolled evaluation of "healing by gentle touch" where seventy-six patients were treated by "noninvasive touch on the head, chest, arms, legs and feet with varying extents of health-related conversation, for approximately forty minutes—usually while the subject lies comfortably on a treatment bed—followed by a ten minute rest."[80] The outcome was evaluated by comparing symptoms on a questionnaire before and after treatment. Ernst points out that the positive results could be explained by the placebo response aided by subjects' desire to please the therapists.[81] Moreover, the fact that subjects with the most severe symptoms fared the best can be explained by regression to the mean. It is surprising that such an unscientific report should appear in a peer-reviewed and esteemed medical journal. The authors, in response to Ernst's criticisms, promised a randomized clinical trial.[82] It will be interesting to see how they design the placebo control.

Citing the difficulty in designing controls, CAM practitioners argue that their treatments cannot be subjected to the scientific method and support their therapies by belief, theories, anecdotes, opinions, and traditions. C. R. B. Joyce states that a major attraction of CAM is that it is directed toward the individual patient.[83] Most CAM begins with a healer-therapist interview that counters the "dehumanization" of orthodox medicine with a personalized explanation for an individual's complaints. Such a customized approach is difficult to test in a controlled trial, and the placebo effect cannot be measured in individuals.[84] Moreover, CAM therapists insist that the results of controlled trials would not help them with their treatment decisions.

There are two reasons why these objections are unsatisfactory. First, such individualization occurs in conventional medicine. Second, the results from properly conducted trials can serve as guideposts informing individual treatment decisions. Ultimately, no modern healer can escape the responsibility to vouchsafe her treatments. If there are other foundations for therapy than science, we must seek and understand them, for belief alone is unconvincing.

The case for evaluating CAM is topical because of increasing pressure on health-care budgets. Many CAM practitioners want to participate in health-care programs. In the United States, Medicare and some health maintenance organizations already oblige some of them. Since resources are finite, authorities must ask, where does CAM fit in health-care priorities? A person waiting many months for a hip replacement might question another's right to homeopathy if both are supported by the finite public purse.

IS CAM A PLACEBO?

This question cannot be answered authoritatively. Those advocating CAM have a duty to substantiate their claims with the requisite research. In some cases, this will be exceedingly difficult as the materials (e.g., herbals) are of uncertain and variable nature, and the "active" element is unknown. It is difficult to design suitable sham treatments for chiropractic or acupuncture, and their varied techniques could mandate many clinical trials. After each trial, advocates may insist yet another variation might work. L. J. Hoffer makes a case for "plausibility building."[85] He suggests that the "more biologically implausible a theory, the higher the bar medical scientists tend to set for crediting evidence supporting its clinical plausibility." Perhaps a treatment such as purified St. John's wort, once its active principle is identified, will follow digitalis from CAM to mainstream medicine. However, some treatments seem implausible by any measure. Reflexology, magnetic bracelets, health stones, paranormal healing, and aromatherapy so strain credulity that no one has even attempted a trial.[86] Homeopathic medicines diluted beyond the last molecule should be implausible to most people. Controls for therapies such as colonic lavage and neck manipulations will tax imaginations, but it is precisely in such cases where controls are most necessary.

Meanwhile, if a CAM therapy is harmless and leaves many clients satisfied, should we be concerned? In a free country, people can choose their therapy. After all, many chronic complaints have no medical solution, and doctors themselves sometimes recommend unproven treatments. "Off-label" use of a prescription drug is seldom science based. There is little evidence that "healthy" diet and exercise help many patients suffering from specific complaints, yet physicians routinely advise them. Their benefit may be placebo as well. In an ideal world, all treatments would be evidence based. While that is logistically impossible, all who propose treatments should strive to ensure that they are at least safe.

CAN CAM BE HARMFUL?

Much is made of the "natural" quality of many CAM treatments, as if "natural" implied safety and purity—"the myth of beneficent nature."[87] Like biomedicine, CAM can sometimes be harmful. Only through careful trials and case reporting can we recognize them. The thalidomide tragedy in the 1960s resulted from a failure of these processes. Some CAM treatments also have a potential for great harm, as in vertebral artery dissection with neck manipulation, colon perforation with hydrotherapy, or liver toxicity with herbals.[88] In the United States and Europe, the herb industry is not required to demonstrate safety or efficacy.[89] Failure to identify and standardize the contents of a product such as kava endangers consumers. Sometimes, diagnosis and specific treatment of a serious disease is delayed while a client pursues alternate treatments of doubtful value. Most troubling, CAM practitioners sometimes practice beyond their métier, by prescribing dangerous diets, manipulating the neck for migraine, or recommending against public-health programs like vaccination. Notorious are those "clinics," often far away, that tout costly and bogus cancer cures (see chapter 16). Only regulation and scientific research can guard against such abuses.

CONCLUSIONS

CAM therapies are so diverse that no definition suits them all. The designations "unconventional," "alternative," and "irregular" fail to acknowledge the unproven therapies to which physicians and CAM practitioners resort daily. T. J. Kaptchuk asks if, for some subjective complaints, "can any of alternative medicine's particular rituals have a greater impact than the rituals of conventional medicine . . . ?"[90] Put another way; is CAM more adept at achieving a placebo effect than biomedicine? For technological triumphs where cures are manifest, it may seem to matter little, but for most therapeutic transactions, art may be the best we have. Just as the border between medical science and the art of medicine is blurred, so is the border between medical practice and CAM. We have seen CAM therapies become biomedicine and medical therapies that are CAM. The CAM professions can learn much from biomedicine's scientific methods in proving their therapies exert more than placebo effects. Biomedicine and its third-party sponsors, by forsaking the art of healing, risk alienating their clientele. Even if CAM's effect is placebo, we all have an interest in understanding how this effect can be mobilized to make ill persons feel and function better. Whether scientifically effective or not, CAM seems adept at eliciting placebo effects, and biomedicine can learn from that.

Chapter 12

The Doctor as Placebo

"One of the essential qualities of the clinician is interest in
humanity, for the secret of the care of the patient is caring
for the patient."

Francis Peabody (1927)[1]

A healer's success depends a great deal upon her personality: her
demeanor, attitude, ability to communicate, and unam-
biguous commitment to an ill person's welfare. Here, we review the
elements of a good doctor/patient relationship and its contribution to
the placebo effect. When it goes awry, the effect may be nocebo. Science-based medicine has vastly increased physicians' powers to heal
disease, but often at the expense of their ability to assuage illness.
There are elements in the professional, societal, and institutional
environment that hinder the doctor as placebo, yet they can help as
well. In the end, the doctor herself must make the difference. This
chapter is not a doctor's manual on the art of medicine. Texts are
available for that. Rather its purpose is to explain the importance of
the healer in healing.

THE SCIENCE AND ART OF MEDICINE
(TREATING DISEASE AND COMFORTING
THE PATIENT)

Medicine's great triumph has been its ability to marshal science to
benefit humanity. Much of this advance is in public health, where
immunization, safe water, and programs to curtail smoking, stop
drunk driving, and promote seat belts prevent much illness or death.
The advancement of science during the Enlightenment led to rational

surgery and the gradual abandonment of dangerous medical procedures such as bloodletting, purging, and cautery with boiling oil. It became safer to see doctors. Aseptic surgery and obstetrics saved lives. Many infections are no longer prevalent in Western countries, and smallpox has been vanquished. The discovery of insulin in the 1920s permitted diabetics an almost normal life. The arrival of sulfonamides and antibiotics in the 1930s and 1940s began to cure previously fatal infections. The list of formerly disabling or fatal diseases that are now curable includes some leukemias, peptic ulcer disease, mitral stenosis, and many others. There is evidence-based prevention of heart disease through control of high blood pressure and high cholesterol, and many cancer patients now live longer. Few organs escape the beams and scopes of medical science. Diagnostics became treatment, so that arteries are cleared by catheter, abscesses drained by ultrasound, and tumors removed by endoscope.

While disease yields to science's advances, illness is another matter. Illness may accompany all disease, and many feel ill with no disease at all. Therefore, healing requires more than scientifically seeking and destroying a pathological process. The art of medicine was practiced long before evidence-based medicine, when doctors and CAM practitioners alike had little else to offer. Around 1900, the charismatic William Osler wrote philosophically about his noble profession and some of his aphorisms are quoted today (see below). In an age when few treatments worked, physicians were beloved because they cared. Art and literature richly portray the kindly doctor presiding over a patient in the family home (see figure 5-1).

Like most nostalgia, the kindly country doctor is part real, part myth. Art also exposed medicine's dark side, such as Shaw's pompous surgeon and Hogarth's quack doctor (see figure 12-1). Dangerous, ignorance-based treatments persisted into the twentieth century, and life could still be brutish and short. It seems ironic that the advent of evidence-based medicine signaled an apparent decline in doctors' stature in society—seeming victims of modern medicine's success.[2] Technology shifts the doctor's focus from the patient's illness to an organ's disease. Each innovation requires experiment, experience, and skill. Medical information so outstrips an individual's ability to cope that many doctors specialize in order to foster their skills and limit their responsibility. Each new cadre of experts mobilizes medicine's scientific power but narrows its view. Patients are parceled out according to their afflicted organ and, as they age, accumulate new doctors for new organ afflictions. Little time or inclination remains to develop a doctor/patient relationship outside the specialty's purview. Who knows the whole patient? Family doctors should be central to patient care, but they are seldom privy to the specialist's endeavors, have heavy schedules, and confront daily technological and administrative challenges of their own. Is it any wonder that many patients seek help elsewhere?

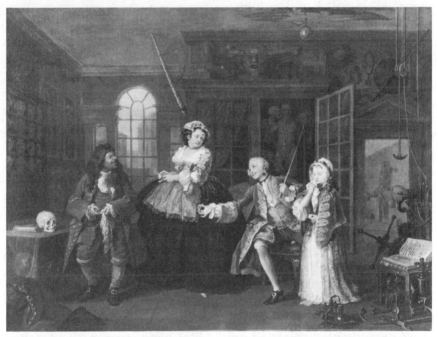

Figure 12-1: *Visit to the Quack Doctor* (also called *The Inspection*). Third scene from "Marriage a la Mode" by William Hogarth (1697–1764). The National Gallery, London (© The National Gallery). The Enlightenment view of the "quack doctor" was not a flattering one. From his young mistress, a recently married and irresponsible nobleman has contracted venereal disease and passed it along to his young bride (on the right). As indicated by the black spot on his neck, he is taking mercury as therapy. He seeks another remedy for her from the doctor, who stands grinning fiendishly at his "patients." The large woman, evidently his assistant, looms menacingly holding a jackknife. Surely, they are not planning to bleed that already pale young girl!

ELEMENTS OF A GOOD
DOCTOR/PATIENT RELATIONSHIP

Doctors are devoted to science, but science alone cannot dictate every action. "Ultimate decisions, the valuations and the choosing of ends, are beyond the scope of science."[3] Since the healer's relationship with her patient is so important to these ultimate decisions and to the placebo effect, we should examine it closely. Interpersonal relationships are complex, and positive or negative impressions color all of life's transactions. Many of the elements that mark a good teacher, salesperson, or leader also describe the successful healer, but the latter is unique. Ill people seek out healers because of fear of the meaning of their symptoms and hope that they can make things better. D. E. Moerman reminds us that placebos are inert and by themselves achieve nothing.[4] Their benefit is to provide meaning for a person's suffering, and a context for dealing with it.[5] Much depends, then, on how well a doctor is able to respond to her patient's fears and hopes. Several essential attributes come to mind.

Appearance and Demeanor

In some societies, perhaps even our own long ago, healers were powerful figures. Their control over evil spirits or their knowledge of the human body were mysterious, austere, and conveyed an aura of healing. The physician teachers who taught my generation were trained by an apprenticeship that predated evidence-based medicine. They typically wore three-piece suits and conducted their hospital ward rounds with dignity and style. These gentlemen-teachers treated patients with respect and were in turn respected and slightly feared. Theirs was the generation that introduced insulin, penicillin, and battlefield transfusions into clinical medicine.

Our own careers spanned the technology revolution where great advances in diagnosis and treatment meant cures or better lives for many. Infections no longer carried off people in their prime. However, people live longer only to acquire other and more chronic diseases. Cardiac disease, strokes, and cancer became more prevalent and new diseases loomed, such as hospital infections, osteoporosis, and AIDS. Meanwhile, great social changes affected the way doctors practiced. Medicare, medical insurance, human rights legislation, greater expectations, litigation, more elderly patients, and the sexual revolution changed doctors' priorities and their public persona.

To some of our students, it no longer seemed important to be professional. Young doctors of both sexes began to wear jeans and T-shirts to clinic and hospital, sometimes as a rebellious statement without concern for their older patients' needs. Authority gave way to familiarity. Patients were addressed by their first names, and bedside manners deteriorated. Team medicine meant that white coats discussed patients' histories and pondered diagnostic options in hushed tones and frightening language outside a patient's room.

The white coat itself has an interesting history. As scientific medicine grew more complicated, patient care occurred less in the home and more in hospitals. Instead of a place for the poor, the abandoned, and the dying, hospitals became citadels of science and hope. To emphasize the notion of the physician scientist, a laboratory coat became his uniform. D. W. Blumhagen alludes to the white coat's association with life, purity, innocence, and chastity.[6] Only doctors and nurses wear white. Other hospital workers are not the healers. The white coat, the stethoscope, the head mirror, and the black bag became symbols of healing power and authority. Now, there are doubts that such symbols are suitable for the new relationships between patients and doctors. There is even evidence of white coat nocebo effects in children and those having their blood pressure taken.

The need to see many patients to meet income objectives or to service a busy clinic more often collided with increasingly shared responsibilities for home and family, so that the time to talk to patients diminished, even as management of their symptoms became more complicated. Many family doctors, estranged from specialists, confined themselves to office practice, seldom visiting their patients in hospitals and nursing homes.[7] Consultations became briefer, often with a different doctor on each occasion. Meanwhile, controversy over physicians' incomes and reports of outrageous malpractices and lurid abuse permeate the news. Societal pressures and lifestyle requirements now steer young doctors to manageable specialties with regular hours, minimal liability, and better pay, and few choose family practice.[8] These developments minimize doctor/patient relationships and cry out for professional and administrative reform. Most doctors are careful and sincere, but many are frustrated by lack of time and strangers bearing guidelines, writs, and regulations into their examining rooms (see chapter 15). None of these pressures encourage the placebo effect. How a healer appears to a patient determines whether trust is to be secured and fears allayed.

However, doctors err if they gaze too nostalgically on their predecessors. Francis Peabody recorded complaints that "[y]oung graduates have been taught a great deal about the mechanisms of disease, but very little about . . . how to take care of patients."[9] That was in 1927, the age of rational medicine, but before evidence-based medicine. Yet it resonates today. Peabody went on to say that doctors learn the art not in medical school, but in the "harder school of experience." Unfortunately, this may be too late for many patients and too difficult a lesson for many doctors who have so little time for "art." Sir William Osler is a medical icon, whose textbook[10] and inspirational writings[11] are often quoted. He wrote of the deportment and attitudes of the good doctor. However, the modern reader might doubt his relevance to our time. Like Shaw's surgeon, there is a certain aloofness or inequality in his tone. He implores his 1889 graduates not to expect too much of the people amongst whom they dwell, and "in matters medical, the ordinary citizen of today has not one whit more sense than the old Romans, whom Lucian scourged which made them fall easy victims of the quacks of the time. . . ." In this short phrase, Osler conveys a haughty distancing between doctor and patient, ignorance of the concept of patient autonomy, a classical reference that would mystify the modern student, and an ironic aversion to "quacks," whose practices were likely no more harmful than the bleeding, cold baths, and strychnine recommended in his own textbook.[12] Osler's eloquence and clinical skills galvanized the medical profession and improved medical education, but we are wrong to regard the profession of a century ago as paradise lost.

Nevertheless, we can seek a better environment in which doctors and patients can interact more favorably. The working ambience affects the physician's demeanor. Osler wrote of the need for physicians and surgeons to be imperturbable,[13] meaning "coolness and presence of mind under all circumstances, calmness amid storm, clearness of judgment in moments of great peril. . . ."[14] *Aequanimitas*, he called it. A calm, unhurried, and confident surgeon can seem like an angel in the emergency room. The operating room can be fearsome but also a temple of healing to a patient well prepared by a caring and confident anesthetist or surgeon. However, most doctor/patient interactions occur elsewhere, where aequanimitas could be mistaken for indifference. In the friendly privacy of a doctor's office, family photos, diplomas, and other examples of her humanity and accomplishments promote a confident healing environment. Compare these symbols and circumstances with the austere impersonality of a hospital clinic or the mumbling team visit in a hospital ward—or even the obscure classical references of Osler. The family doctor's environment, personality, and deportment are important to her sound dispensing of evidence-based advice and healing of illness. Aequanimitas must be accompanied by caring. A confident and congenial demeanor does not demean.

Attitude

A positive attitude is a vital characteristic of a healer. Patients are more likely to experience placebo effects if they like and have confidence in the doctor and if treatment is prescribed enthusiastically.[15] Half the patients in general practice receive no precise diagnosis.[16] K. B. Thomas demonstrated that encouraging such patients with a positive attitude leads to better outcomes than does an indifferent approach and that this can be achieved equally well with and without a pill (see table 5-2).[17] Another study found that patients who were told what to expect after surgery had better outcomes than others who were denied this information.[18] Before surgery, an anesthetist told patients what to expect postoperatively "in a manner of enthusiasm and confidence." He described the pain they could expect, taught them relaxation techniques, and assured them that pain relievers were available on request. Postoperatively, the anesthetist repeated the presentation and visited the patients several times offering encouragement. An independent, blinded observer found these patients to be more comfortable and in better physical and emotional condition than controls. In addition, they consumed fewer narcotics and went home an average three days sooner. The authors of this study remind readers that this caring and reassuring approach required more tact and work (and therefore time) than the usual preoperative visit. When dental patients were given enthusiastic messages about the pain-reducing effects of a placebo prior to local anesthetic injection, they experienced less pain and less fear of the injection than others whose instruction was neutrally presented.[19] Another dental study compared postextraction pain in two groups of patients receiving placebos.[20] Only the doctors knew that the first group, but not the second, might also receive a narcotic. The first group had better pain relief. Clearly, a doctor's positive attitude facilitates a placebo effect.

D. M. Chaput de Saintonge and A. Herxheimer suggest some methods to harness the placebo effect by accompanying effective treatment with specific suggestion and encouragement.[21] Continuity of care, prompt consultation, history taking, examination, prescription writing, and calm, pleasant surroundings reassure patients. Such rituals derive from our primordial programming for healing[22] and encourage compliance that in turn improves outcome.[23] These features are especially applicable to the family doctor who, if equipped with the complete medical record, can guide and monitor her patient's progress through the complexities of modern health care.

These authors go on to caution against promoting perfect health as a realistic goal. A too optimistic approach can be harmful if a treatment goes badly. The patient is disappointed, loses confidence, and suffers nocebo effects. Nevertheless, confidence in the treatment is essential, as is the sense of control over the outcome. The authors remind us that surgical patients who are able to control their postoperative narcotics and women trained to participate actively in the conduct of their labor require less analgesia and have better outcomes than those whose treatments are determined solely by others.

Some patients benefit more than others from science. Thomas demonstrated that about a third of primary-care patients are temporarily dependent.[24] With no treatment other than contact with their doctor, they seldom return. When systematically followed up, most are either better or feel no need for further treatment. Scientific medicine contributes little here. The doctor's attitude and approach are important to most successful outcomes, even with structural disease. Advances in medical science should not retard the very skills that sustained medicine when science was lacking.

It is possible to practice evidence-based medicine, yet have a positive, comforting attitude toward patients, especially those beyond science's reach. The *biopsychosocial* model holds that disease is biological, psychological, and social in origin and that doctors must master all three to be effective.[25] A patient dying of cancer and the temporarily dependent patient reside at opposite ends of the illness spectrum. All patients require tact, empathy, and meaning for their symptoms. Mismanagement of these attributes can be costly. Suppose that the entire one-third of patients seen as temporarily dependent[26] were discontented with their care and sought help elsewhere. About that number resort to CAM.

Communication

The word *doctor* comes from the Latin word *docere*, meaning "to teach." Like teachers, doctors should be skilled in communication. Table 4-1 illustrates a failure of doctor/patient communication. Almost half of adults visiting their family doctor for benign bowel symptoms were worried that their symptoms might mean cancer, yet failed to mention this fear during their visit. We fail to mention our fears to doctors for many reasons: we fear the answer, we are too timid or too rushed, we dislike tests, or we suspect our worries will be belittled. Nowadays, few doctors will say, "It's all in your head," but body language, attitude, and clumsy communication can transmit the message all the same. A doctor's failure to anticipate her patient's fear of cancer in the face of a seemingly trivial complaint negates whatever other good things she may do. Medical successes against disease are headline news, as are warnings of cancer and the diets and nostrums to prevent it. It takes communication skills to undo the damage, calm fears, and temper expectations in a brief visit, yet we seem to value it less than technological skill. Negative tests have great power to reassure patients, but only if the doctor carefully explains the result and dissipates the fear (see figure 5-1).[27] She need not do the test herself to be the doctor. Communication is a doctor's stock in trade, and a responsibility she can neither delegate nor ignore.

The Art of Communication

> "Being able to diagnose correctly is a good test of medical competence. Being able to tell the patient what he or she has to know is a good test of medical artistry."
>
> NORMAN COUSINS

Norman Cousins was a journalist, editor, and author who suffered and overcame debilitating and life-threatening illnesses.[28] Previously concerned with the world's political and social ills, he became an advocate of "holistic" healing and spoke passionately of illness from a patient's perspective. As a communicator par excellence, he served on the faculty of the University of California at Los Angeles School of Medicine where he taught ethics and medical literature. His address to a commencement audience at George Washington University describes the physician as a communicator: "The wrong words can produce despair and defeat or impair the usefulness of whatever treatment is prescribed," and "Proper communication is one of the most difficult undertakings on earth."[29] He went on to cite some consequences of miscommunication. His most important point however, is that we humans are not all the same in how we receive and process information. Yet "[t]he way a patient receives a diagnosis can have a profound effect on the course of the disease." Just as reassurance is valuable to the patient with a benign disease who fears cancer, so malignant disease need not be presented as a death sentence. The art is to enlist the patient as an ally in the struggle to make the best of the circumstances. medical care requires time and patience, rare commodities in the world of increasing demand, economic constraint, encroaching regulation, and the ever-expanding behemoth known as scientific medicine.

The shift from physician paternalism to patient autonomy[30] has made urgent the study and encouragement of doctor/patient relationships. For example, at the beginning of four clinical trials for gastroesophageal-reflux treatments, the supervising doctors disagreed substantially with their 2,674 patients about the severity of reflux symptoms.[31] Poor communication is the obvious explanation. Moira Stewart systematically reviewed twenty-one studies of doctor/patient relationships and found that effective communication improved health outcomes.[32] She found that the patient's education aided the process, but so did the education of the physician. Poor communication is costly. It can result in adverse events, litigation, unnecessary testing, polytherapy, poor compliance, doctor shopping, frequent consultations, and wasteful emergency room visits. These costs are partly due to the lack of time for patients to talk to their doctor. We need to explore the proposition that better communication saves money.

Time

> "You can't see, touch, smell, or taste it, but we spend tens
> of millions of dollars on it every year. To many patients
> and physicians it is precious, maybe the most precious of
> all medical resources."
>
> FRANK DAVIDDOFF (1997)[33]

Time determines communication. Chen-Tan Lin and colleagues reviewed the time spent by patients with primary-care physicians.[34] Ambulatory visits to family doctors averaged 9 to 18 minutes in the United States and only 5 to 10 minutes in Europe. In Great Britain general practitioners allot 5 to 7 minutes to each patient,[35] and the range in one practice was 0.7 to 29.9 minutes.[36] Over the past twenty years, Canadian doctors have spent steadily decreasing time in direct patient care (excluding administration, phone calls, etc.).[37] For internists providing primary care in the United States, new patient visits declined from 29 to 17 minutes between 1980 and 1996, and follow-up visits from 19 to 16 minutes. Data from two national databases found visits to all doctors increased slightly from 20.4 and 16.3 minutes in 1989 to 21.5 and 18.3 minutes in 1998, but how much of this increase was due to administrative work and more complicated illness was not determined.[38] In contrast, homeopaths are reported to spend 30 minutes with their patients.[39] Many wonder if the pressure on doctors within prepaid systems drives patients to seek (and pay for) more leisurely visits to CAM practitioners.[40]

Lin reported that patients' satisfaction was less if the time allocated with the doctor failed to meet their expectations. Brief encounters challenge the doctor's ability to communicate. In five-minute consultations, compared to ten minutes, British general practitioners identified fewer patient concerns, less often recorded the blood pressure, and left their patients less satisfied.[41] The shorter consultation provided less time to explain the patient's problem, propose management, and practice disease preventation.[42] Moreover, shorter visits result in more prescriptions.[43] A Scottish study found that when doctors spent more than nine minutes with their patients who were complaining of an acute respiratory disorder, they prescribed fewer antibiotics than those spending less than six minutes and more likely dealt with psychosocial problems.[44] The same authors subsequently recorded time spent and other data at more than twenty thousand visits to eighty-five GPs.[45] Longer consultations permitted more recognition of psychosocial and long-term problems and more health promotion. As expected, patients were more satisfied with longer consultations.

An example of the importance of good communication is a thirty-two-year follow-up of local patients diagnosed with irritable bowel syndrome at the Mayo Clinic between 1961 and 1963. Notation on the original record of a psychosocial history, precipitating factors, and discussion of diagnosis and treatment were considered evidence of a good doctor/patient interaction and were associated with fewer return visits for bowel complaints. Such interaction requires time, but it is well spent if it saves future consultations for this benign but incurable condition.[46] A system where large patient workloads and increasing administrative duties force ever briefer doctor visits is false economy.[47] If the patient's concerns are neglected, subsequent visits, mistakes, referrals, or CAM treatments will likely result so that any savings are illusory.

Empathy

The above paragraphs make the need for empathy self-evident. Without it, the doctor's demeanor, attitude, and communication skills are stillborn. "The secret of the care of the patient is caring for the patient."[48] While doctors, nurses, and other healers need not suffer with their patients, they can transmit their concern, understanding, and desire to help. The art is to achieve a balance between aeqanimitas and concern for the patient's plight.

THE DOCTOR AND THE PLACEBO EFFECT

Medicine has a foundation in science, yet managing illness is an art. Twenty-first-century medicine is increasingly evidence based, so that in certain circumstances we know what a group of patients' outcomes will be. Yet an individual's outcome is always uncertain. Medicine is not accounting. Even if it were possible to computerize all medical knowledge and feed the machine all an ill person's signs, symptoms, and laboratory data, we could not expect to assemble a perfect management plan. Not only is uncertainty part of every person's future, but his personality, emotional health, societal circumstances, and other less tangible attributes temper a treatment's success. Only an empathetic professional, skilled in science, interpersonal relationships, and communication can weigh all the attributes of a person and his disease, estimate the outcome probabilities, and guide him to the best decisions. Whatever the disease, a good doctor/patient relationship is essential to an optimal result.

What factors foster or hinder this relationship? We will explore these presently, but a few comments are warranted here. Much depends upon the person who wishes to be a doctor. Selection to medical school is a competitive and flawed process. The students are young and there are too few tools to help predict their future behavior. Not only should medical educators foster their students' attitudes and communication skills, but they also must be prepared to guide the insensitive to other occupations. Professional organizations can do more to foster the art as well as the science of medicine. Licensing authorities and health-care organizations can support, rather than complicate, the doctor/patient relationship. The public can help by articulating their need for more time with their doctors. Brody argues that healing power should be vested in primary care from which specialized care is delegated.[49] I will argue, too, that the family doctor should be in overall command and equipped with the necessary resources and time for her to restore the doctor/patient relationship. There will be costs, to be sure, but also savings, and medicare will rid itself of much grief.

Doctors, too, are human. They can be as frustrated, frightened, and intimidated as their patients. Too many react to the stress of their practices with alcohol, drugs, or suicide. Marital discord is common, especially when the demands of medicine conflict with a spouse's own career aspirations. An unhappy doctor is unlikely to be an empathetic one. One whose narrow professional life denies living life itself can contribute little to the doctor/patient relationship and is unlikely to have a satisfactory placebo effect. (In part 3, we will consider more closely the institutional and professional impediments to positive doctor/patient relationships and evidence-based medicine.)

CONCLUSIONS

The healer is the most important element in the placebo effect. Regrettably, as the powers of science-based medicine expand, the demands of technology and administrative restrictions reduce doctors' contact with patients, which weakens the doctor/patient relationship. Even as medical matters become more complex, physicians spend less time communicating with patients. A doctor's ability to make most patients feel better may owe less to her mastery of disease than her ability to deal with the uncertainty and fear surrounding unexplained symptoms. Her appearance and demeanor, the attitude and life experience she brings to the encounter, and the empathy and clarity with which she teaches her patient what he needs to know about his illness contribute to the success of the doctor/patient relationship. These take time—time to learn and time to give. The doctor may not be the placebo, but she is crucial to the delivery of the placebo effect.

CHAPTER 13

THE PLACEBO RESPONDER

I n clinical trials, the number of patients apparently responding to placebo medication, sham surgery, or a switched-off device can be as high as 80 percent. The implications of such data depend upon the observer's point of view. If he is a clinical researcher striving to prove the efficacy of a treatment, he might claim the placebo response is too high. He might even seek ways of minimizing the placebo response in future trials. Others might see this phenomenon as an important component of treatment and seek ways to identify and encourage placebo responses. Here, we shall review the components of the placebo response, attempt to characterize the placebo responder, and explore the determinants and predictability of true placebo effects.

THE PATIENT AND THE DISEASE
(COMPONENTS OF THE PLACEBO RESPONSE)

Natural History

Voltaire characterized a good physician as one who amused his patients until they recovered. In 1800 the German physician Franz Joseph Gall asked, "What is Nature's share and what is Medicine's in the healing of disease?"[1] As noted earlier, Haygarth, in the same year, found that applying wooden rods improved four out of five rheumatic patients. These insights reflect the healer's instinct that if left alone, most ailments will improve. It follows that any treatment will look good if delivered at the right time. However, the natural histories of chronic diseases are poorly recorded. In clinical trials, other factors are in play. In a review of several meta-analyses and trials of painful conditions, Ernst and Resch distinguished the "true placebo effect" from those due to the passage of time.[2] We need to look again at the response of participants to a treatment in a clinical trial (or in real life), expressed in the therapeutic equation first presented in chapter 1:

Treatment benefit = Therapeutic gain + Natural history of
illness + Placebo effect

In some trials, the natural history of the disease accounts for much of a patient's improvement. In the case of a cold, improvement occurs in two to ten days. Therefore, in an uncontrolled environment, any cold remedy inevitably looks good. The trick is to show that an intervention can shorten or lessen the cold's effects. In contrast, patients with terminal cancer have a steadily deteriorating course. While the symptoms can vary a little, the natural history is for them to worsen, so that improvement in a cancer treatment trial will have to overcome the disease's natural history. Different again are most chronic diseases that follow a fluctuating course, with subjective symptoms that naturally tend to improve. Examples include chronic back pain, fatigue, headache, allergies, insomnia, asthma, irritable bowel syndrome, depression, and anxiety.[3] People with these chronic, relapsing conditions are most likely to improve during placebo treatment. Thus, any consideration of the responses of trial subjects to treatment or placebo must consider the natural history of the disease under study.

Other Time Factors

Other changes may occur over the course of a clinical trial (and during a real life treatment period).[4] Many observers include these with natural history, but there are subtle differences. One such phenomenon is *regression to the mean*.[5] In fluctuating disorders such as headaches or constipation, symptoms vary within individuals. Symptoms must be active when subjects enter a clinical trial (or visit their doctor). Otherwise, there would be no point in participating in the trial (or undergoing treatment). Due to the unpredictable nature of headaches, some of the participants will improve naturally (regress to the mean of all those who get headaches) during the treatment period. If we included every person with periodic headaches in a clinical trial, the outcome in the placebo group might then more truly reflect the natural history of headaches (ignoring the placebo effect), but those becoming symptomatic (also regressing toward the mean) would obscure the improvement in those initially symptomatic. Only if the object of the trial were to show that the test treatment *prevents* symptoms from occurring might asymptomatic patients appropriately be entered.

Many things happen when a person gets treatment for, say, constipation. A trial subject (or clinic patient) may alter his diet, get more exercise, amend faulty toilet habits, and so on. Such *parallel interventions* may cause improvement that is due to neither placebo nor natural history. Good trial designers try to minimize this, but in real life, such healthy interventions should be encouraged.

Independent of the test treatment, *environmental changes* might occur during the course of the study that cause measurements to shift between start and endpoint. For example, hay fever and asthma vary in severity according to the season. Changes in personnel or the skill of those making the measurements can alter the apparent baseline. Skill at taking blood pressure improves with experience. We have mentioned "white coat hypertension," where the recordings are higher when initially measured by the doctor. Thus, blood pressure may appear to improve as subjects and investigators become accustomed to each other and to trial conditions.

True Placebo Effect

From the foregoing, it is clear that the true placebo effect accounts for only part of a placebo responder's improvement.[6] To determine the true placebo effect under clinical conditions, we must consider the following equation:

True placebo effect = the change in the outcome measure of subjects
taking a placebo (placebo response),
less the effect of the natural history of the
disease beingtreated,
less the regression to the mean,
less the effect of parallel interventions,
less environmental changes affecting
measurements during the trial.

A physician who knows a disease's natural history and other time-related influences can use the information to estimate prognosis, and instruct and encourage her patient. Moreover, a favorable prognosis can augment the true placebo effect.

Many claim that if we were able to collect the trial data on all the placebo responders with a certain disease, we would know that disease's natural history. Regrettably, this is untrue, as trial conditions are not natural. The symptomatic patients in the trial may not represent all persons with the disease. Regression to the mean, parallel interventions, and shifting baselines confound the data. Subjects are enrolled, processed, given "treatment," and carefully monitored—activities that encourage true placebo effects. Thus, mere participation in a clinical trial can alter the course of an illness.

CHARACTERISTICS OF A "PLACEBO RESPONDER"

In his 1955 review of *The Powerful Placebo*, Beecher was unable to identify characteristics of trial subjects that responded to a placebo,[7] and fifty years later we are little further ahead. A 1954 trial compared postoperative pain relief with morphine and saline (placebo) injections.[8] Responders to the saline injections resembled nonresponders in gender, age, and intelligence. Under blinded circumstances, half the individuals responded sometimes to the placebo and other times did not.

A. K. Shapiro and E. Shapiro studied the placebo effect over many years.[9] This husband-and-wife team attempted to characterize placebo responders by retrospectively examining published data. They were unsuccessful because trial methodologies and recorded characteristics differed from trial to trial. In the 1970s they performed a "placebo test" on 352 subjects with anxiety, 272 with depression, and 129 with both. First, the subjects completed a questionnaire about their symptoms, mood, and attitudes. On the second visit, they rated their symptoms before and after ingesting an inert green capsule with a glass of water, and then guessed whether they had received a drug or placebo. Patients who preferred to be treated by drugs and psychotherapy, as well as those who preferred to leave the decision to the doctor, were most likely to have a placebo effect. The Shapiros concluded that great distress due to symptoms, a favorable attitude toward the doctor, and meeting the patient's expectations that the treatment is relevant to his symptoms are essential to placebo success. (Surprisingly, a positive attitude of the physician toward the patient failed to have an effect in these studies. It seems from these data that for placebo success, the patient must like the doctor, but the doctor need not reciprocate. I suspect this is untrue.)

In an antidepressant trial, control patients had placebo responses associated with short-term, moderate-severity depression, an identified precipitating event, and a good response to previous antidepressants.[10] A later study found contradictory results.[11] C. G. Moertel and his colleagues studied the 112 cancer patients whose pain improved on placebo in a trial of analgesics.[12] They found educated people, farmers, professionals, working women, and singles to be more likely to respond to the placebo. Those less likely to respond were the uneducated, housewives, childless women, and smokers. These authors concluded that normally self-sufficient people unaccustomed to dependency were particularly vulnerable to placebo, while the remainder were already dependent on others.

If we believe that the benefits of alternative medicine are placebo effects (not forgetting natural history and other time factors), then we may learn from the characteristics of those who choose CAM treatments. We know from chapter 11 that those using CAM are white, educated, middle-class people between twenty-five and fifty years of age. Perhaps only they were able to pay for it! Compared to non-CAM users, they subscribe to a holistic health vision and report some transformational experience that changes the way they view the world. They also report poor health status, leading J. A. Astin to suspect that either medicine had failed them or that many were somatizers (those with a propensity to experience and report somatic [bodily] symptoms that have no pathophysiological explanation).[13] Chronic pain and back problems were the commonest complaints for which people sought CAM. Using CAM as a surrogate, placebo responders might be characterized as better educated, embracing CAM cultural beliefs and philosophies, able to afford CAM, subject to anxiety, and suffering chronic painful complaints, sometimes several.

No consistent image of the placebo responder emerges from these and other studies. Nevertheless, the data contradict the popular view that educated, intelligent, imaginative, and self-reliant people are immune to placebo effects. There are reasons why placebo responders' characteristics are so obscure. First, it is possible that no special characteristics exist. Second, diseases vary greatly in subjectivity and prognosis. Third, subjects may improve while taking a placebo because of the effects of time. The fourth and most likely explanation for the unpredictability of placebo effects is that we are all potential placebo responders, and that our changing circumstances determine when we are individually susceptible.

DETERMINANTS OF AN INDIVIDUAL'S PLACEBO RESPONSE

While a placebo responder's character and personality cannot be defined, it appears that circumstances surrounding the treatment can influence placebo responses in a trial situation. The Shapiros concluded that great symptom distress, a favorable attitude to the doctor, and meeting patients' expectations are important to placebo success.[14] C. G. Moertel would add that the normally self-sufficient individual who is rendered suddenly dependent by illness is susceptible.[15] In a dental study, the use of a placebo pill prior to local anesthesia injection reduced the injection pain, lessened anxiety, and reduced fear of subsequent injections. These effects were associated with the enthusiasm, faith, attitudes, and expectations that accompanied the giving of the placebo pill.[16] The authors conclude that the quality of the information the patients received with their placebo pill determines the placebo effects.

The patient's expectations of a treatment are also important. If you expect to get well, you are more likely to do so. However, unreasonable expectations may be counterproductive. We saw earlier that success with acupuncture is best if expectations are modest, so that modest improvement will not be disappointing.[17]

We discussed the significance of the doctor's demeanor, attitude, and behavior in the generation of placebo effects. Symbols of the doctor's accomplishments and healing power can also contribute. We have noted that the color of pills could alter treatment responses, and it appears that branding accounts for a third of branded aspirin's therapeutic effect.[18] Surroundings, appearances, and healing associations augment treatment and placebo effects. Satisfaction is greatest if the doctor examines the patient, provides the relevant information, and listens carefully. These virtues depend on the time allotted to the visit.[19] In a systematic review of thirty-eight treatment trials for ulcerative colitis, Alexandra Ilnyckyi and her colleagues determined the rates of remission and benefit in the patients who received placebo (see table 13-1).[20] These data show that the placebo improved endoscopic and microscopic appearances of the colon as well as symptoms. The more follow-up visits there were, the greater the placebo effect. This makes sense. Patient satisfaction and treatment adherence are best when the patient perceives that he is allotted sufficient time.[21]

TABLE 13-1
Placebo Responses* in Ulcerative Colitis[22]

Endpoint	Percent Well	Percent Benefited
Clinical (symptoms)	16	35
Endoscopic (appearance of the colon)	11	20
Histological (microscopic appearance of the colon)	8	14

*Placebo responses include placebo effects plus those due to natural history, regression to the mean, parallel interventions, and shifting baseline.

Adherence (Compliance)

The manner and quality of treatment information has other effects. Adherence is the extent to which a person's behavior coincides with medical advice.[23] During a placebo-controlled trial of lipid-lowering drugs after a myocardial infarction (heart attack),[24] the five-year mortality was the same for men taking the drug as those taking placebo— a negative trial. Using pill counts, investigators found that those taking the lipid-lowering drug at least 80 percent of the time (adherers), had a five-year mortality of 15 percent compared to 25 percent in nonadherers. We normally would expect this improvement. However, among the placebo group, adherers also had an advantage, with a mortality of 15 percent against 28 percent for nonadherers. Another trial compared the mortality after myocardial infarction in those taking a drug called propanolol versus those on placebo.[25] In both groups of patients, adherers had much better outcomes than did nonadherers. Poorer outcomes after noncompliance with placebo in these and other examples cannot be explained by associations with disease severity, psychological traits, or high-risk health behaviors such as smoking.[26] It seems that adherers do better than nonadherers do, even if the treatment is a placebo.

The reasons cited for lack of adherence to treatment include fear of drug side effects, forgetfulness, and low expectation that the treatment will help. Since adherence estimated through self-report and pill counts is unreliable, some trial managers install electronic monitors in the pill dispensers. Right out of the "Ministry of Truth," these devices spy on subjects' pill taking, reporting "pill dumping," or "catch-up" in the days before clinic visits. A now-abandoned maneuver was to monitor adherence during a run-in period and drop nonadherers from the trial. This is unrealistic, since the resulting study population would not be "generalizable," and in the trial nonadherence occurs anyway. Nonadherence to placebo likely indicates unknown characteristics (perhaps including lack of placebo responsiveness) that cause poorer outcomes and is probably greater in practice than in trials. It is a fact of the practicing physician's life and underscores her responsibility to explain the treatment properly.

Why Do Some Patients Seek CAM?

Astin surveyed a random sample of Americans and found that 40 percent used some form of CAM in the previous year.[27] Over 95 percent of these also saw doctors. A few said they used CAM because it made them feel better, rather than because they were dissatisfied with doctors. Therefore, it appears that CAM supplements rather than displaces many patients' medical care. In the United States, Medicare and other medical plans insure only some CAM. It is ironic that in Canada, where medicare insures every citizen for conventional medicine, citizens will pay to supplement or replace this free benefit with CAM. Payment implies a contract, a commitment on the part of both practitioner and patient to the success of the encounter. Could it be that such a contract or that paying for a health-care service amplifies the benefit? We know too little about this possibility.

ONCE A PLACEBO RESPONDER . . .

A half century ago, some doctors often gave placebos to difficult patients or suspected malingerers as a test of the validity of their complaints. An example was a person, usually a young woman, presenting with hysterical paralysis of a limb. A saline injection often "cured" such a person, thereby ruling out serious brain disease. Sometimes young doctors or nurses gave placebos for obscure pain,[28] and if it vanished, concluded that the patient was faking. This was a false conclusion. Pain trials have high placebo responses whatever the source of the pain. Using the placebo response as a diagnostic test can obscure an important disease. Now, such tests are considered unethical.

In 1973 Stewart Wolf gave an emetic drug (ipecac) to twenty-three young healthy subjects on two occasions.[29] On each occasion, all were nauseated and most vomited. On seven subsequent occasions, a placebo preceded the ipecac and often lessened or prevented the nausea and vomiting. All subjects had this placebo response at least once, but based on several exposures it proved impossible to predict who would respond in the later placebo/ipecac treatments. Wolf did not explain how he found twenty-three young people repeatedly willing to ingest this disgusting drug, but he did demonstrate that they all were sometimes susceptible to placebo effects.

Because responses to placebo in clinical trials are so high, there have been attempts to reduce it. A two-week period of placebo therapy prior to a trial was meant to identify and eliminate placebo responders. However, some nonresponders become responders in the subsequent trial. Randomized clinical trials of selective serotonin reuptake inhibitors (SSRIs) that excluded patients who responded to placebo in a two-week run-in period were compared to those that did not employ the run-in technique.[30] No difference in therapeutic effect was observed. In the ipecac study mentioned above, subjects responded to placebo on some occasions and not on others. While there are few longitudinal data of placebo responsiveness in individuals, the data presented here suggest that it varies from time to time and from situation to situation. It is also likely that no one is immune. Is it not likely that at a vulnerable moment, anyone with a worrying symptom who consults a caring physician can have benefits that go beyond practical treatment? We are all "temporarily dependent" occasionally, and so are all potential placebo responders. The notion that only some of us have such a "weakness" is absurd.

CONCLUSIONS

Research has failed to identify the characteristics of a placebo responder, perhaps because from time to time everyone can be one. Moreover, in individuals it is difficult to separate changes associated with a true placebo effect from those due to natural history, regression toward the mean, parallel interventions, and a shifting baseline. The nature of the illness determines the likelihood of a placebo response. Chronic, painful, and benign disorders that have no pathology are most likely to respond to sham therapy. Colds get better anyway, and terminal cancer is least susceptible to improvement on placebo. Attributes that seem to encourage a placebo response include communication, patient expectations, enthusiasm for the therapy, and sufficient time for the doctor to talk to the patient. However, predicting a placebo response is unreliable, and it seems that the same person may react differently to the same placebo on different occasions. Understanding why this is so should help doctors learn how to optimize their treatments. Insufficient time to encourage their patients hampers physicians' treatment of chronic disorders and encourages people to look beyond their health-care system for healing relationships.

CHAPTER 14

THE ETHICS OF USING PLACEBOS

"[A]s the terms of reference change to efficiency and management, there has been more than a noticeable lack of
concern with medicine as a humane institution and with
the motivations and ethics that govern its endeavors."

DAVID MECHANIC (1975)[1]

The use of inert pills or sham treatment at any time is fraught
with ethical and philosophical considerations, and in clinical
practice it is seldom, if ever, justified. Nevertheless, without the use of
placebos as controls in clinical trials, evidence-based medicine would
be severely limited. Our medical predecessors understood a placebo
to be an inert pill, liquid, injection, or sham treatment that might
make the patient feel better without doing harm. Now, a placebo is
more commonly understood to be an inactive substance, treatment,
diet, or sham procedure used to control for placebo and time effects
during clinical trials. Here, we shall consider the ethics of using
placebos in clinical trials and then their possible use in practice.

THE ETHICS OF USING
PLACEBOS IN CLINICAL TRIALS

When Are Placebos Justified?

Anecdote, case series, clinical impression, and other uncontrolled data
usually provide little information about a treatment's effectiveness.
The use of placebo-controlled, randomized, double-blind clinical
trials over the last half century has laid most of the foundation of evidence-based medicine. However, is a placebo control always justified
in clinical trials? The answer is not an easy one.

When randomized clinical trials were pioneered in the 1940s and 1950s, little thought was given to the ethics of using placebos as controls. Up to then, there were few proven treatments and their benefits were so obvious that no trial was necessary. During World War II, the solution to several medical problems was deemed essential to the war effort.[2] This involved trials of drugs to prevent dysentery, malaria, and influenza—diseases that could disable large numbers of troops. Supervised by the Committee on Medical Research set up by President Franklin D. Roosevelt, government-funded investigators conducted medical research on orphans, mentally incompetent people, and prisoners. Many felt these trials were justified as part of the war effort. The end justified the means. After the war, the success of wartime research, and the profound benefits of the miracle drug penicillin prompted the United States Congress to generously fund the National Institutes of Health. This led to a productive expansion of medical research, mainly at universities and veterans' hospitals, but also at the NIH itself. David Rothman claims that wartime philosophy and ethics carried over to the postwar period, a time of rapid progress in evidence-based medicine.[3]

In reaction to the atrocious Nazi medical experiments before and during World War II, the 1949 ten-article Nuremberg Code was drafted.[4] This document set out the rules for human experimentation, emphasizing human rights and the principles of informed and voluntary consent. Since randomized trial technology was in its infancy, the code made no mention of placebo controls. However, two transatlantic randomized trial pioneers, A. Bradford Hill[5] and H. K. Beecher[6] began to discuss when it was necessary and proper to use placebos. In 1963 Hill, designer of the innovative British streptomycin trial, declared that if there was an available "orthodox" treatment, the question of placebo control "will not arise, for the doctor will wish to know whether a new treatment is more, or less, effective than the old, not that it was more effective than nothing." "Orthodox" was a euphemism for anecdotally accepted treatments, and, of course, we now know that placebo treatment is not "nothing." On the other side of the Atlantic, Beecher cited twenty-two egregious examples of unethical trials, urging that there be clinical trial guidelines.[7] In one example, despite knowledge that penicillin prevented poststreptococcal rheumatic fever, five hundred patients with streptococcal throat infections were randomized to sulfadiazine or to "no treatment." In each group, about 5 percent suffered rheumatic fever, a serious disease that often leaves a damaged heart. To have placed these subjects at such risk by withholding penicillin was unethical. In another study, investigators infected mentally defective children in an institution in order to follow the course of hepatitis. In a 1971 study after Beecher's article, seventy-six Mexican American women seeking contraceptives were randomized to hormone pills or placebo.[8] Neither they nor their physicians were informed. Seven in the placebo group became unwillingly pregnant and were offered no compensation. Such studies would be forbidden today.

In response to such concerns, the World Medical Association in 1964 expanded on the Nuremberg Code by drafting the Declaration of Helsinki.[9] This document has had five subsequent revisions. Earlier versions said little about placebos. The declaration seemed to forbid their use by specifying that in any medical study subjects, including those in a control group, "should be assured of the best proven diagnostic and therapeutic methods."[10] After Beecher's 1966 editorial, the NIH and particularly the Food and Drug Administration made informed consent of competent individuals a requirement for participation in clinical trials. These initiatives mandated an explanation to prospective trial subjects that they might be treated with a placebo and what the implications of that would be.

In 1994 K. J. Rothman and K. M. Michels wrote uncompromisingly that if an effective treatment exists for a disease, then a new drug must be compared to it, rather than a placebo.[11] In this case, an effective treatment must have been proven so by a prior placebo-controlled trial. Nonetheless, others have found Helsinki's and Rothman and Michel's views too restrictive. R. Temple and S. S. Ellenberg argue that in a clinical trial the equivalence of a test drug with an existing "effective" drug does not prove the test drug's efficacy if: the comparator is not consistently effective in all populations; its benefit is marginal; or the disease studied is fluctuating in course.[12] Statistically, equivalence is more difficult to prove than difference, and it requires many more patients to avoid a type II statistical error. All agree that if the patient would suffer because of withheld treatment, especially in the case of a fatal disease, then the best effective treatment should be the control, even if its benefit is marginal. In addition, all agree that if there is no effective treatment, placebo control is necessary to establish a new treatment's efficacy. What they disagree about is the grey area in between. E. J. Emanuel and F. G. Miller seek a middle ground that permits placebo controlled studies even if effective treatment exists, but only when there are convincing methodological reasons for their use and patients would not be harmed if existing treatment were withheld.[13] If investigators do choose to use a comparator drug, the comparison must be fair. The dose, duration of treatment, and other conditions that prevailed when the comparator drug was shown to be effective should be recreated in any new trial.[14]

The 2000 version of the Helsinki Declaration addresses this issue in article 29 (see table 14-1). This document was severely criticized by members of the Department of Bioethics at the National Institutes of Health[14] for its contradictions, poor wording, and lack of precision about the use of placebo controls. In particular, the best current treatment in some populations may be unavailable, or inappropriate in others. The Food and Drug Administration has not accepted these new regulations, despite the World Medical Association's claim that the Declaration of Helsinki has priority over national regulations. In recognition of the controversy, the World Medical Association added the following footnote to article 29 in 2002:

> The WMA hereby reaffirms its position that extreme care must be taken in making use of a placebo-controlled trial and that in general this methodology should only be used in the absence of existing proven therapy. However, a placebo-controlled trial may be ethically acceptable, even if proven therapy is available, under the following circumstances:
>
> —Where for compelling and scientifically sound methodological reasons its use is necessary to determine the efficacy or safety of a prophylactic, diagnostic or therapeutic method; or
>
> —Where a prophylactic, diagnostic or therapeutic method is being investigated for a minor condition and the patients who receive placebo will not be subject to any additional risk of serious or irreversible harm.
>
> All other provisions of the Declaration of Helsinki must be adhered to, especially the need for appropriate ethical and scientific review.

The Helsinki declaration and its national counterparts are works in progress and the last word on the ethical use of placebos in clinical trials is yet to come.

Informed Consent

Informed consent is another important theme of the Declaration of Helsinki (see articles 22–26, table 14-1). But these articles say nothing about informing subjects about placebos. Nevertheless, investigators must inform potential subjects that they may receive a sham treatment as a control for a new treatment to be tested and that they will not know the truth until the end of the trial. In chapter 7, we suggested that there were several advantages of entering a clinical trial, even if the participant received the placebo. Nevertheless, investigators and review committees must ensure that the risk of placebo therapy is minimal and that participants are truly informed.

TABLE 14-1
Declaration of Helsinki 2000
Articles 22–26 and 29: Regarding Informed Consent and Placebos

22. In any research on human beings, each potential subject must be adequately informed of the aims, methods, sources of funding, any possible conflicts of interest, institutional affiliations of the researcher, the anticipated benefits and potential risks of the study and the discomfort it may entail. The subject should be informed of the right to abstain from participation in the study or to withdraw consent to participate at any time without reprisal. After ensuring that the subject has understood the information, the physician should then obtain the subject's freely-given informed consent, preferably in writing. If the consent cannot be obtained in writing, the non-written consent must be formally documented and witnessed.

23. When obtaining informed consent for the research project the physician should be particularly cautious if the subject is in a dependent relationship with the physician or may consent under duress. In that case the informed consent should be obtained by a well-informed physician who is not engaged in the investigation and who is completely independent of this relationship.

24. For a research subject who is legally incompetent, physically or mentally incapable of giving consent or is a legally incompetent minor, the investigator must obtain informed consent from the legally authorized representative in accordance with applicable law. These groups should not be included in research unless the research is necessary to promote the health of the population represented and this research cannot instead be performed on legally competent persons.

25. When a subject deemed legally incompetent, such as a minor child, is able to give assent to decisions about participation in research, the investigator must obtain that assent in addition to the consent of the legally authorized representative.

26. Research on individuals from whom it is not possible to obtain consent, including proxy or advance consent, should be done only if the physical/mental condition that prevents obtaining informed consent is a necessary characteristic of the research population. The specific reasons for involving research subjects with a condition that renders them unable to give informed consent should be stated in the experimental protocol for consideration and approval of the review committee. The protocol should state that consent to remain in the research should be obtained as soon as possible from the individual or a legally authorized surrogate.

29. The benefits, risks, burdens and effectiveness of a new method should be tested against those of the best current prophylactic, diagnostic, and therapeutic methods. This does not exclude the use of placebo, or no treatment, in studies where no proven prophylactic, diagnostic or therapeutic method exists.

Physicians should explain the proposed trial to participants in plain, nontechnical language and in a manner that suits their understanding. Although one should strive to make each participant understand, one cannot guarantee that he will fully comprehend the information. G. Screenivasan points out that a participant's comprehension would be difficult to ascertain, and it places all the responsibility for the comprehension on the physician, a notion ironically contrary to that of patient autonomy.[16]

Conflict of Interest

The task of recruiting subjects for clinical trials usually falls to physicians. However, a doctor's primary duty is to her patient. A secondary responsibility to further medical science rests uncomfortably beside that primary duty. In asking a patient to enter a trial, she is also asking him to suspend individualized care for its duration.[17] Explaining randomization is difficult enough, but reconciling the notion of placebo treatment to a patient's overall care can be even more difficult. Entering a trial for headaches demands little treatment sacrifice for most patients. However, if the disease is more serious, consent may imply frank discussion of negative issues such as prognosis and current "lack of effective treatment." A patient may prefer not to know this, and frank discussion may undermine the hope and optimism that the doctor has carefully cultivated. Thus, doctors may agree to participate in trials but balk at entering any patients.

This reticence has led to the appearance of for-profit contract research organizations (CROs) in patient-care clinics. Some of these set up clinics to participate in clinical trials. Others pay doctors finder's fees to persuade patients to enter trials, or in some cases, they pay the subjects themselves. Not only do these practices risk conflicts of interest and selection biases, but they risk the recruitment of unsuitable and ungeneralizable subjects that can undermine the study's validity. These problems can only exacerbate with the increasing demands to validate treatments through large clinical trials.

Ethical review committees, also recommended by Helsinki and required by organizations such as the NIH, are essential for institutions where clinical research occurs. Among their duties are the detection of conflicts of interest, and assurance of full disclosure and patient safety.

Clinical Trials as Duty?

Against these difficulties, one should imagine modern medicine without randomized clinical trials. While enlightened thinking and basic science would have likely rid us of the most outrageous treatments like venesection, we would have learned little about the placebo response, and much useless medicine would remain on formularies. Prescription drugs produced by a wealthy pharmaceutical industry would flood the market, unrestricted by the need to show efficacy. Approval would be based solely upon the drug's effect in animals or the results of uncontrolled physiological experiments on humans. We would know little of the possibly harmful effects of combination hormone replacement therapy or the benefits of antihypertensive medication. Medical-plan managers would have no means of determining which drugs to insure. As a result, medication would proliferate on theoretical grounds and marketing prowess. Surgeons would still believe that internal mammary artery ligation relieved angina pectoris or that a lavaged knee benefited osteoarthritis. In short, we would have no tool to evaluate the usefulness of any treatment or diagnostic test. Given that we do have the means to prove efficacy and safety for many treatments, is it ethical to permit public funds to support useless and possibly harmful ones?

There is much yet to do. Many prescription drugs are "grandfathered" from a previous era. Over-the-counter drugs and CAM therapies are largely untested. Much of surgery and psychiatry remains based on tradition, theory, and anecdote. We need improved trial methods and a more systematic approach. We must have a repository of clinical trials that maintains data in the public domain. As citizens, patients, health-care workers, and managers, we all have a duty to understand the placebo effect and promote evidence-based medicine.

Publication

Article 27 of the Helsinki Declaration states, "Negative as well as positive results should be published or be otherwise publicly available." Chapter 7 includes a discussion of the many reasons why trial data go unpublished and the resulting risks of publication bias. Some pharmaceutical firms have been known to suppress data that is unfavorable to their product.[18] Even regulatory authorities keep pharmaceutical company data confidential.[19] Scientific reasons aside, participants enter a trial partly on the strength of their doctors' persuasion that the results would improve medical treatment. Even if the trial fails to meet the investigator's expectations, its methods and data should be in the public domain—a subject we return to in part 3. If the trial was flawed, the information can help future trial design. If there were unwanted effects in the trial, that surely should be known. Failure to ensure that data resulting from volunteer participants' efforts are published is a breach of trust.

THE ETHICS OF USING PLACEBOS IN CLINICAL PRACTICE

Several authors have credited Harvard professor Robert Cabot as the first to ponder the probity of placebos in practice. In 1909 he admitted, "I used to give them by the bushels."[20] When a patient caught him substituting water for morphine, he realized that placebos worked only if he deceived his patients. He believed that deception harmed the doctor/patient relationship and could bring the profession into disrepute. He advocated avoiding "falsehoods, lies and deception," recommending the truth, even if it requires more time. "Placebo giving is quackery," he declared. His epiphany seems a little quaint a century later, yet it long anticipated the realization of the placebo effect through placebo-controlled trials and demonstrated an appreciation of the doctor/patient relationship. As recently as 1974, writers were decrying the prescribing of sugar pills for the deception and the mistrust they engendered.[21] Few physicians would knowingly give a fake treatment today. Still fewer recent medical graduates would recognize or sympathize with the original paternalistic use of a sham treatment "to please the patient."

However, as discussed in chapter 1, there are at least three categories of placebo use. The first is the deliberate dispensing of a fake treatment. Most contemporary doctors would eschew such a practice and regard it as the province of charlatans. Nevertheless, 60 percent of eighty-nine Israeli specialists, family doctors, and head nurses used placebos in this way.[22] Among users, most prescribed a placebo as often as once a month or more and told patients they were receiving actual medication. Almost all reported that they found placebos generally or occasionally effective.

The second category is the dispensing of a drug that either has no proven effect on the condition being treated or is used in insufficient dose to have any pharmacological effect. However harmless the proffered drug might be, or however its use is rationalized, the practice is still paternalistic, deceptive, and not in the patient's best interests. There is great pressure for physicians to prescribe. Patients expect a treatment and may even have heard of a certain drug in the media. Reaching for the prescription pad is a time-honored method of terminating the visit. Even Cabot admitted that talking to the patient and explaining that no medicine is needed takes more time, and that was a century ago! Time or lack of it affects our health in many ways.

A third category of placebo use occurs when neither healer nor patient knows the treatment is useless. Doubtless, many patients benefit through a placebo effect. But such double deception can be harmful if it perpetuates dangerous therapies or employs expensive treatments to no avail. This is not charlatanism as the deception is due to ignorance and is unintentional. Such unconscious employment of placebos is more common than healers would like to admit. In orthodox medicine, examples include the use of antihistamines for an established asthma attack or vitamin B_{12} for tiredness. Many CAM practices appear to fit this third category.

Many critics have discussed how using placebos might undermine trust. In one parable, a physician orders a saline injection for a hypochondriacal patient.[23] The nurse caring for the patient gives the injection with an actual or implied lie. Whatever the patient's reaction, the nurse must continue to care for him, live with the lie, and feel guilt. She loses respect for the doctor and his authority is undermined. When the patient or others learn of the deception, medicine itself is undermined. The deliberate use of an ineffective drug or an insufficient dose of a drug is less obviously a fake but ethically just as troublesome.

All three types of placebo administration exploit the placebo effect, and all defy the precepts of evidence-based medicine and trusting doctor/patient relationships. While we cannot and should not limit patient choice of treatment, we can be scrupulous about what treatments are worthy of medical authentication and support through the public purse. To do otherwise impairs the probity and ethical standing of medicine, and the health-care organizations that fund it.

Mobilizing the Placebo Effect

We know that the placebo effect is often more effective than a drug. We also know that the placebo effect along with the natural evolution of most diseases greatly enhances the outcome of any treatment, whether that treatment is effective or not. We have learned that a positive attitude helps many patients even if no treatment is given.[24] Can doctors not ethically harness the placebo effect with their treatment?[25] Brody believes so, "because some element of the placebo effect exists in every clinical encounter even when no placebo is used .... [A] clinical approach that makes the illness experience more understandable to the patient, that instills a sense of caring and social support, and that increases a feeling of mastery and control over the course of the illness, will be most likely to create a positive placebo response and to improve symptoms."[26] No deception is necessary. Patients look for a cure, or relief of their symptoms, but they also want time with their doctors—time to get an explanation, to understand the meaning of their sufferings, and to know what it means for their future. If by providing that, physicians elicit a placebo response, then all the better. "To cure sometimes, to relieve often, and *to comfort always*" presents no ethical dilemma.

CONCLUSION

The ethical employment of the placebo effect requires no deception. Subjects recruited for clinical trials must be told about the aims and methods of the trial and of their likelihood of being in the placebo group. Investigators must honestly explain the benefits and risks of being in the trial. Placebo-controlled trials are ethical if there is no proven therapy, and if other measures are sufficiently and equally applied to all subjects. If a trial-proven, very effective therapy already exists for a disease, then that treatment should be the control for proposed new treatments. In chronic, fluctuating, but non-life-threatening disorders without a proven treatment, placebo controls are desirable. This is so even if a moderately effective treatment exists, providing that withholding it results in no harm. It is seldom, if ever, justified to give a placebo to a patient without his consent, since deception ultimately may harm all parties. Modern physicians eschew deliberate placebos in practice because deceit is required. More common are treatments that both healers and patients falsely believe to be useful. It seems possible that useless treatments will become unethical as we accumulate more comprehensive medical evidence. Meanwhile, a placebo effect, devoid of deception, elicited by a caring, positive physician in conjunction with proven therapy or even during a supportive encounter with no specific treatment is not only ethical, but also good practice.

PART 3

DOCTOR/PATIENT RELATIONSHIP, EVIDENCE-BASED MEDICINE, AND HEALTH CARE

If as a patient, you are convinced of the importance of placebo effects, and that care should be as evidence-based as possible, you will want to be assured that your doctor can provide them both. Your primary-care physician needs time, continuity, and authority to establish a therapeutic relationship with you. She must be able, with the help of consultants and other health-care workers, to apply medical evidence judiciously and compassionately in accordance with your circumstances, needs, and desires. These two tasks should neither be delegated nor usurped, and administrators and other disciplines involved in health care need to support rather than interfere with them.

Modern physicians must deal with many outsiders. Some seek to help, others to control, but all take time and influence the doctor/patient relationship. Physicians themselves seem more distant from their patients. If medical care is to be evidence based, physicians must be able, through accessible information technology and expert evaluation, to distinguish medical evidence from theory. Health-care systems help determine doctor/patient relationships and influence how well medical evidence is applied, not the least by controlling the resources and time allotted for therapeutic encounters. Our national health-care debates should pay more attention to these issues. Meanwhile, despite their current disillusionment, physicians must supplement their technological skills by seeking better therapeutic relationships and by judiciously applying evidence to your treatment.

***

If these two functions were optimal, more efficient health care and greater patient satisfaction would result and ultimately save money. As those managing health care contemplate reforms, they should keep these tasks in mind. Without their effective deployment, more money, more regulation, and more choice will not satisfy your expectations.

CHAPTER 15

STRANGERS IN THE CONSULTING ROOM

"The image of a physician alone with a patient is being supplanted by one of an examining room so crowded that the physician has difficulty squeezing in, and of a patient surrounded by strangers."

D. J. ROTHMAN, *STRANGERS AT THE BEDSIDE*[1]

To the Shapiros, the strangers were "lawyers, judges, journalists philosophers, bioethicists, clerics, community people, federal and state legislators, hospital administrators, insurance clerks, institutional review boards, and committees to ensure adequate informed consent."[2] They characterized medicine and demoralized physicians as "increasingly enmeshed in bureaucracy, committees, forms, regulations, contracts, and procedures," and feared "the death of a noble profession." However, D. J. Rothman goes beyond the foreign invasion metaphor to describe the transmogrification of doctors from patients' confidants to strangers themselves. Both the strangers and the estrangement threaten doctor/patient relationships and the placebo response. Technology and societal changes have altered medicine irrevocably. While technology enhances medicine's power to help and heal the sick, strangers and estrangements compromise the attributes that previously sustained the profession.

THE DOCTOR AS A STRANGER

Rothman traces the changes in medical practice since the 1930s.[3] Until a few years after World War II, North Americans embraced the notion of the friendly, ever-available, and hard-working general prac-

217

titioner. This Norman Rockwell vision was never entirely true, especially for the poor, but doctors occupied a special position in Western society. Moreover, they were of the patients they served. That is, they lived among them and often shared social backgrounds. In such a milieu, they knew their patients, who in turn usually trusted them. Familiarity and trust strengthened doctor/patient relationships. When migration was less than now, families could count on their GPs to be present at their lives' great events and crises: births, bereavements, and illness. Treatment of illness often occurred in the home. Tales of kitchen table surgery and other lore entertained medical students even in the 1950s, although by then such exploits were vanishing from all but remote communities. The irony is that until the availability of sulfonamides, penicillin, and (earlier) insulin, the GP's effective treatment repertoire outside surgery and obstetrics was meager. Like the shamans of old, much good that he did rested less on science than on the magic of time and the placebo effect.

The local hospital also was located among the people. Often run by ethnic or religious groups, it was staffed by local GPs. Such hospitals might have a surgeon (sometimes an itinerant one), or at least a GP who did some surgery. Nurses or GPs performed anesthesia. Later a specialist in internal medicine might join the hospital staff. These specialists had private practices in the community, and like GPs, they knew, and were known by, their patients. Hospitals were not pleasant places to visit, but their personnel were local and chances were that a patient had acquaintances working there.

In 1930s America, only 19 percent of doctor visits were to specialists—mainly surgeons, obstetricians, and pediatricians—many of whom were GPs as well.[4] Even in 1940, 70 percent of American doctors were GPs, and specialists outside urban centers were scarce. The war and postwar periods saw remarkable advances in medical science, and new methods of treatment exceeded the GP's capabilities. Specialization and medical centers began to grow, and small community hospitals closed for the sake of efficiency and economy. As the use of institutionalized subjects for wartime medical research became postwar scandals, trust in physicians lessened. In the United States, the press publicized the use of institutionalized subjects for research without their consent, and Congress intervened. By the 1960s congressional investigation and oversight into medical research extended to medical practice as well. Mandated oversight of issues surrounding death and birth required lay participation.

After the war, specialists grew apace and soon outnumbered GPs in the United States. The Royal College of Physicians and Surgeons of Canada now lists fifty-nine specialties. Medical advances and sophisticated technology attracted specialists to large city hospitals. GPs became remote from hospitals and specialists, and so found it increasingly difficult to keep up with rapidly expanding information. Their interest and involvement in hospitals waned and they became strangers to their specialist colleagues. Efforts to reestablish GPs' status through their reinvention as "family doctors" seemed to isolate them further from the rest of the profession, and their diminished status led an increasingly affluent and insurance-covered population to shop around or see specialists directly if they could. The decline of primary care has resulted in transient encounters with walk-in clinics, overcrowded emergency rooms, the proliferation of CAM, and the disintegration of the patient's medical record.

Meanwhile, hospitals became less sectarian, responding to government mandates for public ownership and the needs of an increasingly mobile, less religiously divided population. Administrations sought to increase the status of their institutions by setting up advanced specialty units, and recruiting "world-class" doctors like sports stars, who were not rooted in the community. Rothman, a non-physician introduced to hospital medicine, was "unprepared for the grueling and continuing pace of medical practice."[5] He noted the long working days and the ongoing rush from crisis to crisis. The frenetic pace, the inability to pursue outside interests, the professional fraternization, and shoptalk further isolated physicians from the people they served. The monklike devotion of training for professional qualifications often had untoward consequences for doctors' personal lives. Unhappy doctors are not comforting doctors.

These changes accommodated incredible technical advances that saved many lives, but something was lost along the way. Family doctors' place in society declined, but more important, they became less familiar with their peoples' lives in health and disease. Despite efforts by universities and governments to foster special family practice programs, a primary care doctor shortage occurred,[6] especially in Canada, where provincial governments, equating doctors with costs, cut back on medical students and postgraduate training.[7] By the 1990s more than 50 percent of the graduates of many medical schools were women. While they make just as excellent physicians as men, they work fewer hours.[8] Moreover, compared to the previous generation, male physicians are more likely to have professional spouses, and they work fewer hours as well.[9] These changes are occurring in the face of an aging population that will depend more and more on sophisticated technology. Many students now avoid general practice and seek "jobs" that command predictable hours such as dermatology or an emergency roster. Doctors working part-time or in walk-in clinics have less longitudinal patient interaction. Records are decentralized, and no professional knows a patient's complete medical history. Hence, many doctors are strangers to their patients.

As Rothman puts it, "Practically every development in medicine in the post–World War II period distanced the physician and the hospital from the patient and the community, disrupting personal connections and severing bonds of trust."[10] He implies that these developments underlie the division between the profession and the laity, and prompted the strangers to the patient's bedside. I would add that these developments have led everyone to ignore the importance of the doctor/patient relationship that is now too often fleeting and impersonal. The isolation, pace, and restraints of medical-care systems work against thoughtful primary-care/patient/specialist interactions. Medical encounters have become commodities or isolated service packages, and who keeps track of an individual's overall well-being? That is not to say that specialists cannot generate placebo effects. Of course they can. Moreover, a well-orchestrated referral to an expert can be very reassuring, meaningful, and hopeful. Equally, an unfocused referral of an ill, frightened, and unprepared person to a stranger in an alien institution can have nocebo effects.

The developments of the past half century that diminish the doctor as a placebo rob us all of a basic human interaction. A medical-care system, institution, or caregiver operating in ignorance of this crucial relationship between the healer and the ill risks many nocebo effects—and money alone will not fix them.

OTHER STRANGERS

The strangers that Rothman described are legislators, lawyers, journalists, administrators, "health-care economists," and many more who seek to influence the doctor/patient relationship. Some are desirable and socially necessary, but they have costs. Our concern is the extent to which they compromise the doctor/patient relationship and their placebo/nocebo effects on patients' health outcomes.

Legislators

By the 1960s and 1970s, there was a strong impetus to change the practice of medicine from an autonomous solo enterprise governed by its own ancient code of ethics to a more collective one with rules imposed from without. The reasons for this are complex, but include the research scandals such as those exposed by Beecher, the inadequacy of medical ethics for the modern world, the isolation of doctors from the people they serve, and the gulf between family doctors and specialists.

In 1962 a sedative known as thalidomide caused serious birth defects after approval in Canada and Europe. In the United States, the FDA deferred approval because of concern over the drug's safety, but experimentally, more than twenty thousand Americans had already received the drug. The Kefauver Senate hearings learned that many people had received this and other drugs without their consent. This information and Beecher's 1966 editorial describing the unethical use of institutionalized subjects for human research[11] led the National Institutes of Health and the FDA to introduce institutional review boards and requirements for informed consent. These developments and the 1964 Declaration of Helsinki embedded a new standard of ethics into medical research (see table 14-1).[12]

In 1967 Christiaan Barnard performed the world's first heart transplantation in South Africa, making medical ethics a public concern. It was urgent to define brain death, in order to determine when a dying person could become an organ donor. Similar concerns arose in neonatal units because of highly publicized life or death decisions concerning "defective" newborns. Brain surgery to modify "abnormal" behavior was also scrutinized. According to Rothman, the highly publicized case of Karen Ann Quinlan was a test for medical ethics in the United States. Quinlan was brain dead and her parents wanted her respirator to be discontinued. Her doctor refused on moral grounds. Public discussion over who should make such a decision was a harbinger for change. The United States Senate hearings and commissions headed by Senators Walter Mondale and Edward Kennedy led to federal oversight of human research and eventually the life and death decisions of medical practice. What is surprising in

Rothman's account is the bitter opposition of doctors to *any* lay participation in medical decisions.[13] Prominent medical researchers, including Barnard himself, arrogantly opposed the notion that anyone but them could make such decisions. Their behavior only seemed to compromise their public esteem. Professional attitudes against outside participation in medical decision making illustrate how isolated many physicians had become. They had become strangers to their patients and to the community. Today, informed consent and lay participation in medical decision oversight are facts of daily practice.

The notion of oversight and informed consent also lagged elsewhere. As a young Canadian doctor seeking research experience in England, I was able (with negligible documentation) to see patients in the clinic, and, if I wished, could even recruit them for research projects. However, my project involved animal research and for that, I required a bureaucratic, three-month-long application, with references, to the Home Office in order to conform to the Cruelty to Animals Act of 1867. The irony seemed to escape my colleagues. Today, most Western countries have adopted principles of medical licensure and human experimentation similar to those in the United States.

Medical tradition and the Hippocratic Oath charged the doctor to be his patient's advocate and admonished him to "do no harm." It became clear in the 1970s that tradition and Hippocrates' ethics were inadequate for the life-and-death dramas of modern medicine (see table 15-1). The traditional invocation to speak no ill of colleagues and to spare patients from bad news defied modern ideas of full disclosure. New ethics were needed and outsiders played a leading role.

While these developments were inevitable and desirable, they complicated medical practice. The need for informed consent prompted the legal necessity to prove that informed consent had taken place. This required more bookkeeping, a formal consent form, an explanation of possible adverse events, and a witnessed information process, all of which consumed more time. In many cases, unexpected outcomes are extremely rare, and physicians feared fully informed consent could cause an anxious patient to reject the procedure and be deprived of its benefits. Doctors have had to learn to compromise their optimism and need to reassure with a catalog of frightening possible calamities. Whatever readers might think of these requirements, they take time and have implications for doctor/patient relationships. If not deftly executed, they can mitigate the placebo effect.

TABLE 15-1
Hippocratic Oath—Classical Version

I swear by Apollo the Physician and Asclepius and Hygieia and Panaceia and all the gods and goddesses, making them my witnesses, that I will fulfill according to my ability and judgment this oath and this covenant:

—To hold him who has taught me this art as equal to my parents and to live my life in partnership with him, and if he is in need of money to give him a share of mine, and to regard his offspring as equal to my brothers in male lineage and to teach them this art—if they desire to learn it—without fee and covenant; to give a share of precepts and oral instruction and all the other learning to my sons and to the sons of him who has instructed me and to pupils who have signed the covenant and have taken an oath according to the medical law, but no one else.

—I will apply dietetic measures for the benefit of the sick according to my ability and judgment; I will keep them from harm and injustice.

—I will neither give a deadly drug to anybody who asked for it, nor will I make a suggestion to this effect. Similarly I will not give to a woman an abortive remedy. In purity and holiness I will guard my life and my art.

—I will not use the knife, not even on sufferers from stone, but will withdraw in favor of such men as are engaged in this work.

—Whatever houses I may visit, I will come for the benefit of the sick, remaining free of all intentional injustice, of all mischief and in particular of sexual relations with both female and male persons, be they free or slaves.

—What I may see or hear in the course of the treatment or even outside of the treatment in regard to the life of men, which on no account one must spread abroad, I will keep to myself, holding such things shameful to be spoken about.

—If I fulfil this oath and do not violate it, may it be granted to me to enjoy life and art, being honored with fame among all men for all time to come; if I transgress it and swear falsely, may the opposite of all this be my lot.[14]

Specialists

Doctors can themselves intrude in other doctors' examining rooms. Specialty societies and others seek to exert their influence in primary care, of which they know little. Primary care is perhaps the most burdened and misunderstood branch of medicine. The very fact that we have so many specialists attests to the burgeoning volume of medical knowledge and to young doctors' aversion to primary care. No one can audit the thousands of medical journals, let alone determine what is nonsense and what is not. Primary-care doctors, including GPs, family doctors, and internists, must get their information from their journals and from the refresher courses that their societies oblige them to attend.

Specialists with little experience in primary care provide much of this education, and their advice can be esoteric or irrelevant. Some specialists are critical of the lack of expertise of doctors who refer them patients. Academics advise that the proper management of a disease requires a certain procedure, thereby ensuring that a patient with that disease must be referred to them to have it done. This manifests a misunderstanding of the family doctor's role. In a general practice study in the United Kingdom,[15] we found that only 8 percent of adults had a gastroenterology problem, usually a self-limiting one such as gastroenteritis, that was managed without referral. In addition, the British GPs cared for children, expectant mothers, and engaged in disease prevention programs. Thus, gastroenterology is a small part of the GP's daily experience. It is naive to expect them to be minispecialists in gastroenterology as well as the fifty-eight other "official" fields of medicine.

As a result of this experience, I helped organize two symposia to develop management guidelines in a gastroenterology subject.[16] To avoid the above pitfalls we invited family doctors to participate and formally criticize the specialists' recommendations. The result was an exchange of views that enlightened both sides of the medical divide. The ideal world met the art of the possible. Education efforts, guidelines, and even specialists' reports should be suitable for primary care. If primary-care doctors knew everything, there would be no need for consultants! If consultants engaged in primary care, they would no longer *be* consultants!

Industry

Many voices lament the conflicts of interest and the uneven attention to medical diseases that physicians encounter when dealing with the pharmaceutical industry.[17] The industry's estimated US marketing expenditures for 2001 were between $8 billion and $12 billion, or about $8,000 to $15,000 per physician.[18] Armed with enormous resources, companies dispatch ninety thousand detail personnel to hospitals and doctors' offices across the United States to promote their products—about one per five office-based doctors. Pharmaceutical representatives are therefore familiar strangers in the examination room, and are well briefed about the benefits of their product and its principal side effects. Few have pharmacology training, and fewer still have any notion of the practice of medicine. Detailing is a continuing source of irritation to academics who think they, not salespeople, should be the source of knowledge about drug efficacy. However, primary-care doctors are busy people. Few specialists are around to help, but a pharmaceutical representative often lingers in the waiting room.

Primary-care organizations require their members to maintain their competence by attending educational sessions that are often sponsored by drug companies. The programs are usually laudable and conform to guidelines but have a commercial object. Directly or indirectly, medical journals, national meetings, clinical trials, and other professional enterprises are overwhelmingly supported by industry.[19] Academics serve as guest speakers at specialty and primary-care events that are directed toward subjects of commercial interest, but other treatments or diseases with no drug interest get short shrift.

Thus, not only do pharmaceutical representatives demand an inordinate portion of a family doctor's time, but they also distort her continuing education. There must be unbiased countervailing efforts to present the vast amount of evolving medical knowledge that is not addressed by the drug industry (see chapter 16).

Media

Western democracies cite the free press as an essential component of their citizens' freedom. Anyone should be free to publish anything that is not hateful or libelous. However, no statute decrees that television, magazines, and newspapers must publish material that is thoughtful or reliable. Many health reporters study their subject carefully, but too many others tout magical diets, fanciful treatments, and miracle drugs with little attention to the truth or public consequences. Personal testimony, anecdotes, and blanket advice that fails to account for individual circumstances are of little value in the examining room. A doctor, when faced with a patient's interpretation of a media report of a treatment, has inadequate resources to find the truth behind the headline. We may not think of the media's presence in the examining room, but it is there all the same. Doctors must deal with such information and misinformation, yet lack the time to do so effectively.

David Sackett cites the arrogance of preventative-medicine advocates who aggressively tell asymptomatic individuals what they must do to remain healthy.[20] He speaks of prevention interventions that are unsupported by scientific data. Citing observational data that confuses coincidence with cause, "experts" recommend certain nostrums for everyone. The ever-changing healthy-diet fads and recommendations for vitamin therapy often derive from observations, anecdotes, and theories rather than science. Reporters urge the public to comply, and doctors must advise confused patients. Clean water, sanitation, vaccination, aspirin (for some), antihypertension drugs, seat belts, and bans on smoking and drunk driving are science-based activities that save lives. Many other putative prevention programs do not. They may seem like good ideas, but so did seawater for scurvy, kava for anxiety, and leeches for almost anything. Medicine by media can have nocebo effects.

Administration

After World War II, comprehensive health-care systems evolved in developed countries, each with its own rules. A result has been removal of one part of the doctor/patient relationship—payment for services. In its place, administrators with their forms, regulations, and cost containments have invaded the examining room. In many jurisdictions, these strangers are the most troublesome of all (see chapter 17).

Lawyers

No group generates more consternation for physicians than lawyers do. The legal necessity for confrontation is alien to the way most doctors think and function, and certainly the antithesis of a caring relationship. Moreover, malpractice issues distort medical care. In Miami an obstetrician pays an annual malpractice insurance fee of $200,000.[21] Such premiums increase the overall cost of health care. In many places, obstetricians choose to practice only gynecology to lower their risk and their premiums. Family doctors avoid obstetrics for similar reasons. In Las Vegas a trauma center closed for ten days because its doctors could not afford insurance. The blame for the longstanding malpractice crisis is difficult to pin down—malicious patients and lawyers, obsolete tort law, incompetent doctors, and bad investments by the insurance industry are suspect, but they are not the whole story.[22] What is certain is that litigation is an inefficient way to compensate patients harmed by a medical treatment. Legal and court fees take much of the award, and most who are injured but do not litigate receive no compensation at all.

Malpractice litigation is a double nocebo (see chapter 6). Not only does the issue at hand have a nocebo effect, but there are downstream nocebo effects as well. Protracted legal proceedings suspend the lives of the accused and accuser. The litigating patient may so focus on recompense or retribution, that he further endangers his health. Other physicians, hearing of the complaint, may be unwilling to care for him or do so with unseemly caution. The accused physician's behavior and attitude may change in unconstructive ways.[23] These include the practice of defensive medicine (the ordering of treatments, tests, and procedures for the purpose of protecting the doctor from criticism rather than diagnosing or treating the patient). Superficially, this may seem beneficial to patients because more tests are good, are they not? Not so! Unindicated tests can have unintended consequences. Some procedures that irradiate or penetrate the body are potentially harmful. Others may generate false-positive results mandating repetition or more tests. Not only does this cause unnecessary anxiety and risk, but it also distracts attention from the care of the original complaint. From a health-policy standpoint, defensive testing (as distinct from scientifically justified public-health measures such as screening colonoscopy for colon cancer or tuberculosis testing) is expensive and diverts precious resources needed by others. Of course, defensive medicine can be constructive if it improves communication with the patient and promotes appropriate referrals.[24] More patient-centered care is an obvious strategy.[25]

The threat of litigation harms doctor/patient relationships. Sensationalized media reports of malpractice cases damage the trust that is essential to a healing relationship. Litigation burdens the health-care system, yet does little to correct medical error or help most of the aggrieved.[26] Many experts call for tort reform,[27] but observers do not expect it soon.[28] This is disappointing, as the malpractice threat casts a malevolent shadow in the examining room. The crisis, while inter-national, is particularly troublesome in the United States. I lack the temerity to suggest a solution, but reform should embrace the princi-ples of proper compensation for patient injury without needing (if there is no incompetence) to always to attach blame or render punish-ment. Timely mediation and settlement are preferable to destructive legal confrontation. When damages are not due to malpractice, com-pensation should be possible without jeopardizing doctor/patient relationships. The most important strategy is the prevention of unnecessary claims. For that, doctors need sufficient time to establish the doctor/patient relationship, and properly explain the aims and limitations of medical treatment. Only then can an autonomous patient give informed consent.[29]

CONCLUSIONS

There is no going back. Strangers are in medical practices to stay. However, doctors, especially primary-care doctors, should be better equipped to deal with them. They need more time to interact with their patients as well as cope with the strangers' agendas. They must have easier access to information that is evidence based, relevant, and impartial. Dealing with the strangers in examination rooms should be simplified and expedited. Mediation, not litigation, should rule on medical mishaps where no malpractice has occurred. The strangers should help the doctor help her patients, not complicate her job.

Most important, physicians must strive not to be strangers them-selves. For this, too, they need more time with their patients. Good doctor/patient relationships maximize therapy and minimize nocebo effects. When properly exploited, this relationship should increase patients' well-being, reduce the need for consultations and tests, and ultimately save money.

CHAPTER 16

THE BURDEN OF PROOF

"[W]hile the individual man is an insoluble puzzle, in the aggregate, he becomes a mathematical certainty. You can, for example, never foretell what any man will do, but you can say with precision what an average number will be up to. Individuals vary, but percentages remain constant. So says the statistician."

SHERLOCK HOLMES[1]

In part 2, we discussed the judicious application of evidence-based medicine to medical treatments and explored its special challenges in surgery, psychotherapy, and complementary and alternative medicine. Hitherto, evidence-based medicine has been of most concern to academics, pharmaceutical firms, and regulatory agencies. We must now consider how to apply this principle more generally to health care. There are two burdens of proof. The first is to prove that treatments are safe and effective. The second is to apply this proof to medical practice. Practical, evidence-based information should be conveniently available to health-care professionals.

THE SCIENTIFIC BURDEN

While clinical trials permit scientific judgments about the efficacy of many treatments, much of medical practice remains unscientific. The proliferation of treatments and the rising costs of medical care force us to evaluate them carefully. Beliefs, medical fads, media sensationalism, and biased research effort undermine the evidence-based ideal. We need to combat these obstacles and ensure safety and efficacy for medical tests and treatments.

Safety and Efficacy

Safety

Randomized trials testing the efficacy of a treatment also determine its safety. In the treatment of mortal diseases such as cancer or heart disease, doctors and patients must weigh the efficacy of a drug against the risk of drug toxicity. For chronic, deforming diseases such as rheumatoid arthritis, nonsteroidal anti-inflammatory drugs reduce joint inflammation and pain, but in some people they cause bleeding stomach ulcers. Both the doctor and her patient must decide if the severity of the arthritis justifies this risk.

Ongoing observations and postmarketing surveillance supposedly guard against long-term adverse effects, but they failed to alert the public to an increased incidence of myocardial infarction among patients taking the COX-2 anti-inflammatory drug rofecoxib (Vioxx). This was blamed on overzealous marketing of the drug and unpredictable effects on large numbers of people, lax regulators, overlooked basic pharmacology, and the hype that outstripped reason in prescribing.[2] The FDA will now be advised by a Drug Safety Oversight Board with access to FDA and other government databases, but some doubt that this new board is sufficiently independent for the task.[3]

For treatment of the nonfatal, nondeforming, chronic, painful disorders we sometimes call functional, no risk is acceptable. In 2000 the FDA approved *alosetron* for the treatment of women with diarrhea and irritable bowel syndrome based on well-conducted clinical trials.[4] However, reports of bowel ulceration and severe constipation prompted the drug's withdrawal. (It is now available with strict precautions only in the United States.) In this example, IBS is nonfatal and nondeforming, and safety concerns trump efficacy. Many observers insist that complementary and alternative medicine treatments should submit to similar safety standards. Strict regulation of pharmaceuticals and laissez-faire with CAM is a double standard.

Efficacy

Randomized, controlled clinical trials determine a treatment's efficacy. Anecdote, observation, and experience are inadequate. Evidence-based medicine is more satisfying if there is a scientific rationale for a treatment. For example, an antibiotic that kills organisms in a laboratory dish provides a rationale for its use to combat that same organism when it infects humans. Scientific rationales do not exist for acupuncture, homeopathy, herbal medicines, or many older prescription drugs. Some practitioners of CAM and psychotherapy protest that controlled trials are antithetical to their treatments, which depend upon belief and individualization. Nevertheless, belief and anecdotes are not proof.

Within medicine, the burden of proof is awesome. There are so many existing treatments to be tested, so many diseases to treat, and so few researchers that medicine can never be completely evidence based. There is also the great task of studying CAM. Clinical trials of CAM and psychotherapy must account for the variations within each treatment. The active principles and dosages of most herbal medicines are a mystery. Homeopathic treatments are "individualized." Acupuncture has many contact points and methodological variations such as moxibustion and electroacupuncture. Psychotherapy also embraces many techniques. Proponents should agree what constitutes their optimal treatment and then submit it to randomized, clinical trials.

Once the legitimacy and safety of therapies are determined, societies need to decide which treatments—indeed, which illnesses—are of sufficient health importance to warrant public subsidy. To many peoples, traditional healing is part of their culture. Acupuncture has been part of Chinese culture for millennia. To challenge culture-based healing is to challenge the culture itself.[5] Similarly, faith healing is often rooted in religion. Science may find no truth in the healing claims of culture or religion, but these have no place for science. Beliefs are individual rights, but, in most societies, not likely to be publicly funded.

Obstacles to Proof

Dealing with Uncertainty

Scientists seldom stumble on medical discoveries, as Fleming did with penicillin. Rather, a belief or hypothesis must be tested by experiment. In therapeutics, experiment usually takes the form of a clinical trial. However, as so cleverly stated by Sherlock Holmes, we can prove how the average among a group of patients is likely to behave, but the individual's response is uncertain. Thus when treating a patient, an evidence-based decision is one based on probabilities. A patient is most likely to improve if we choose a treatment shown to benefit most similar patients. Seldom can a doctor be 100 percent certain of the outcome. She usually has time and the placebo effect on her side, but by choosing an evidence-based treatment, she adds a chance that the patient will do even better. Nevertheless, like repeatedly flipping a coin, using the treatment in successive patients will eventually fail.

Perhaps we can understand this uncertainty better through the "number needed to treat" (NNT). You will recall from chapter 8 that the NNT is one, divided by the therapeutic gain. In a series of patients treated by a drug, many will improve because of time and placebo effects, and an additional few will improve because of the drug's effect. Some will not improve or will become worse. The NNT expresses the number of patients one must treat before an improvement occurs due *solely* to the drug's effect. Thus, for an individual patient, improvement on the drug is more probable than improvement with a placebo, but it is still not certain.

Doctors are familiar with probability, having long diagnosed disease in this way. In the nineteenth century, surgeons and pathologists through operations or autopsy, described anatomic diagnoses. Gradually, physicians learned to predict these diagnoses in life through physical examination and history taking. An enlarged liver discovered by examination of the adult abdomen is abnormal. By correlating that finding with other evidence, physicians learn to select a few disease possibilities. Medical students consulting textbooks are likely to include a great many possible causes of a large liver, but experience teaches them to narrow the possibilities quickly and order appropriate tests. For example, a large liver in a young person abusing drugs is likely to be due to hepatitis that blood tests can confirm. In a middle-aged person with a large liver, any suggestion of alcohol abuse will prompt the doctor to look for signs of cirrhosis. A large liver in an elderly person is assumed to be due to cancer until it is disproved through a biopsy. Probabilities may differ where parasites or other exotic infections are common. By narrowing the possible causes of a physical finding or a set of symptoms, a doctor can select the test most likely to secure the correct diagnosis. With experience, doctors can make educated guesses. Acute shortness of breath in a patient bedridden after hip replacement is probably due to a blood clot in the lung. When a measles epidemic exists in the community, high fever in a child suggests that probability to a family doctor.

Similarly, a doctor weighs the probabilities when choosing a particular treatment. She has recognized the patient's disease through diagnosis, she knows his personal history, and she has evidence from clinical trials that a certain medicine usually helps improve the condition of similar patients. The process of examination, precise diagnosis, and (when available) evidence-based treatment is almost unique to medicine and dentistry. It works best when the physician observes an anatomical or chemical marker of the disease such as a large liver or low serum iron content (a sign of blood loss). However, we have already noted that for many complaints, doctors find no such abnormality. It is in chronic and functional disorders that diagnosis and treatment become less scientific, and medicine is more dependent upon theory, belief, and judgment.

Medicine attempts to overcome diagnostic uncertainty by classifying disorders according to symptoms and then relating the classified disease with other facts. For example, psychiatrists have classified mental disorders through a consensus process reported in the *Diagnostic and Statistical Manual of Mental Disorders* (DSM).[6] When a patient has a DSM diagnosis of depression, his physician can select an antidepressant that is trial-proven for that diagnosis. Since the diagnosis of many chronic, painful disorders—including most headaches, bellyaches, and backaches—is imprecise, there is no treatment target other than the symptoms. Using the DSM model, physicians classify such complaints into syndromes such as irritable bowel, chronic fatigue, and fibromyalgia. Identification of a syndrome prompts the doctor to judiciously select an appropriate evidence-based treatment, if there is one.

Few would disagree that the treatment of mortal and disabling diseases is the domain of orthodox medicine. The placebo effect is important but often overwhelmed by the certainly effective treatments afforded by technology. No wise person will consult a CAM practitioner for an acutely blocked coronary artery or pneumococcal pneumonia. However, CAM might be a competitor with medicine in treating chronic painful disorders of uncertain treatment where time and placebo effects may be the best anyone can offer. Eventually, evidence should overtake belief in most treatment decisions, but uncertainty will always haunt therapeutics.

Healing Fads and Obsolescence

A reappearing theme in medical history is the healing property of magnets. The best known magnetizer was Franz Mezmer, a flamboyant Austrian who introduced *animal magnetism* to the prerevolution Paris of Louis XVI.[7] He arranged his patients around a vat filled with water, waving a wand over them while they held magnetic rods that protruded from the vat. Soon he skipped the magnetic rods and just waved the wand. Like homeopathy, the treatment was reduced to nothing. Benjamin Franklin, the electricity pioneer and then US delegate to Paris, wryly surmised that *mesmerism* worked because it diverted people from Paris's dangerous orthodox physicians. Louis appointed Franklin and the pioneer chemist Antoine-Laurent Lavoisier to a royal commission investigating Mezmer. Through a series of tests where subjects believed they were receiving Mezmer's treatment when they were not, and others received the treatment but believed they had not, the commission discredited Mezmer. Thus exposed, he returned with his wands to Vienna. Magnetic healing has resurfaced in several guises such as magnetic "tractors" discredited by Haygarth in 1800, Cumming's electrogalvanism in 1849, and recent "biomagnetic" therapy in which magnets are strapped to injured muscles.

Healing fads commonly appear and disappear. Homeopathy declined as an independent profession after joining the American Medical Association a century ago but resurfaced in recent years. Colon laundries pop up periodically in the Paris of Louis XIV, nineteenth-century London, and twenty-first-century North America. Diets come and go as gurus live and die.

Medicine itself is not immune to fads. Novel treatments are embraced enthusiastically, only to disappear as time proves them ineffective or something newer (perhaps no more effective) displaces them. Hence, colonic irrigation preceded and succeeded colectomy for autointoxication. Over the last half century, doctors have successively treated irritable bowel syndrome with anticholinergic drugs, high-fiber diets, bran, commercial bulking agents, psychological treatments, prokinetic drugs, antidepressants, and, most recently, drugs acting on the serotonin system.[8] As a rule, a long list of treatments for a disease suggests that probably none of them work well.

Past approval by regulatory authorities is an unreliable guide to authenticity. Dicyclomine, approved for bowel symptoms a half century ago, remains on some formularies despite the absence of evidence that it is effective.[9] Each European country maintains a unique formulary of obsolete and unproven drugs for gut symptoms,[10] some the products of local industry. Archaic tests linger as well. Flexible instruments using fiber optics or microchips were available to examine the sigmoid colon by 1970, but some doctors still use the obsolete and far less useful rigid sigmoidoscope. Radioisotope liver scans persisted long after they were rendered obsolete by other imaging techniques. How do we decide which treatments and tests are legitimate or, at best, harmless? What should be insured with public funds? How do we withdraw support when the item becomes passé?

The Sensationalism of Medicine

> "The danger of magazine medicine is that it selects the sensational and eschews the Humdrum."
>
> RICHARD ASHER (1959)[11]

A *Lancet* article reported that vaccination against measles, mumps, and rubella (MMR) was associated with autism in a few children.[12] Despite an editorial urging caution lest an important public health program be compromised, many parents denied their children vaccination. Doctors, reporters, and parents confused association with causality—a classic misinterpretation. The editor discovered that one of the authors was a paid advisor of parents with alleged vaccine-damaged children.[13] The report might not have been published had that information been declared. This potential conflict of interest surfaced too late to prevent many children from missing an important disease-prevention program. Such experiences should caution anyone who would base decisions on a single uncontrolled report, especially when the phenomenon makes little medical sense and was not the study's primary outcome measure. Health policy should not depend upon coincidence or belief!

Two spectacular examples reinforce this point. In the 1990s an eighty-five-year-old Italian former physiology professor named Luigi Di Bella promoted an "antineoplastic regimen" to treat cancer.[14] The treatment cocktail contained somatostatin, melatonin, vitamin C, very low doses of cyclophosphamide (the only component with any anti-cancer activity), parathormone, corticotrophin, bromcriptine, and retinoids. The international press hailed this "miracle drug," and desperate patients flocked to Di Bella, some abandoning evidence-based treatments. Public demonstrations demanded "freedom of treatment." An Italian judge ordered the health authorities to pay a patient US$6,000 monthly for the Di Bella treatment.[15] Yet examination of Di Bella's records provided neither rationale nor scientific support for his treatment. The authorities ultimately conducted a trial that discredited the drug,[16] but not before the media had lost interest, thousands had aggravated their personal tragedies, and money was diverted from more useful treatments. The trial, which should not have been necessary, cost US$5 million.[17]

Lest readers imagine that this is a "foreign" phenomenon, they should recall the Laetrile story.[18] Amygdalin is an unstandardized herbal ingredient, rich in cyanide, used to treat various diseases for two millennia.[19] In 1952 a homeopathy student named Ernest Krebs Jr. registered amygdalin as *Laetrile* with the United States Post Office. Combined with a "metabolic treatment" of diet, enzymes, and vitamins, it was promoted as a cancer cure. For twenty-five years, Laetrile was in the news, a miracle drug and civil rights issue to some, but to others a cynical fraud. A cast of shady characters somehow kept it in play among patient advocates, lawsuits, legislative approval in twenty-seven states, and celebrity endorsements. In detective novel fashion, enforcement agencies raided doctors' offices and some proponents fled to Mexico to escape regulation and prosecution. Amid much publicity, a Mexican clinic treated the actor Steve McQueen. I recall one young man with colon cancer who mortgaged his house to try Laetrile in Mexico. He died shortly thereafter, having burdened his young widow with considerable debt. No reasoning could counter the media hype. It took a Supreme Court decision, a Senate committee hearing, Steve McQueen's death, and a National Cancer Institute (NCI) clinical trial[20] to end the Laetrile fantasy. The drug cured or stabilized none of 178 cancer patients in the NCI trial, and several of them showed signs of cyanide toxicity.

These are textbook cases of how not to go about legitimizing treatments. It is noteworthy that the trials that ended the Di Bella and Laetrile frauds were single-blind. No controls were necessary to demonstrate that the treatments offered no help or solace to terminal cancer patients. A sophisticated electorate, wiser officials, attention to medical evidence, and less sensational media reporting can prevent such travesties.

Biased Research Effort

While new prescription drugs require evidence for their approval by regulatory agencies, few other treatments undergo stringent testing. Over 90 percent of new chemical agents approved by the FDA were developed by the pharmaceutical industry.[21] The research bias toward new pharmaceuticals distorts medical care by ignoring established medical treatments and CAM. Moreover, disproportionate resources are devoted to benign conditions that command a large market.[22] A drug called omeprazole is very effective in treating heartburn and gastroesophageal reflux disease. The costly addition of "me too" formulations adds little to the repertoire. There are too few innovations for deadly or rare diseases.[23] Despite the urgent need for antibiotics for resistant organisms, antiviral agents for AIDS, and effective treatments for malaria and other killers, many fewer new drugs are approved now than formerly,[24] and few randomized trials address the world's major diseases.[25] Once approved, a drug may be used "off-label" for other conditions, a non-evidence-based practice that competes unfairly with noncommercial advice. Julio Montaner and others argue that some pharmaceutical companies introduce bias by delaying or suppressing publication of unfavorable data or designing trials likely to favor their product.[26] In 2004 a company was fined $480 million for fraudulently marketing an antiepileptic drug for other diseases where it had no better than a placebo effect.[27] Why not subject CAM to the same standard?

Applicability of Observational Trials

Randomized, controlled studies can prove the efficacy of a new drug. However, for many treatments they are impossible or ethically forbidden. An observational trial is an uncontrolled observation of a population undergoing a treatment. While observations make important contributions to medical science,[28] they are controversial and sometimes at odds with randomized controlled trials.[29] For example, observational studies suggest that antioxidant vitamins prevent cancer and cardiovascular disease, but randomized trials fail to confirm it.[30] Observations are a common source of misleading information. Since they are uncontrolled, known and unknown biological and social factors that affect the observed subjects may bias the results. Nevertheless, they can detect adverse events and often are the only feasible sources of information. Debbie Lawler urges more careful attention to confounding factors in such studies.[31] Doubtless, we would benefit from new methods of conducting and analyzing patient-oriented research.[32]

THE BURDEN TO EDUCATE

Only proof will permit doctors and other healers to choose optimal therapy. Then government and private insurers can decide what society should pay for. For such decisions to occur, healers and managers must educate themselves in evidence-based medicine. Just as the examining room strangers and lack of time undermine the therapeutic relationship, so doctors' lack of ready and reliable information compromises evidence-based decision making.

It is impossible for doctors to audit the estimated twenty thousand medical journals. Most of the information they contain is of little value to them anyway. Throwaway journals and advertisements litter doctors' mail. Published recommendations cannot compete with pharmaceutical marketing. For example, British guidelines recommending a certain type of hip replacement device failed to change subsequent practice.[33] Doctors need assistance in finding evidence-based gold among the dross, and the time and incentive to extract and apply it.

By directly or indirectly financing most physicians' continuing medical education, drug companies have inordinate influence.[34] Nongovernmental organizations cannot compete with pharmaceutical largesse. Nevertheless, universities and medical associations can help individual doctors provide their own continuing education. Academic detailing by clinical experts,[35] use of information technology, and more university-sponsored programs would help. If health-care managers supported independent and manageable information for the practicing doctor, and allowed her the time to deal with it, they should improve patient care and save money.

Continuing Medical Education

What is to be done? Well, academics can try to explain science-based medicine, the natural history of disease, and placebo effects in terms the public can understand. Reviewers can thoughtfully criticize health "discoveries" in the medical and popular press, rather than proclaim "breakthroughs." Medical editors can urge critical comment on controversial research, and temper the claims and fads that override sensible interpretation. However, broadening the reach of evidence-based medicine requires the support of industry and the media, as well as the creative use of information technology.

Industry

Medicine would not have accomplished most of its great advances in the last half century were it not for the pharmaceutical industry. While individuals may discover some drugs, only industry can develop them through the required scientific, production, and regulatory hurdles. Industry claims that high drug costs support the research and development of new drugs. Others claim that much basic research is subsidized by taxpayers, and the research budget includes marketing through advertising and educational programs that ignore other medical needs.[36] Yet central planning is no solution. No government will risk $800 million over a decade to bring a drug to market.[37] Only firms with large capitalization can raise sufficient money, and the lenders expect a return on investment. "Big Pharma" is here to stay, but it needs managing.

The pharmaceutical industry has serious production and public relations problems.[38] They squander their successes by the self-serving image they cultivate with the medical profession, the media, and the public. To be sure, there would be little drug innovation without healthy pharmaceuticals, and no one benefits if they go out of business. However, their products are not luxuries. They have responsibilities to the public as well as shareholders. Many people protest their monopolistic patent protection and their behavior in the developing world. Here we are concerned about their contribution to bias in medical education.

A pharmaceutical firm's scientists depend upon the academic medical community for scientific and clinical advice. Physician/industry cooperation is productive and mutually beneficial until the drug is ready for marketing. The personnel charged with selling drugs often have sales backgrounds and care little for science or medical care. Marketing events for doctors are lavish and narrowly focused. Physician advisers find themselves morphed from experts to "opinion leaders" who endorse the product by association. "Medical education" events celebrate the product's official launch. New opinion leaders appear and an audience is assembled. The program focuses on the drug, not on the patient with the disease. Doctors are put in conflicting positions, and if they balk, more pliant replacements are recruited. Many argue that these activities are educational. This would be true if the disadvantages of the drug were prominent; if prevention, diet, and lifestyle advice were part of the package; and if other diseases and other treatments were given equal time. Marketing focuses on the few patented drugs that command the highest prices, ignoring important older and off-patent drugs such as ranitidine, hydrochlorothiazide, or digoxin.

How can a conscientious company compensate its shareholders and remain socially aware? To restore public confidence, they should rethink their educational policies.[39] Educational events should be managed in-house, assisted by independent expert physicians who are sensitive to professional and health-care issues. Events should address all aspects of disease management including the doctor/patient relationship. Evidence-based medicine would advance if various companies collaborated with medical experts and regulatory authorities to solve industry-wide problems related to trial-entry criteria, data management, placebo effects, and outcome measures.

The pharmaceutical industry will find itself increasingly in conflict with governments who must regulate and pay, and the public who perceive great profits, lavish promotion, and conflicted physicians as insufficient justification for their drug costs. An ethics ombudsman could sensitize marketing personnel to public, professional, and humanitarian issues. A broader view of medical care, respect for physician/patient autonomy, and cooperation in issues of general interest would do much to restore the industry's troubled image.

Media

In a 2004 year-end article, a health reporter turned a critical eye on how the media report health news.[40] Citing the fact that most people get their health information in the media, he recognized the responsibility that places on reporters. Among twenty shortcomings he included the lack of sufficiently dedicated and educated health reporters, obsession with "cute" stories and technology, lack of balance between sensational breakthroughs and the serious health problems that threaten people, and a lack of healthy skepticism. His suggestions need codification and could become a "Hippocratic oath" for all health reporters. Alas, such ideals seem distant, and the public can expect continuing tales of "blockbuster drugs," "scientific breakthroughs," and "cures" that are destined to be heard from no more.

In a democracy, the media must be self-regulating, so only journalists can ensure responsible reporting. They should supplement medical reports and researcher interviews with peer opinions. A science education and an understanding of medical evidence should inform a reporter's judgment. Health pages of newspapers and magazines should include in-depth panel discussions of medical issues, like those routinely offered for politics, business, and sports. They should eschew sensational cures or diet and lifestyle fads without evidence to support them. Such evidence should not confuse coincidence with causality, and reporters should understand the need for controls in most biological and health experiments. Dramatic headlines and human-interest anecdotes are biased and have no legitimate place in medical reporting. Health care is not a celebrity.

Information Technology (IT)

Medical libraries are quiet places now, and their permanent collections are contracting.[41] Many people expect them to be superseded or transmogrified by personal computers or handheld devices connected to the Internet.[42] However, no computer chip or antispam program performs peer review. Rather than filter out the intellectual noise, the Internet simply turns up the volume. If IT is to live up its promise, means must be found to authenticate the information and produce it in a digestible form for its application at the point of doctor/patient contact. Administrators, policy advisers, and the public also need access to reliable information. Peer review, imperfect as it is, helps ensure quality for the published medical literature, but who will serve that function in the ether? We come back to the role of IT in the next chapter.

CONCLUSIONS

National health-care systems share two burdens of proof: the need to support research proving the efficacy and safety of tests and treatments, and the task of educating doctors, managers, and the public so that such evidence informs patient care. Uncertainty, medical fads, sensational cures, and biased research hamper judicious evidence-based medical decision making. The scientific burden in clinical medicine is to supply the evidence, usually through randomized clinical trials. As Holmes reminds Dr. Watson, we know little about how an individual will respond to a treatment, but science can help us determine how most will behave.[43] The educational burden is to provide better, convenient, and independent continuing education so that physicians' decisions are judicious and evidence based. For this, information technology is a surprisingly underused resource.[44] Managers and the public must understand the difference between evidence and belief. The pharmaceutical industry, media, governments, private insurers, and physicians themselves must share these burdens.

CHAPTER 17

HEALTH-CARE SYSTEMS AND THE PLACEBO EFFECT

> "[F]or every problem, there is a neat, simple solution and it is always wrong."
>
> H. L. MENCKEN

Developed countries' health-care systems differ significantly. While they provide care to their citizens with considerable success, they all face swiftly rising health-care costs, increasing demand for services, and limited resources. Here we briefly explore some national systems, and the public and professional disillusionment that seems to be international in scope. Each system is flawed and needs reform, but for different reasons. Reformed systems must embrace the doctor/patient relationship and the judicious application of evidence-based medicine as core values, along with proper understanding of the placebo effect. Otherwise, more money, more regulation, and more managers will be futile, and opportunities to provide better health care more efficiently will be lost.

A BRIEF COMPARATIVE ANATOMY OF NATIONAL HEALTH-CARE SYSTEMS[1]

At social evenings in Canadian living rooms, the discussion inevitably turns to health care. After hockey, medicare is our national passion. It seems that no amount of money can reduce waiting periods or satiate booming demand. Eventually, a visitor suggests that private investment might be a solution. Then, someone cries, "That's two-tier medicine!" and a chill silences the group until, thankfully, the host changes the subject. Visitors in a similar living room in the United States worry about increasing insurance fees, lack of physician choice, or even the inability to obtain insurance,[2] and there may be concern that almost forty-five million Americans lack health-care benefits. "Maybe we need a national system," ventures one guest. Then, someone cries, "That's socialized medicine!" and a similar chill ends that discussion, too. As it was with religion and sex, it seems that serious health-care discussion is taboo in polite society. Few politicians will express views contrary to their national myths, for it is a sure vote loser. Thus, the two polarized North American nations blunder on with flawed and increasingly expensive systems, united in their status quo, their mutual schadenfreude, their ignorance of European solutions, and their disdain for each other's programs. They are also both wrong. Each system has much to admire, but both need reform. Similar xenophobia characterizes national health-care systems elsewhere. European systems face rapidly rising costs, aging populations, stretched resources, and unhappy patients and doctors. With fewer immigrants entering the work force compared to North America, their fiscal future looks ever starker. The following discussion briefly describes four health-care designs: the Bismarck, Beveridge, entrepreneurial, and state models.[3] Our concern here is how these systems affect doctor/patient relationships and evidence-based medicine.

The Bismarck Model

In 1881 the German chancellor Otto von Bismarck introduced the Sickness Insurance Act to the Reichstag, in which workers and employers contribute to sickness funds regulated by the federal government. Through many upheavals over the last century, the system has grown to 453 funds covering 88 percent of Germans. Private insurance or the government provide for the remainder. The funds are very generous and include dental care. To cut costs, the government has tinkered with unpopular reforms such as reduced benefits and user fees to control doctor visits.[4] Throughout its history, the German system has had troubled relations with its physicians, who have frequently gone on strike. Moreover, the job-related premiums are seen as a tax on labor.[5] Civil servants, retired citizens, and the unemployed contribute nothing, yet must be increasingly covered by the state. Fewer workers threaten to worsen matters. It's too early to see what form it will take, but it seems inevitable that reform will detach benefits from employment and the venerable system founded by the "iron chancellor" will more closely resemble the Beveridge model described below.[7]

Nevertheless, the employer-based system redistributes wealth to provide universal health coverage, as have similar systems in France, the Netherlands, and Japan. Life expectancy and other health measures are very good in these countries, and all citizens have guaranteed health care. Expenditures are about 10 percent of each nation's gross domestic product (GDP) except for Japan, which spends less (see tables 17-1 and 17-2).

TABLE 17-1
Health Expenditures in Several Countries, 2002[7]

Country	Health-Care System Model	Expenditure per Capita (US$)	Expenditure (% GDP*)	Expenditure (% Public Funding)	Doctors/ 1,000 Persons
Australia	Beveridge	1,741	9.2	68	2.5
Canada	Beveridge	2,058	9.5	71	2.1
Cuba	State	185	7.2	86	5.3
France	Bismarck	2,102	7.6	76	3.3
Germany	Bismarck	2,412	10.8	75	3.6
Japan	Bismarck	2,627	8.0	78	1.9
Russia	Ex State	115	5.3	68	4.2
Sweden	Beveridge	2,150	8.7	85	3.0
United Kingdom	Beveridge	1,835	7.6	82	2.0
United States	Entre-preneurial	4,887	13.9 (18.4 by 2013)[8]	44	2.7

*GDP: Gross Domestic Product

TABLE 17-2
Some Health Indicators in Various Countries, 2000

Country	Health-Care System Model[9]	Life Expect-ancy (Years)[10]	Infant Mortality (per 1000 Live Births)[11]	Child Mortality <5 years (per 1000)[12]	Immunization with DPT[3] (% Population)[13]	Maternal Mortality (per 100,000)[14]
Australia	Beveridge	79	6	6	93	8
Canada	Beveridge	79	5	7	97	6
Cuba	State	77	7	9	99	33
France	Bismarck	79	4	6	98	17
Germany	Bismarck	78	4	5	97	8
Japan	Bismarck	82	3	5	95	10
Russia	Ex State	66	18	21	96	67
Sweden	Beveridge	80	3	3	99	2
United Kingdom	Beveridge	77	5	7	91	13
United States	Entre-preneurial	77	7	8	94	17

Beveridge Model

The British health-care system is rooted in the Poor Law of 1834 and rural "friendly societies" that pooled health-care resources. There were adjustments as people moved to cities during the industrial revolution, but the first major legislation was Lloyd George's 1911 National Health Insurance Bill that provided general-practitioner care for poor workers. This echoed, but failed to match, the Bismarck system. By the 1940s, half of British citizens were insured, despite the workers' objections to payroll deductions. The GPs, fearing unequal money distribution, opted for a capitation system (where the physician receives a flat fee for each patient on her "list") that survives today. In 1942, with German bombers overhead, the Beveridge report recommended a major postwar overhaul of British social services and the introduction of the National Health Service (NHS).[15] The Labour Party's defeat of Winston Churchill's Conservatives led to its implementation in 1948. According to the NHS act, citizen's rights are:

- to be registered with a general practitioner;
- to be referred to a specialist acceptable to him or her where the GP thinks it is necessary; and
- to receive emergency care at any time.

The GPs have lists of citizens for whose medical care they are responsible along with their medical records. Virtually every citizen is on a list. A GP's pay is scaled according to the size of her list (capitation). Specialists are hospital based and salaried. Their contracts permit a minor portion of their time for private practice, to which about 10 percent of Britons subscribe through private insurance.

In practice, a patient with hip pain may consult his GP within the NHS.[16] The GP refers him to a specialist, who indicates that necessary surgery will be done a year hence, or longer.[17] However, the service is expedited if the patient chooses to "go private," where the expenses are paid by himself or his insurance company. The GP remains in charge of continuing care and the medical record. Referrals require a GP's letter and the consultant must respond with a report.

There have been innumerable attempts to reform the NHS, through competition between hospitals, regional authorities, and GP trusts where the GP controls the budget for her patients. The government even awards stars to hospitals that reach its objectives—a controversial practice that according to the editor of the *Lancet* demoralizes staff and undermines community confidence.[18] Some even suggest that individual physicians be rated publicly. Despite worries about cost and internal competitiveness, the NHS has been successful, combining respectable health data such as infant and fetal mortality with the lowest expenditure among developed countries (see tables 17-1 and 17-2). Much of the NHS success seems due to a tightly managed GP system. Ironically, the government seeks to compromise primary care with promises of choice and competition, while countries such as Canada, Germany, and France seek to restore it. Australia, France, Sweden, and Canada have adopted the Beveridge model, which is characterized by universal coverage, state funding, and state control of most health services. Health outcome indicators are similar to countries using the Bismarck model, for roughly equivalent expenditures (see tables 17-1 and 17-2). The British NHS seems to do the most with the least.

Canadian health care is sufficiently different from the others to warrant special mention. Federal legislation guarantees universality, accessibility, portability (between provinces), comprehensiveness, and public administration for all Canadians. There is only one payer, the provincial government, which retains a mainly fee-for-service payment system and permits some physician autonomy within the system. Uniquely, doctors cannot "extra bill" or practice outside the plan, unless they perform unlisted services like dentistry, cosmetic surgery, and removal of tattoos. (Physicians could practice independently and forgo all public payment until a recent change in Ontario regulations removed even that privilege.)[19] Patients are free to see as many GPs as they wish, and referral to specialists is informal. Hence, the medical record is fragmented, and often no one is in total charge of a person's health care. Medicare has been extremely popular, and Canadian health data are among the best (see table 17-2). However, in recent years, the thirteen Canadian provincial and territorial governments that run the plans have faced rapidly increasing health budgets, and patients experience long waiting periods for elective procedures. In the 1980s, on the dubious premise that doctors were the main cost generators, governments reduced the provincially funded medical school enrollments by up to 10 percent. Predictably, the critical shortage of doctors and rapidly aging population has resulted in long waiting lists, and many citizens cannot find a family doctor.[20] An estimated four hundred new orthopedic surgeons are required to service a population the size of California.[21]

ENTREPRENEURIAL MODEL

Among developed countries, the United States' health-care system is the only entrepreneurial model. In this system, "the goals of efficiency, increased productivity and cost containment take precedence over equal access to health services and equal treatment by medical personnel."[22] An American representative to an international conference on health resource allocation explained to other delegates, "The difference between you and us is that you guys believe in equity and we don't. In the US people are less interested in making sure everyone gets care than that those who can get it get great care. . . . People in the US want opportunity, not equity."[23] In line with this philosophy, the United States is the only developed nation where private financing of health care exceeds public funding (see table 17-1). Nevertheless, per capita public funding itself is similar to that of other countries and there are national programs for the elderly and disabled (Medicare) and, in conjunction with the states, for the disadvantaged (Medicaid).

While work-related health insurance and Blue Cross plans covered many Americans up to the 1960s, many were unprotected. Since then, health maintenance organizations (HMOs) deliver a list of services to an enrolled population and employers usually pay the fees. By 1998, 651 HMOs had enrolled sixty-five million members. When the Clinton Health Security Act failed in the early 1990s, for-profit managed-care organizations embraced many HMOs and set limits on individual medical encounters. Typically, HMOs contract doctors for their services, but staff-model HMOs such as Kaiser Permanente in Southern California, and Group Health of Puget Sound own their facilities, and doctors work exclusively for the organization.[24] Called a nonprofit "multispeciality group practice," Kaiser compares favorably with the British NHS.[25] Unlike the NHS, it is funded by employer-subsidized premiums and individual subscriptions, and makes no claim to universality. Most Kaiser members have an ongoing primary-care doctor, but integration with specialists and other services permits the organization to provide competitive health care with one-third of the hospital use of the NHS and at similar cost.[26] Kaiser and similar nonprofit plans provide care to less than 5 percent of the United States population.[27] Ownership and integrated care characterize the Kaiser organization, but subscribers accept an egalitarian philosophy and limited choice.[28] Systematic reviews indicate that nonprofit private hospitals such as Kaiser have lower mortality rates and costs than for-profit private hospitals.[29] Given the many competing health plans in California, a less than 3 percent subscriber turnover indicates Kaiser's success.

No brief summary can begin to characterize the many ways that Americans insure themselves for health care. However in 1998, 16 percent of Americans were enrolled with public plans only, 69 percent with private insurers and various health-maintenance plans, and 16 percent (44 million people) were uninsured. The uninsured are expected to be 60 million by 2008.[30] Many more are underinsured, as employers seek ways to reduce premiums, and insurers avoid risk by

limiting coverage to healthy organs. Not only do the poor have difficulty obtaining health-care insurance, but self-employed people face
high premiums or may even find themselves uninsurable if they have
an affliction as minor as hay fever.[31] In 2001 almost 1.5 million American families filed for bankruptcy.[32] A sample of 931 filers were interviewed and almost half cited medical causes, even though 75 percent
had insurance at the beginning of their illnesses.

The cost of medical care in the United States is about twice that of
most other developed countries (see table 17-1). Much of this difference is accounted for by overhead costs.[32] In 1999 the United States'
administration cost US$1,059 per capita compared to US$397 per
capita in Canada. Between 1964 and 1999, health-care administration's
share of the United States health-care labor force grew from 18 percent
to 27 percent compared to 16 percent and 19 percent in Canada (insurance company employees excluded). Similar differences are reported in
Australia, which provides universal insurance with a blended public and
subsidized private system.[34] There, private administration accounts for
12 percent of premiums compared to 0.6 percent in the public system.

The entrepreneurial system exists in some developing countries
such as the Philippines, Thailand, and Bangladesh. In China, free
enterprise serves the increasingly wealthy middle class, but not eight
hundred million farmers or the urban poor.[35] The costs, complexities,
and inequalities of the United States' system need reform. Debate
seems frozen, as it is for different reasons in France, Canada, and elsewhere. In no national debate do the proponents of reform address the
issues that motivate this book—the need for good doctor/patient relationships and the importance of evidence-based medicine.

State Model

Canada and other developed countries do not have "socialized medicine." That term characterized medical care delivery in communist
countries. While the Soviet states guaranteed universal access to health
care, they restricted patient and professional freedoms, and failed
because of inadequate funding. By 2000 the former Soviet Union's
health-care budget had fallen to US$115 per citizen compared to
US$185 per person in Cuba and $4,887 in the United States (see table
17-1). Most Russian health indicators, including life expectancy, have
worsened since the 1960s. Former Eastern Bloc countries will likely

adopt systems similar to those of western Europe.[36] Cuba anachronistically clings to the state system with expenditures that are less than 10 percent of developed countries. Nevertheless, some Cuban health indicators compare reasonably well and are much superior to those of the Russian Republic (see table 17-2).

PRIMARY-CARE REMUNERATION

If the GP or family doctor is to manage an individual's care, society needs to think carefully how he should be remunerated. There are three basic systems: *capitation, fee-for-service, salary*, and combinations of these.

Capitation

In a capitation system, the doctor receives a fixed amount for every patient on his list. Physicians are rewarded according to the size of their lists, but the system is relatively noncompetitive. In countries such as the Netherlands[37] and Great Britain,[38] where capitation is the norm, everyone is on a list and therefore theoretically everyone has a GP. Among the advantages of this system are continuity of care, no incentive to overservice, centralization of the medical record, and an institutional gatekeeper system where access to specialists is through the GP. From the payer's viewpoint, the costs are predictable and controllable. Disadvantages include limited choice. Although one can change his GP, it must be done formally with transfer of the medical record. There are also incentives to limit the availability of appointments, keep visit times to a minimum, and maintain an office-only practice.[39] As discussed earlier, capitation in the NHS permits very short patient/doctor interactions. In the United States and Canada a few family doctors and GPs are paid in this way.[40] There is some concern that capitation's lack of incentives and competition leads to inefficiency, and one commentator calls it a "haven for Laziness."[41]

Fee-for-Service

Fee-for-service is the normal means of remuneration in Canada (85%),[42] the United States, and several European countries.[43] The incentive under this system is to see as many patients as possible, an important consideration where family doctors are in short supply. In general, this system is more competitive and responsive to patient's demands. In Belgium fee-for-service permits 46 percent of GP-patient encounters to occur in the home,[44] while the service is negligible in the Netherlands where capitation is the norm. Many see disadvantages. Primary-care physicians are rewarded for seeing many patients briefly and discouraged from employing other health professionals for appropriate services.[45] Several visits earn more than one "good" visit, and in chapter 12, we learned that short visits are associated with overprescribing, less preventative medicine, and little time to discuss psychosocial issues. Governments and many health-care economists dislike fee-for-service but must tread lightly in the current climate of increasing demand and declining doctor supply. Fee-for-service makes sense when you personally pay the doctor for what he does (as for your plumber). However, when a third party pays, even if it is your own insurance company, the usual market forces do not exist. When a patient pays for a visit that is delayed, too short, or otherwise unsatisfactory, he blames the doctor. When others pay, they share the blame.

Salary

There are salaried physicians responsible for the care of workers or the members of companies and institutions. In the United Kingdom, salaried consultants are the norm. Salary was how physicians in the now-discredited and disbanded state systems were paid. Now, many physicians wish to work part-time and/or be uninvolved in practice management. In many countries, entrepreneurs pay doctors a salary. From a health perspective, salary can be similar to capitation except for the profits of the entrepreneur, but in many countries, salary-based walk-in clinics fail to provide continuity of care. About 35 percent of British GPs are salaried.[46] In Canada about 15 percent receive a salary for all or part of their income.[47] Salary may support the doctor/patient relationship no better than capitation or fee-for-service, but it lessens the need to crowd too many patients into an appointment schedule. Ideological rigidity serves us ill. Only by experimenting with various forms of payments and incentives will we learn what works best.

Blended Systems

Some governments explore ways to capture the best features of different systems. There are attempts to combine capitation for basic payment, and fee-for-service to achieve certain objectives. In the United Kingdom[48] and Australia,[49] there are financial incentives for certain programs such as vaccination or cancer screening. However, such blends can also capture the worst features of both, as doctors, being human, will seek activities that maximize income, while governments and insurers overreact with bureaucratic regulations. France, New Zealand, and others blend private and public funds to remunerate doctors, while in the United Kingdom, some citizens who can afford it choose private care.

Sadly, governments and health-care administrators focus mainly on cost containment, with some lip service to the sometimes contradictory notions of risk management and quality assurance.[50] In Canada and the United Kingdom, long waiting lists rightly capture the public's attention. Seldom mentioned are effective doctor/patient relationships and the judicious employment of medical evidence. Without these, no health service can efficiently satisfy patient demands, ensure quality health care, and reduce waste and medical error. No existing payment plan guarantees compassion and judicious use of medical evidence, yet without these, unnecessary tests and treatments, repeated consultations, and misdirected resources are inevitable. Such waste may be exacerbated if there are incentives or restrictions that reduce the time a doctor spends with her patients.

DISILLUSIONMENT

Before 1965, when Canada implemented national health insurance, physicians depended on their patients' fees. Those who practiced among the poor were often unpaid or were paid in kind. As an unmarried GP in a rural community, I received eggs in lieu of my $4 fee for a house call. (I learned to boil them.) Much city hospital work was charity, where clinicians taught medical students in clinics caring for indigent "public" patients. With the introduction of medicare in Canada, there were no more bad debts, and physicians' incomes rose comfortably. The pejorative "public patient" disappeared from the vernacular, and eggs ceased to be currency. The 1970s in Canada were the golden years of health care when physicians' financial worries receded, yet their autonomy remained. People who remembered the past were grateful for free doctor's services, and the system worked well. Gradually, however, costs and demand for services grew. Physicians' fee schedules failed to keep pace with inflation. Governments attempted to control costs by manipulating physician manpower and behavior. Now, few remember the pre-Medicare days, and free medical care has become a right, not a privilege.

Health costs consume 46 percent of Ontario's budget and are increasing at 8 percent annually at the expense of education, roads, social services, and other provincial responsibilities.[51] While the system is judged to be "unsustainable," ideas of reform invite derogatory rhetoric such as "taxing the sick" and "privatizing the system," or worse, "US-style medicine." Rising public expectations and doctor shortages compound the problem and doctor/patient contact suffers accordingly—no support for placebo effects or evidence-based decisions here. Open-minded discussion is required to equip Canadian medicare to meet the needs of retiring and increasingly ill baby boomers.

This sequence was echoed in Australia, which introduced medicare a decade later.[52] Now only 19 percent of Australians express satisfaction with the health service.[53] In the United Kingdom 69 percent are dissatisfied with their NHS.[54] Similar unhappiness is rife in Germany[55] and France,[56] where the specter of declining ratios of workers to retirees threatens future benefits. In Germany patients can see specialists without a GP referral, and doctor shopping is common. The government's cost-containment plans for copayments and increased GP control of patient care provoke angry protests. In France the 2003 heat wave was associated with fifteen thousand deaths, and it exposed weaknesses in their system, just recently rated the finest in the world by the World Health Organization (WHO). French patients are happy. Doctors make house calls, waiting lists do not exist, and mothers remain in the hospital five days after delivery. French men and women can go to as many physicians (GP or specialist) as they wish, a practice known as *nomadism médicale*.[57] The French use more drugs than other countries, in a system of rampant consumption that the minister of health describes as "mad." Rising costs, a doctor shortage, incentives to use the system, and a legislated thirty-five-hour workweek for health-care personnel all contribute to a financial crisis that is compelling unpopular reforms.[58] Reforms introduced in 2004 and 2005 are described as introducing state-led managed care where patients must register with a single family doctor (gatekeeper), and make a small copayment with each visit.[59] The French see doctors twice as often as Americans,[60] and have better indicators of health status (see table 17-2). No data measure the length of the doctor/patient relationship, nor the application of evidence and placebo effects during therapeutic encounters.

National medical care is experiencing difficulties throughout the developed world. Many say that more funding is the solution, yet Britain has maintained comparable health-care results with the least funding. Clearly, funding is not the only health determinant. Britain's relative cost containment may be due to its GP system, which theoretically establishes more long-term primary care doctor/patient relationships than exist elsewhere. Kaiser Permanente builds on this model and by integration of primary, secondary, and hospital care is able to achieve better outcomes and less hospitalization at a lower cost than the NHS. In light of this, it may be counterproductive for the British government to offer more choices.

In the United States, hopes for a primary-care revival were thwarted by third-party interference and the need for large corporations to control costs.[61] In the early 1980s health maintenance organizations mandated family doctors to expand services and reduce costs through "managed care." They were to act as "gatekeepers" controlling access to expensive specialists, and sometimes forbidden to mention expensive treatments or tests to patients ("gag rules"). Bonuses awaited practitioners who kept services down. This placed family doctors in a conflict of interest, yet uncooperative physicians could have their contracts terminated without cause.[62] A class-action lawsuit reflects the tensions between physicians accused of overbilling and managed care organizations alleged to delay or obstruct payments to improve their bottom line.[63] Low pay, strains in the doctor/patient relationship, declining respect, and decreased enrollment in family practice programs led one commentator to lament the "end of primary care."[64] Meanwhile, HMO members were told which physicians they could see. Patients and physicians sensed that managed care was harming the quality of medical care.[65] In one survey, over 75 percent of respondents described the medical-care system as a nightmare to navigate.[68] This caused a backlash, and by 1996 there were fifty-six state laws passed attempting to regulate the HMOs.[67] By the late 1990s some claimed that the needs of the uninsured and cost containment were beyond the capabilities of managed care,[68] and that it was a "failed experiment."[69]

In no other developed country do others interfere as much in the doctor/patient relationship. Direct access to specialists has long been a feature of American medicine, but managed care has thrust many GPs into the conflicted "gatekeeper" role, which appears to be ineffective.[70] There are media "horror stories" of payment denials for emergency room visits, for more than twenty-four-hour postpartum care, or for expensive lifesaving procedures. HMOs have been sued. Reports of egregious executive salaries and the retention by some HMOs of up to thirty cents of every premium dollar aggravate public unease.[71]

Because people who are healthy and insured are generally satisfied despite high premiums, and those who are uninsured tend to be poor and politically inarticulate, there is little incentive for fundamental change. As in Canada, an unwillingness to abandon or modify outmoded ideology inhibits reform.[72] Few politicians are willing to take on the $1.6-trillion health-care industry,[73] so it seems likely to continue to be "a paradox of excess and deprivation."[74] Meanwhile, HMO attempts to reduce services or increase premiums will be resisted by the public and employers,[75] and companies are seeking to reduce their health-care costs.

The data in tables 17-1 and 17-2 suggest that America is not getting value for its money, and Hillary Clinton contends that liberals and conservatives alike would not "fashion the kind of health care system America has inherited."[76] The triad of having the world's highest health-care per capita budget by far, 15 percent of its people uninsured, and health indicators that are no better, or worse, than other developed countries suggests that indeed something is amiss. Not only does administration consume $300 billion,[77] but there is evidence that some of those who are insured may be getting too much care, which is detrimental to their health.[78] Per capita Medicare spending is $10,550 in Manhattan, where practice is more in-patient and specialist oriented, and only $4,823 in Portland, Oregon, with no difference in illness, price, or outcome. In addition, the Department of Veterans Affairs achieved better care and better outcomes by decreasing hospital beds and focusing on high-level primary care.

More is not necessarily better,[79] and, as we have seen, unnecessary testing and treatment can be hazardous.

UNHAPPY PROFESSIONALS

Medical associations greeted the introduction of national health insurance in Canada and Australia with bitter strikes. In both protests doctor "refugees" from the British NHS led the resistance to perceived assaults on physician autonomy. However, once Medicare was in place, most doctors accepted the guaranteed fee payments and there was great public satisfaction. Interference with physician autonomy was slow to materialize. By the late 1980s, cost controls began to restrict physician incomes, and physician unrest returned. Primary-care doctor shortages began to hamper medical care in some countries, aggravated by early retirements. In Canada the government ordered cutbacks in medical graduates just as baby boomers began retiring. This, along with fewer working hours[80] caused a doctor shortage, which a recently increased medical school enrollment will take years to correct.[81] The shortage is compounded by fewer graduates choosing family practice[82] and a declining involvement of family doctors in hospitals, nursing homes, house calls, emergency medicine, and obstetrics.[83]

Sixty-one percent of British medical school admissions are women, sparking a debate of the future of the medical workforce in Britain.[84] In 2004, 81 percent of the incoming medical class at Laval University in Quebec were women, and more than half of Canadian and medical graduates are female.[85] This is a good thing, but a 1980s champion of women doctors now notes that "men are no longer embracing medicine because the profession is devalued, both financially and socially. Doctors don't get as much respect as they used to, they earn much less than businessmen and engineers, and their autonomy is shrinking in an increasingly bureaucratized system."[86] Worldwide, men and women are working fewer hours,[87] making it even more difficult to see a doctor.

Strikes in support of better pay and working conditions occurred throughout the long history of many European health systems. Recent strikes in Italy and protests in Germany and France continue this tradition. Among Europeans, only British doctors accept their fate without industrial action, but their erstwhile possibility of escape to the colonies looks to be less attractive now.

After World War II, Americans saw the introduction of effective treatments, and medical insurance covered many people. Amidst general prosperity, physicians enjoyed a golden age of professional independence, with admiring assistants, loyal patients, respectful colleagues, and financial security.[88] By the 1980s all that changed. Managed care intruded deeply into doctor's professional lives. Primary-care doctors found "gatekeeper" duties competed for their attention with patient care.[89] Since then, there have been pressures to see more patients and to refer or prescribe less frequently. As in Canada, fewer graduates choose primary care.[90] Some specialists find themselves bidding for inclusion in HMO rosters, a process that erodes their incomes. Doctors must deal with Medicare, Medicaid, and the myriad insurance and managed-care plans each with unique rules and payment schedules. In some cases, specialists must check with the insurer before providing a service, and the decision may lie in the hands of a clerk. Many physicians complain of their inability to meet their patients' ever-rising expectations.

The irony is that the American Medical Association (AMA) vehemently opposed any government-sponsored universal medical-care plan as a threat to physician autonomy. It only reluctantly accepted Medicare and Medicaid.[91] Yet private-system bureaucrats are often more troublesome to physicians than their government counterparts in Canada, where the single-payer system is straightforward and electronic. The AMA has shifted its position to favor universal medicare,[92] but the conversion is late. Like sister associations in Canada, Britain, and elsewhere, the AMA has a diminished influence on health-care policy.

Physicians are disillusioned. Surveys show that, if able to choose again, 30 to 40 percent of American physicians would not now choose medicine as a career.[93] Even more would not recommend the profession to their children or another young person. A quarter of final year physicians-in-training said that they would not choose medicine again. In a Canadian survey, only 20 percent of doctors are very satisfied with their lives, and almost a quarter are planning to retire or leave practice.[94] Despite the French people's happiness with their unparalleled freedom of access to a very responsive system, doctors feel underpaid and experience increasing difficulties with administrators and government (*les étrangers?*). Italian doctors are striking against new restrictions on their practices,[95] and German physicians are unwillingly becoming "tax collectors."[96] Thus for different reasons, doctors in developed countries are unhappy. A *British Medical Journal* commentary asked why,[97] and received responses all over the world citing overwork, lack of support, loss of status, demanding patients, and negative media attention.[98] According to an Australian doctor, intrusive bureaucratic paperwork forces GPs to practice "consultio interruptus."[99]

DOCTOR/PATIENT RELATIONSHIPS AND HEALTH-CARE ORGANIZATION

This unhappiness should not be dismissed as the justified humiliation of a proud profession. The changes bode ill for doctor/patient relationships and the compassionate care of patients. One should expect physician dissatisfaction to breed poor clinical management, and evidence supports it.[100] The rapid turnover of doctors and patients within plans leads to discontinuous care, and lack of physician authority impairs patients' compliance with treatments. Doctor shortages, a record number of retirements, and decreased time spent with patients aggravate doctor and public dissatisfaction.

If we believe that positive attitudes and placebo effects are important to citizens' well-being, then the intrusions in doctors' examining rooms can be health hazards. A nation's health-care system may not itself be a nocebo, but physicians' dissatisfaction with its bureaucracy can have nocebo effects. While the media, administrators, and politicians focus on waiting lists, the number of magnetic resonance imaging machines per population, or the need to cope with out-of-control drug costs, they ignore the very interface of medical care where these problems are rooted: the interaction of patients with doctors, nurses, and other health-care professionals. Whatever ideology prevails, individual healer/patient encounters remain medicine's front line. As any good general knows, morale, support, and supplies for the troops are essential to success. Functioning doctor/patient relationships must be encouraged—they can save money in the end.

EVIDENCE-BASED MEDICARE

Where possible, medical care should be evidence based. The placebo effect has a dual personality. On the one hand, it is the key ingredient of the art of medicine. On the other, its effect is the standard against which treatments must be judged. In part 2 we discussed placebo controls as a key element in the evaluation of diagnosis and treatment. However, the evidence seldom fits the patient exactly. Indeed, almost half of patient visits in family practice permit no medical diagnosis,[101] and the patients are "temporarily dependent."[102]

Some physicians' vague distrust of the evidence-based movement reflects the day-to-day uncertainty of patient outcomes. Many object to subordination of clinical judgment to the dictates of evidence-based enthusiasts and fear becoming tyrannized by evidence, as interpreted by managers or clerks. Professional opinion is placed at the bottom of the evidence hierarchy, and patients' preferences are given short shrift.[103] However, the definition of evidence-based medicine specifies the "*judicious* use of current best evidence," and "more effective and efficient diagnosis and . . . more thoughtful identification of individual patients' predicaments, rights and preferences. . . ."[104] Doctors must use individual clinical expertise *and* best evidence—neither alone will do.

Who can make the diagnosis, find out the patient's preferences, know his unique circumstances, and judiciously present him with the options and their probabilities of success? Not the strangers! Surely this is the role of the family doctor and her specialist advisors. The front lines of evidence-based medicine are in doctors' examining rooms and at hospital bedsides, not departments of health or HMO boardrooms. Health-care organizations that fail to permit and equip practitioners to judiciously apply medical evidence at the point of contact are doomed to unsatisfactory service and ultimately, greater costs.

Yet there is little understanding or support for the family doctor in most systems. Freedom of choice often means that no one is fully in charge of the patient's care, and the medical record is fragmented. In Canada and France, patients are free to doctor shop, with no unified record to ensure coherent treatment. In Germany, France, and the United States, direct access to specialists for a single-organ problem compromises total care, especially if a second problem lies outside the specialist's purview. In contrast, coordinated care provided by multispecialty group practices such as Kaiser Permanente or the revamped veterans' systems in the United States offer continuing primary-care relationships with ready access to specialists, who share the patient's electronic medical record.[105] In the United Kingdom, the Netherlands, and at Kaiser Permanente, general practitioners play a central role.[106] Ideally, the family doctor should coordinate medical care, while ensuring the "judicious" application of evidence-based medicine and a continuing doctor/patient relationship.

The media and television glorify the drama of acute illnesses and spectacular cures. Most systems respond well to emergencies since they are in the public eye and since physicians usually drop everything to deal with them. However, 75 percent of direct health-care costs are for chronic illnesses that affect 46 percent of Americans.[107] Few reporters or artists dramatize primary care management of the chronically ill, where cures and rescues are rare. We can determine the costs and morbidity benefits of diagnostic tests[108] or cancer screening from society's perspective,[109] but know little of the value of tests to a person's well being (see figure 5-2).[110] We can work out the utility of a new drug,[111] but not that of a good family doctor's placebo effect. Economists can estimate the cost of liver transplants for the very few, but who can fathom the complexities of daily encounters of the many with nurses, doctors, and dentists. As an American Medicare spokesman put it, "[W]e will probably approve . . . billions of dollars for biventricular pacing, yet we still don't know how to pay for someone to have their own doctor."[112]

Investigators supported by the RAND Corporation interviewed Americans in twelve cities about 439 "indicators of quality of health care."[113] After reviewing the medical records, they found that the participants received only 53 percent of the recommended evidence-based prevention and treatment options. This illustrates the need to bring evidence to doctors' examining rooms and provide sufficient time to deploy it. None of the 439 indicators concerned the doctor/patient relationship, yet without it, evidence-based decisions will fail to attain their potential.

INFORMATION TECHNOLOGY

There must be better ways of providing information to doctors, particularly family doctors. The entire patient record should be available electronically. With controls to protect patient confidentiality, a doctor could review drug history, previous surgeries, and other information without relying on the vagaries of memory. (In a survey, 40 percent of Swedes on a national registry forgot broken bones they had suffered nine to fourteen years before.)[114]

Equally important, primary-care physicians need access to usable information about medical evidence. Just as too much care can be harmful, so can too much information. The Cochrane Collaboration is a start, but the reports need to be continuously updated and the conclusions made more primary care–friendly. In the United States, the federal Agency for Healthcare Research and Quality sponsors systemic reviews to assist public- and private-sector health-care organizations. However, these are too comprehensive to be digested by time-challenged family doctors. Collecting and evaluating medical evidence should be an international effort, perhaps sponsored by the WHO,[115] utilizing Cochrane expertise and coordinating national initiatives.

We have observed that patients have too little time to talk to their doctors, and that many with chronic or benign disorders seek solace with CAM. What does this cost? Who will address the paradoxes of medical-insurance plans that exclude dentistry, or FDA regulations that do not apply to CAM, or free choice that fragments care and leads to redundant, excessive, and sometimes harmful treatments? How will we deal with the biases in evidence and education that follow from pharmaceutical largesse? How can medical evidence best be translated into action in doctors' examining rooms? These questions have yet to be addressed by those who would organize medical services.

CONCLUSIONS

National health-care systems evolved independently, with unique histories, philosophies, and management practices. Nevertheless, they share rising costs and demands, complaining patients, and unhappy doctors. Missing from national discussions of the nature and future of medical care are thoughtful considerations of the art of empathetic doctor/patient interaction and the healing placebo effect on the one hand, and the judicious application of medical evidence on the other. In an otherwise thoughtful essay about the US health-care crisis, Hillary Clinton omits these two themes entirely.[116] When health care was raised in the 2004 national election campaigns in the United States and Canada, politicians clung to their national myths, avoiding serious discussion of these complicated health-care issues. The results are ill-informed electorates in both countries.

The family doctor has a central role to play in the successful execution of these tasks. For her to do so the profession must afford her sufficient status, and health-care authorities must provide her with the tools and incentives to do the job. Expel the strangers from the examining room and assign them a supporting role, rather than a merely regulatory one. Give the doctor more face time with her patients, and place less administration between them. Provide her with electronic access to the patient record as well as independent and reliable information about medical evidence. Devise remuneration formulas that reward patient care quality, not quantity or gatekeeper responsibilities. Put family doctors in charge of the patient's electronic medical record, which could promptly, formally, and legally be transferred when the patient changes doctors. Make it part of her duties to visit her patients when they are in the hospital so she can truly be her patients' advocate and counsel, and provide continuity after discharge. Family doctors at least must not be strangers to their patients. Insist that specialists become consultants in the original sense of the word, not transiently engaged technicians. A health-care system built around a properly prepared and equipped family doctor maximizing the doctor/patient relationship and judiciously applying medical evidence and specialist expertise will require many changes. Nothing less ambitious can restore public confidence and provide economies in our fragmented, wasteful, and expensive medical-care systems. Unlike the guests in North American living rooms, we need to discuss the taboos, stop disparaging other systems and learn from one another. As Mencken implied, the solution of health care's problems will be neither "neat nor simple," but if based on good doctor/patient relationships and reliable evidence, it cannot be "wrong."

CHAPTER 18

PHYSICIANS, HEAL YOURSELVES

> "What has become of our calling? The answer depends upon
> whom we listen to . . . licensing boards, credentialing com-
> mittees, peer-review organizations, and insurance carriers,
> but they do not define us. . . . The one person who will chal-
> lenge us the most, who will deliver us to our finest hours,
> who will talk to us through every moral conundrum, is the
> patient, who we thought needed *us*."

> DAVID LOXTERCAMP[1]

A merican doctors are described as a profession in retreat, plagued by bureaucracy, loss of autonomy, diminished pres- tige, and deep personal dissatisfaction.[2] One metaphor describes unhappy doctors "mourning the passage of a beloved profession with the full cascade of denial, anger, bargaining, depression and accept- ance."[3] Physician disillusionment is not unique to the United States— physicians from the Netherlands,[4] the United Kingdom,[5] Canada,[6] and elsewhere have eloquently written of their sense of loss. The *British Medical Journal* attracted correspondence from disaffected physicians from around the world.[7] Unhappy doctors deliver inferior health care and certainly little placebo effect.

Trained during the "golden years," many older physicians are dis- appointed with their careers. Many young doctors are unhappy as well. Medical graduates shun general practice.[8] Disappointment is none the better for realizing that the profession itself is partly respon- sible for its own decline, through resisting medicare and lay participa- tion in medical decisions, generating unreasonable expectations, over- reliance on technology, and estrangement from patients. Nonetheless, realizing past errors may help doctors deal with the future. Students usually enter medicine to help people, but other priorities draw them away from such idealism, as if "[w]ith what [they] most enjoy con- tented least."[9]

Although many doctors seem discouraged today, things are not as bad as they seem. Certainly, their predecessors' practices were not

Nirvana. Before the postwar "golden years," many doctors found it difficult to make a living. While sophisticated diagnosis was common by the 1930s, treatment for most diseases was ineffective. Few modern doctors would wish to return to the horse-and-buggy house call, the bad debts, and the appalling infant and child mortality that preceded the era of antibiotics and effective immunization. Physician autonomy usually meant physicians were on their own financially as well as professionally. The golden age is the anomaly, not what went on before.[10] To rescue the medical profession from its current international funk, physicians will need to develop new attitudes. Primary-care doctors, consultants, and academics can do much to reorient health care to compassion and cognition rather than hardware and anecdote. Pills, procedures, and other technology are merely tools to help doctors help patients, not ends in themselves.

By recapturing the idealism that once attracted them to medical school, physicians can find joy in their noble profession. Talking to patients, sharing their triumphs and sorrows, and providing empathy with the best that medical evidence can offer are what a doctor should aspire to.

THE NEW PROFESSIONALISM

Some call for a new medical professionalism.[11] The British General Medical Council (GMC) developed a regulatory framework for a "new professionalism" for doctors.[12] Malaise among British doctors and scandals including professional misconduct in a children's cardiac surgery unit and a general practitioner who was a serial killer prompted this initiative. The GMC promotes the teaching of medical humanities, communication, and clinical skill. Regular assessment of physicians' fitness to practice will involve government and lay representatives—more strangers in the examining room. In every developed country, physicians are engaging in mandatory continuing medical education and some form of professional "relicensure."

Is "professional" correct? Dictionaries turn up terms like "expert," "vocation," "engaging in a given activity as a source of livelihood or as a career." Each fails to convey what we mean. David Rothman is especially scathing in his assessment of medical "professionalism" in the United States, where he claims it must be invented, rather than restored.[13] Such criticisms are important but not the main subject matter here. The critics and the term "professional" fail to embrace the ideas central to this book—that compassionate doctor/patient interaction can independently help people, and that judicious, evidence-based clinical decisions are essential to good medical practice. Here we consider how to exploit these unique attributes of the good doctor.

WHAT DOCTORS CAN DO

Physicians' associations have decreasing influence in health-care policy, sometimes functioning more like trade unions than promoters of professional values. Nevertheless, individual doctors can do much by exploiting the placebo effect and embracing evidence-based principles in their daily practice. Academics can provide leadership through research and continuing medical education to inspire their students with the human and scientific sides of medicine.

Primary-Care Physicians

Most primary-care doctors instinctively understand the placebo response and the importance of having an ongoing therapeutic rapport with their patients. To many, that is what primary care is about. However, this role is constrained by the demands of modern life. Family doctors lack sufficient time to nurture their relationships with patients or pursue the ever-changing world of medical evidence. Many prefer to work part-time or locate in storefront locations where continuity of care is minimal, and the medical record is someone else's responsibility. The personal reasons behind such choices are understandable, but family doctors and their associates should seek to manage this better. They should regard their patients' total medical care and its record as *their* responsibility, and insist on communication with and reports from the specialists they consult. They should keep electronic medical records and ensure that other doctors covering their practices maintain them in their absence. The family doctor, medicine's human face, should know the patient as a person.

Family doctors can pressure their associations and academic colleagues to produce unbiased and more efficient continuing medical education. Dependence on industry-sponsored information is not in patients' best interests. Drugs cost most health systems more than physician services. Self-interest, if not lack of supporting evidence, should prompt physicians to prescribe wisely, lest their share of the budget should further diminish. Tempering the positive attitudes of the doctor/patient relationship with skepticism of treatments seems a contradiction. However, skepticism is not cynicism, and demanding the evidence is not a negative attitude. Indeed, the ability to say, "I don't know" when appropriate should inspire confidence, not despair.[14] That is why there are consultants.

Specialists should serve as consultants, not as those to whom care is permanently transferred. It should be clear that the family doctor is in charge of ongoing care, and a consultant's report to her should state the precise diagnosis, prognosis, and treatment plan. Chronic painful disorders such as fibromyalgia, chronic back pain, or irritable bowel may overlap several specialties and be diagnosed according to the specialist the patient happens to see.[15] When symptoms blur specialty lines, the primary-care doctor, knowing the patient and his family, is best positioned to supervise. When there is no specific problem to solve, referral can invite unnecessary procedures and inappropriate therapy.

In hospitals, many consultants, each with his priorities and retinue, confuse patients. Hospitals, health-care organizations, and specialists working in separate silos[16] communicate poorly with each other, the patient, and the primary-care doctor. In many North American institutions, "hospitalists" manage inpatients, but this is only a partial solution.[17] No one is in charge of the patient's total care, and continuity of care discontinues upon discharge. Doctors are strangers to patients and to each other. If we are to have a team approach to medical care, then we must have a team leader who transcends the artificial borders that divide specialties. The patient's family doctor must return to visiting the hospital, assume responsibility for coordination of the patient's care, and be the human face of medicine. She will periodically need to delegate care to specialists, but be there when the patient is discharged.

Consultants

Many consultants risk making technology an end, rather than a means to an end, thereby diminishing their value as consultants. It is a paradox that specialists must spend ten or more years learning science and analytical thinking, while their professional time and income may be largely dependent on technical skills they learned in the last few months of their training. A further paradox is that society rewards doctors most for technical procedures that sometimes could be done by well-trained and supervised technicians, and reward them least for the more challenging tasks of formulating evidence-based opinions and achieving positive interactions with patients.

Technical skill is important to be sure, but judging *when* it is useful is even more so. A surgeon must not only know how to operate but also *when*. Unnecessary surgery is costly and harmful. The rates of eleven common operations on Medicare patients from 306 regions of the United States were found to vary greatly.[18] Some, including restoring blood flow to the lower extremity or to the brain, back surgery, and radical prostate surgery were performed ten times more frequently in one region than in another. Fee-for-service surgeons in North America perform more elective gallbladder surgery than their salaried counterparts in the United Kingdom. Do these data mean that some patients have unnecessary surgery, or that others fail to get necessary surgery? Patients with irritable bowel are prone to unnecessary operations.[19] Decisions to operate should be evidence based, and time should be spent talking to patients.

Many specialists do diagnostic and therapeutic procedures such as cardiac catheterization, colonoscopy, bronchoscopy, and stress tests. At first, such procedures are time consuming and require innovative skills. Powerful specialty societies secure high fees, but as equipment and experience improve, the test becomes safer, easier, and less time consuming. Yet the fee remains high compared to taking a history, performing a physical examination, establishing a diagnosis, and planning treatment in a caring, positive, and therapeutic manner. If physicians are to create positive patient relationships and ensure that their activities are evidence based in the patient's best interests, technology must be subordinate.

Another of modern medicine's many paradoxes is the call for physicians' assistants. Some propose that nurse practitioners or technicians take the medical history, prescribe treatments for "minor" illnesses, and thereby cheaply replace otherwise busy doctors, who presumably are doing things that are more important. Such a proposal illustrates what the profession has lost. What can be more important than taking a patient's history, establishing a therapeutic relationship, thinking of the humane and evidence-based options, and managing all dimensions of an illness? The paradox is that no one suggests that physician assistants do some of the mechanical, repetitive, and highly remunerative procedures that require lesser skills.

For example, gastroenterological associations (rightly) propose colon cancer prevention for all citizens at a certain age. (This is available to American Medicare beneficiaries.)[20] Timely removal of colonoscopy-discovered precancerous lesions can prevent colon cancer more reliably than smoking cessation prevents lung cancer. The impediments to screening colonoscopy are that it is expensive, and that there are insufficient facilities or gastroenterologists to screen everyone. The proposal would be more credible if other medical societies with no financial interest endorsed it, and if gastroenterologists proposed that supervised technicians do the screening. A precedent exists in diagnostic imaging, where technologists take the pictures, while doctors interpret them and perform any necessary interventions. Technicians command less pay, yet soon develop the necessary technical skills. Nurse endoscopists certainly do so safely.[21] Of course, physician endoscopists must supervise and must deal with any disease found by the technicians. Nonphysician endoscopy programs exist in Britain,[22] and some suggest them in Canada[23] and the United States.[24] Such physician-supervised programs would require fewer specialists, who would then be freer to concentrate on consulting.

Consultants are the family doctor's natural teachers. The learning objective should not be to make them minispecialists in every organ system, but rather to present evidence in digestible and usable packages. To do so, the consultant must better understand the challenges of primary care, where many interests compete for the family doctor's time.

Academic Medicine

For leadership, professionals must look to the medical schools. However, academic medicine is itself buffeted by the illogical economics of modern medicine. Traditionally, physicians in teaching hospitals donated their time to care for the poor and teach medical students and interns. This was not entirely altruistic, as the rewards were kudos and enhanced reputations. Still, as practicing general physicians and surgeons, they were role models and taught the basics of the clinical interview, examination, and therapeutic decision making. They would not use the term "placebo effect," but most achieved the effect nonetheless through their autonomy, authority, and singular relationships with patients. Now, everyone at a teaching hospital is a "professor,"[25] yet few are devoted to a clinical academic career. Equal status trumps excellence in clinical skill, teaching, and research. The need for physicians to fund their institution through their clinical earnings is an absurd feature of North American medical schools.[26] Required earning quotas and involuntary contributions are incompatible with a thoughtful academic mission. Medical schools need adequate public financing and a cadre of committed academic clinicians if they are to create, teach, and exemplify doctor/patient relationships and evidence-based medicine.

Whereas the professor of medicine was a role model and focus of medical education in the 1960s, his modern counterpart is virtually unknown to students. Rather than appointed for inspirational skills as a physician or teacher, the paramount attributes of the professor have become the "research profile" and the ability to garner funds for his institution. If medical schools attach such low priority to clinical skills, no wonder the profession is troubled. Professors of medicine and surgery should be in charge of, and engage in, education and *clinical* research, rather than become consumed with fiscal and management issues.

Medical schools should balance the humanities and sciences of medicine. Both are vital to the quality of patient care and the future happiness of the profession. By training the family doctor to be in charge of a person's health, we improve her status and interactions with her consultant colleagues. Then the patient will have an advocate, a friendly face familiar with his background, preferences, and psychosocial requirements. Training programs should promote consultant understanding of the broad social issues that affect patient care and force them to think and act outside their organ silos. They should also train technicians to lessen consultants' manual work in favor of the more difficult challenges of diagnosis and patient care.

Not only must academic clinicians in all specialties address a reorganization of medical practice, but they must also foster a clinical science. In yet another paradox, medical schools seek physicians who are laboratory researchers. After an aspiring academic completes the ten years of training as a doctor, he must spend several more years acquiring laboratory skills and care for rats and guinea pigs. When such a person joins the medical school, he must reconcile his duties to teach students and care for patients, with the need to compete for research grants with doctors of science who have no such duties. Clinicians are devalued, and clinical research is subordinated to the misplaced emphasis on clinician careers in basic science—a paradox indeed.[27]

While newer career paths of clinical epidemiology and clinical teaching help give academic physicians self-confidence, neither initiative necessarily addresses doctor/patient relationships and evidence-based clinical decision making. Clinical epidemiologists have brought us meta-analysis and the systematic review but also the shortcomings of armchair research. Practicing doctors should provide new medical evidence in partnership with informed patients. Clinical teachers should be role models and foster doctor/patient relationships, imparting a sophisticated understanding of the placebo effect's dual personality. The ideal is the clinician educator and investigator who teaches students not in the classroom, but in the examining room, and who addresses clinical problems scientifically with patients, not rats. Such persons can exemplify and teach the twin missions of medicine made implicit by the placebo effect—positive, humane doctor/patient interaction and the judicious application of medical evidence.

HUMANITIES IN MEDICINE

Medical training is based upon what the *Lancet* calls the "hard" sciences such as anatomy, physiology, and pathology.[28] Medical schools must prepare doctors to cope with a massive amount of scientific information, while they ignore the humanities. Students master the medical sciences. Then, once in practice, they must cope with the not-so-scientific business of caring for patients, where "the quasi-rational human psyche is continually colliding with the scientific method."[29] Evidence-based medicine can indicate what large groups of patients might do under certain circumstances, but not what an individual may do. To help an individual, a doctor must know her patient's personality, his psychosocial predicament, his fears, his preferences, and his ability to cope with a treatment.

Prodded by patient complaints and increasing litigation, most schools provide formal courses on medical ethics. However, doctor/patient relationships, mind-body interactions, medical sociology, and behavioral science are left to the informal teaching of the many individual clinical teachers, who may themselves have little training in these "soft" sciences.[30] There is no easy remedy for this omission. Students and faculty will be unhappy to add more courses to the already overburdened curriculum. Nevertheless, academic leaders need to consider how to integrate the humanities into medical training during and after medical school. The future of medicine will depend as much on how wisely and articulately doctors help individual patients cope with their illnesses as on their mastery of medical science.

COPING WITH THE STRANGERS

Strangers are in the examining room to stay. It is undeniably difficult to work and establish a meaningful doctor/patient relationship with so many looking over one's shoulder, yet physicians must do it. Were Osler still among us, he would counsel aequanimitas,[31] although even he might struggle to cope with an American HMO, a Canadian manpower planner, or a British hospital trust.

Government and Plan Managers

Collectively, physicians should remind those who manage health care of the importance of doctor/patient relationships and the need for doctors to spend more time with patients. Managers must be convinced that clinician-generated medical evidence will improve patient experiences with doctors, maximize well-being, prevent adverse events,[32] and ultimately save money. Good decisions can reduce the need for expensive technology. Physicians can temper the rhetoric of politicians and managers by explaining the limitations of evidence-based medicine and reminding them that most patients have a chronic disease or worry for which spectacular technology has little to offer. Medical care needs clinical research to produce the evidence and educational programs to make the evidence available to doctors.

Organized Medicine

Physicians have the power to change the attitudes of those who are the profession's public face. The American Medical Association did the profession and the public a disservice by long opposing a universal medical care plan. The former editor of the organization's journal, George Lundberg, accused it of putting the needs of doctors before patients, describing it as a "disastrous severance of trust."[33] He points out that more than two-thirds of American doctors do not belong to the AMA, indicating their disregard for it.[34] Echoing Loxtercamp's lament (above), Lundberg wants doctors to take back their profession. No one can be happy with the expensive, patchwork, and uneven system that now exists.[35] Local Australian and Canadian medical associations were also initially reactionary and lost public credibility by appearing to be more concerned with doctors' incomes than patients' welfare. Members of these organizations should ensure their leaders are in tune with public as well as professional opinion, so they can credibly influence developments.

Medical associations can champion many of the issues discussed in this book. For example, a consortium of general and specialty organizations could negotiate a convention establishing rules for relations with industry, and seek educational programs from sponsors that go beyond their commercial horizons. They can support public clinical trial registries to prevent publication biases,[36] as have the AMA[37] and several prominent journal editors.[38] Specialty organizations should emerge from their organ silos and concern themselves with medicine and society as a whole. Promotion of specialty initiatives must be in context with medical need and available resources. Greater understanding and collaboration with primary-care doctors will make specialty organizations more relevant to their patients and the public. Doctors need not be strangers to each other.

Industry Representatives

It is essential that those who develop treatments are advised by, and work closely with, doctors. Who else will identify the diseases that need treatment, select patients that are likely to benefit from it, design and execute the necessary clinical trials, and provide ongoing surveillance of the treatment? This cooperation is a public good and attracts little controversy. Conflict occurs with the company's marketing personnel, who see a newly developed drug through the prism of maximum sales rather than maximum patient benefit.

Sales personnel alter the collaborative atmosphere. Seamlessly, lavish and narrowly focused marketing co-opts consultants. Academic physician advisors morph from experts to "opinion leaders" who, by association, endorse the product. "Medical education" events are organized, new "opinion leaders" found, and an audience assembled. The focus is on the product, not the patient with the disease. Occasionally, an unfavorable press forces companies to make token ethical adjustments, but fundamental conflicts remain.

A broader view of medical care, greater respect for academic and physician/patient autonomy, and cooperation in education and research about issues of general interest would do much to restore public confidence in industry and doctors. Rather than squander consultants' expertise in ill-advised marketing roles, companies should seek their advice with initiatives that would make the product known but also achieve objectives in the public interest. Medical organizations, were they to collaborate, could negotiate the following objectives with the industry:

- Physicians should independently organize educational events for physicians, ensuring that all elements of the disease for which the drug is marketed are on the program and that the material is unbiased, patient centered, and relevant to the audience.
- To remedy the pharmaceutical bias in continuing medical education, elements of company-sponsored events could be devoted to topics that are unlikely to be supported otherwise. For example, an asthma program could include sessions on exercise and smoking cessation.
- Companies could design educational programs with in-house staff and consultants, rather than with expensive organizers whose expertise and showmanship is not necessarily relevant to the subject at hand.
- Independent physician educators could help drug representatives broaden their comprehension of disease and medical evidence.

Industry-physician collaboration is essential to medical progress, and rules of "ethical" conduct must not stifle it. Nevertheless, rules are necessary. Cooperation among doctors, companies, regulators, and health-care organizations may all benefit as long as the welfare of patients is paramount. How successfully physicians and company representatives clarify their relationship will determine the value of their future collaboration and public respect. Failure invites less public esteem for doctors as well as companies, more regulation, and more strangers into the examining room.

Lawyers

In the United States the malpractice phenomenon limps from crisis to costly crisis,[39] doing irreparable damage to doctor/patient relationships. Litigation is increasing worldwide. Doctors have two powerful weapons to avoid needless lawsuits. Good communication is an essential ingredient of the placebo effect (see chapter 14). There is evidence that, even after an adverse event, treating patients with respect and communicating the facts in an unhurried, open, and, empathetic manner can reduce legal risk.[40] Moreover, the more a physician's treatments are evidence based, the more defensible they will be. Wise managers should see that providing time for these activities will save money and prevent complaints.

Media

The media can often frustrate physicians. Journalists should rethink the sensationalizing of medical malpractice, miscasting of doctors' incomes, misinterpreting of medical information, and uncritical broadcasting of medical fads and fantasies. Doctors can best counter reporting bias by teaching, practicing, and publicizing evidence-based medicine. Researchers should be more guarded in the interpretation of their data and explaining their results to reporters.[41] Organized medicine can help journalists get their stories right.

CONCLUSIONS

Many physicians are unhappy with those who interfere with their practice. However, they can do much to strengthen their role. A reorientation of medical practice should put the family doctor in charge of a patient's care so that consultations and lab results flow to and from her office where the medical record resides. Specialists who function more as consultants, and defer expensive but repetitive procedures to lower-paid technicians, will have time for the intellectual and societal challenges of their discipline. Professional organizations could act as one to reduce the pharmaceutical bias in continuing education. Physicians in academic centers can lead the restoration of public confidence in the profession by restoring the art of medicine alongside the science.[42] As independent institutions, only medical schools can direct clinical education and research to counter industry bias. It is not enough to espouse the use of medical evidence or even to review it systematically; clinicians in medical schools should create it. By example and by persuasion, professors of clinical medicine and surgery can lead a shaken profession to collaborate with the strangers in their examining rooms—and promote positive doctor/patient encounters founded in compassion and clinical science. Then, physicians will rediscover their calling.

CONCLUSION

The three themes of this book interrelate (see figure C-1). The placebo effect is the concept underlying evidence-based medicine and, through healer/patient interaction, is a vital component of healing. Placebo-controlled, randomized clinical trials indicate evidence-based medical care and provide insights into the nature of the placebo effect. Health-care systems influence the placebo effect by controlling the circumstances of doctor/patient interactions, and they are most efficient when they promote and employ evidence-based practice. It follows that this integrated triad should animate health-care policy.

PLACEBO EFFECT

There can be no doubt that a true placebo effect exists and that it is distinct from the effects of time. Where naysayers err, it is in their confusion of the placebo with the effect. The placebo effect depends upon the circumstances, expectations, experience, and temporal susceptibility of the ill person and the empathy, personality, and positive attitude of the healer. It answers a human need to be cared for when feeling ill, and can be achieved without deception or prejudice—nor indeed a placebo.

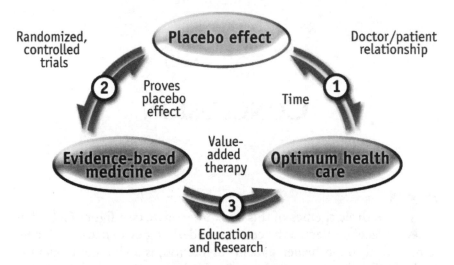

Figure C-1: Three Themes: (1) The *placebo effect* contributes to optimum health care, if the doctor/patient relationship is given sufficient time. (2) It is also the yardstick against which a treatment is measured in the randomized clinical trials that underpin *evidence-based medicine*. In turn, the trials illustrate the placebo effect. (3) Evidence-based medicine adds value to therapy by indicating the *optimum health care*, and an enlightened medical system supports research and education to generate and disseminate the evidence. Successful interaction between these three themes determine the quality of a nation's health care.

Furthermore, no one should doubt that placebo effects resulting from a therapeutic relationship are a good thing. A healer's attitudes and interpersonal skills are necessary requisites for optimal care. Politicians and health-care managers must understand that when those who are ill are comforted and satisfied, their care will cost less in the long run. Conversely, mistreated, unhappy patients cost a great deal through second opinions, poor compliance, and litigation. Patients' search for alternatives is a measure of failure.

The placebo effect merits scientific study. Physicians and managers must know how best to deploy it. Some fear that too close an examination might undermine it, that mystery is a component of its success. Nevertheless, secrecy is an improper solution that mires us in an authoritarian and ethically dubious position. The best recourse is to understand it. We must study the placebo effect as a product of a good doctor/patient relationship and as a foil against which to measure all treatments.

EVIDENCE-BASED MEDICINE

There is little disagreement that medical care should be as evidence based as possible, but there is disagreement over what that means. Experience, anecdotes, traditions, or beliefs are insufficient evidence. Health-care programs should support treatment practices that are scientifically proven to produce better results than a placebo effect. Numerous surgeries, tests, psychotherapies, and ancient remedies have never been submitted to randomized clinical trials, yet are inextricably woven into our health-care fabric. In most cases, complementary and alternative medicine operates outside medicare plans, some might say as refuge from the hurried, impersonal service of contemporary medicine. CAM practitioners knock at medicare's door for recognition and admission. How can society decide what treatments are a patient's rights?

There are many explanations as to why much of medical care itself is not evidence based. Clinical trials are expensive and difficult to design and execute. While new drugs are meticulously tested for their prime indication, their off-label use and the use of many other therapies are beyond regulatory purview. Countless older drugs, diets, and procedures have never been tested, because of tradition or lack of interested personnel. Worse, many treatments are sustained by poorly conducted or uncontrolled trials—shoddy evidence that cannot be improved by armchair meta-analysis. The acquisition of clinical evidence should be public policy, and support of independent clinical research should be a priority. Every citizen has a stake in the scientific foundation of healing. Many recognize this through their participation in randomized trials.

Medical evidence is of little use if it fails to guide the delivery of care. Thousands of medical journals, Web sites, and media programs produce abundant data and opinions. Even in respected medical journals, much of this information is random or irrelevant, and its magnitude is beyond the capacity of any doctor to assimilate. Yet an Internet-skilled patient within minutes may consider himself an expert on his own illness, often on the basis of scientifically inadequate material. Thus, there needs to be a repository of accurate, updated, and digestible information at the physician's fingertips. How this is accomplished will require much thought, for unrealistic guidelines or Orwellian regulations are likely to do more harm than good.

The Cochrane database is a fine start, but its maintenance depends upon volunteers, and their conclusions often leave the clinician with little guidance. The Cochrane ideal could be the basis of an international project perhaps under the aegis of the World Health Organization. Electronic provision of the best usable medical evidence at the point of health-care delivery is a major challenge.

However, having the evidence is not the end of the story. In primary care, as many as half the patients have complaints that do not lend themselves to a medical diagnosis and many more have features that are different from the original subjects from whom the evidence was derived. A doctor must judge how to apply existing evidence to her individual patients. To do so, she must know them well.

HEALTH-CARE DELIVERY

As potential patients, we want a health policy that encourages and promotes placebo effects and evidence-based medicine. Medicare should promote these themes and support the professionals who must execute them. Those managing or attempting to influence medical-care programs share with physicians a desire for satisfied patients and good evidence-based health outcomes. Family doctors with ready consultant advice are most likely to make these realities. By seeing a patient over many years and maintaining the medical record, a family physician can know his previous illnesses, his job, his family, and his fears—a strong background upon which to develop a healing relationship. She is the best person to collaborate with him in the choice of tests, treatments, and referrals, while protecting him from adverse events.

For this to occur, some attitudes must change. Family doctors must equip themselves (and be equipped) to assume the central role and return to visiting their patients in hospitals to ensure continuity and advocacy. Specialists must see themselves as consultants prepared to accept responsibility for care when needed, but in touch with the family doctor and ready to return care to her when their responsibility is complete. Medical schools should set the example and educate doctors to fulfill these roles, no longer strangers to each other and to their patients. Managers and others must desist from micromanaging and instead support medical care. Those reporting medical evidence should be modest in their claims and insist upon accurate reporting by the media. Most "breakthroughs" are not. The public must sacrifice some choice to work with their family doctor. Everyone has an interest in the production and dissemination of accurate medical evidence for compassionate implementation by primary-care doctors and their consultants.

***

Medical care is rich in irony and paradox. In the past, doctors lacking effective treatment could console, encourage, and adjust attitudes, but seldomly could they cure. Most were respected, even loved, for their time and compassion, and in many cases, these were all they had to give. Now, effective, evidence-based treatments can often improve or cure, yet if delivered without time and compassion can also alienate, dehumanize, and anger. The nocebo effects of a bad medical encounter may cancel any evidence-based benefits. Physicians, health-care managers, and an enlightened public must find ways to restore healing relationships *and* ensure that health care is as evidence based as possible.

GLOSSARY

Absolute benefit increase: *see* **therapeutic gain**.

Aequinimitas: philosophical essay by Sir William Osler (1849–1919) that promotes a calm and rational approach to illness: "coolness and presence of mind under all circumstances, calmness amid storm, clearness of judgment in moments of great peril. . . ."

Active placebo: a drug with pharmacological effects to achieve a placebo effect. For this purpose, it may be given in inadequate doses and/or for a condition for which it is not indicated (*see* **impure placebo**).

Adherence (compliance): the extent to which a person's behavior coincides with medical advice.

Amygdala: an almond-shaped mass of gray matter in the anterior (front) portion of the temporal lobe of the brain.

Analgesic: pain reliever.

Angina pectoris: chest pain due to blocked coronary arterial blood supply to the heart.

Anecdote: a particular or detached incident or fact of an interesting nature; a biographical incident or fragment; a single passage of private life. In medicine, a very limited source of useful knowledge.

Anthropology: the scientific study of the origin, the behavior, and the physical, social, and cultural development of humans.

Antisepsis: destruction of disease-causing microorganisms to prevent infection.

Anxiety: a state of apprehension, uncertainty, and fear resulting from the anticipation of a realistic or fantasized threatening event or situation, often impairing physical and psychological functioning.

Arrythmia: abnormal rhythm of the heart.

Articular: referring to the joint surface where the bones meet or articulate.

Arthralgia: pain in the joints.

Arthritis: inflammation of the joints.

Arthroscopy: examination of the interior of a joint, such as the knee, using a type of endoscope that is inserted into the joint through small incisions.

Autointoxication: a nineteenth-century notion that the contents of the colon were toxic and could cause maladies including headache and arthritis. This nonsensical theory led to ritual purging and even colectomy.

Baseline: the period just before or at the beginning of a clinical trial where investigators record "baseline" measurements to which the outcome measurements are compared.

Bias: any factor or process that deviates the results or conclusions of a trial away from the truth.

Binary response or outcome: a response to a question or a trial outcome where there are two options: "yes" and "no."

Bioavailability: the amount of a drug that reaches the blood stream regardless of how it is given. For example, some drugs are poorly absorbed from the intestinal tract, or are destroyed by digestive enzymes so that only a fraction of the orally administered drug is "bioavailable."

Blinding: where participants in a clinical trial are not aware which treatment they are receiving. When only the subjects are blinded in a randomized controlled trial, it is said to be *single-blind*. When both subjects and investigators are blinded, the trial is said to be *double-blind*.

Bloodletting (venesection): removal of blood from a vein, usually from the arm. Used for centuries to treat many diseases.

Cartesian: refers to the philosophy of René Descartes—in this book specifically to the separation of mind and body.

Charlatan: a person who makes elaborate, fraudulent, and often voluble claims to skill or knowledge; a quack or fraud.

Clinical trial: a carefully and ethically designed experiment with the aim of answering some precisely framed question (Bradford-Hill).

Cognitive: from cognition, the process by which knowledge is acquired. Cognitive behavioral therapy aims to correct faulty perception of symptoms.

Compliance (adherence): the extent to which a person's behavior coincides with medical advice.

Conditioning: a process of behavior modification by which a subject comes to associate a desired behavior with a previously unrelated stimulus.

Continuous outcome: mean of a range of values in a group of subjects that is compared to the mean at the baseline or against the mean in another group.

CNS: central nervous system—the brain and spinal cord.

Concealed allocation: randomization where investigators and subjects are unaware in what treatment group the subject is.

Cyclosporine: an immunosuppressant drug used in organ transplantation.

Debridement: surgical excision of dead, devitalized, or contaminated tissue, and removal of foreign matter from a wound.

Defensive medicine: the ordering of treatments, tests, and procedures for the purpose of protecting the doctor from criticism rather than diagnosing or treating the patient.

Delta: *see* **therapeutic gain.**

Delusion: a false, fixed, odd, or unusual belief firmly held by the patient. The belief is not ordinarily accepted by other members of the person's culture or subculture. There are delusions of paranoia (others are plotting against them), grandiose delusions (exaggerated ideas of one's importance or identity), and somatic delusions (a healthy person believing that he/she has a terminal illness).

Double-blind: condition in a clinical trial where neither the trial subject nor the investigator knows which treatment the subject is getting.

Dropsy: edema, fluid in the tissues.

Dyspepsia: upper abdominal pain or discomfort that may be due to a peptic ulcer or have no known cause (functional dyspepsia).

Edema: fluid in the tissues.

Effectiveness: the extent to which a treatment achieves its intended purpose.

Efficacy: the ability of a drug to control or cure an illness. Efficacy should be distinguished from activity, which is limited to a drug's immediate pharmacological effects.

Endorphin: a neurochemical occurring naturally in the brain and having analgesic properties.

Emetic: a drug that causes vomiting that is sometimes used to treat poisonings.

Empirical treatment: that which is ". . . guided by mere experience, without knowledge of principles," or ". . . without scientific knowledge."

Endoscopy: examination of the intestinal tract through a flexible tube that transmits an image via fiber optics or microchips.

Endpoint: the time in a clinical trial when the outcome is determined.

Enlightenment: a movement in the eighteenth century that advocated the use of reason in the reappraisal of accepted ideas and social institutions (Age of Reason).

Erythema nodosum: inflammatory skin lumps over the shins, often associated with inflammatory disease elsewhere.

Exclusion criteria: criteria by which certain subjects are excluded from participating in a clinical trial.

Exercise tolerance: a measure of heart health. Usually the individual is tested on a treadmill with electrocardiograph equipment in place.

Extinction: the end of a placebo effect induced by a certain treatment.

Food and Drug Administration (FDA): United States federal agency responsible (among other things) for the approval and safety monitoring of prescription drugs.

Fibromyalgia: a syndrome characterized by chronic pain in the muscles and soft tissues surrounding joints, fatigue, and tenderness at specific sites in the body.

Fistula: an abnormal communication between two body cavities, e.g., enterovesical fistula, a communication between the bowel and bladder resulting from a chronic inflammatory disease such as Crohn's disease.

Functional disease: disorder of function, not due to any known cause.

Generalizability: the ability of data from an experiment or a clinical trial to be accurately applied to a larger population. Implies that the subjects of the experiment were representative of the target population.

Hallucination: a sensory perception (seeing, hearing, feeling, and smelling) in the absence of an outside stimulus. For example, with auditory hallucinations, the person hears voices when there is no one talking.

Hawthorne effect: changes of the behavior of subjects in a trial or experiment that are attributable to their knowledge that they are being observed.

Hematocrit: the percentage by volume of packed red blood cells in a given sample of blood after centrifugation.

Hypochondria or **hypochondriasis:** the persistent conviction that one is or is likely to become ill, often involving symptoms when illness is neither present nor likely, and persisting despite reassurance and medical evidence to the contrary.

Immunosuppressant: a drug that reduces the body's immune response.

Impure placebo: a placebo that has pharmacological properties that may work for certain conditions, but is inappropriate, or given in insufficient dose for another condition (after Shapiro).

Iritis: inflammation of the iris (colored membrane in the eye).

Irritable bowel syndrome: abdominal pain and altered bowel habit in the absence of structural or biochemical cause.

Laparoscope: a slender tubular endoscope that is inserted through a small incision in the abdominal wall and used for viewing the abdominal or pelvic cavities and performing surgery.

Laparotomy: a surgical incision through the abdominal wall.

Ligation: to tie off or occlude; to tie off an artery with a suture or ligature.

Litigation: the act of suing (lawsuit); to engage in legal proceedings.

Locum: someone (physician or clergyman) who substitutes temporarily for another member of the same profession (syn: locum tenens).

Medicare: United States government program to cover medical expenses for disabled people and citizens over sixty-five. When not capitalized in this volume "medicare" refers to any nation's medical-care program.

Meta-analysis: the process or technique of synthesizing research results by using various statistical methods to retrieve, select, and combine results from previous separate but related studies.

Mitral stenosis: narrowing of the mitral valve between the left atrium and ventricle of the heart, which eventually fails. Usually a long-term consequence of poststreptococcal rheumatic fever, it can be corrected surgically. Since penicillin cures streptococcal infections, rheumatic fever and mitral stenosis are now much less common.

Moxibustion: the burning of moxa or other substances on the skin to treat diseases or to produce analgesia.

Myocardium: heart muscle.

Naloxone: a drug that blocks the effects of narcotics.

Natural history of a disease: the course or outcome of a disease if there was no intervention.

Neuroendocrine: pertaining to the anatomical and functional relationships between the nervous system and neurotransmitter substances.

Nitroglycerine: not in this case used as an explosive! A drug formulated in a small soluble pill that when placed under the tongue improves coronary blood flow and relieves angina pectoris.

Nocebo: like its antonym, placebo, is difficult to define. The causation of sickness (or death) because of the expectation of sickness (or death) and by certain emotional states. The expectation is induced by the action of a healer or priest.

Nosology: the classification of diseases.

Normotensive: a person with normal blood pressure.

Null hypothesis: statistical hypothesis that for a given measure there is no difference between two groups. Experimental and statistical testing is designed to prove or disprove this hypothesis.

Number needed to treat (NNT): number of patients that need to be treated for one additional good outcome to occur (1/therapeutic gain).

Ordinal scale: scale of verbal responses to a question where the distance between them is imprecise.

Organic: a term for a disease that has a known pathology.

Outcome measure: the value(s) determining the outcome of a trial usually compared to the baseline.

Placebo: an inert pill, injection, sham incision, or otherwise harmless and ineffective treatment (*see* chapter 1, table 1-1).

Pharmacokinetics: the process by which a drug is absorbed, distributed, metabolized, and eliminated by the body.

Placebo control: the use of a placebo to control for placebo and time effects in a clinical trial.

Placebo effect: a beneficial effect on a patient's symptoms or a pathological abnormality that is not accounted for by the properties of the treatment itself, nor by the natural history of the symptom or abnormality (true placebo effect).

Placebo response: a response to a treatment that is the sum of the placebo effect, the natural history of the disease being treated, and time-dependent factors such as regression to the mean.

Pneumococcal pneumonia: infection of the lung by the pneumococcus bacteria, initially very sensitive to penicillin.

Primary care: (not easily defined) the first physician a patient encounters upon entry to the health-care system outside of the hospital. Called general practitioners (GPs) in Europe and North America and family doctors (North America). In many countries, specialists in gynecology, pediatrics, and internal medicine practice primary care within their specialties.

Psychoneurosis: a mental or personality disturbance not attributable to any known neurological or organic dysfunction. Also called *neurosis, neuroticism*. Other terms are *anxiety neurosis, disturbance, hysteria, hysterical neurosis, mental disorder, mental disturbance,* and *psychological disorder*.

Psychosis: describes severe mental disorders that are characterized by extreme impairment of a person's ability to think clearly, respond emotionally, communicate effectively, understand reality, and behave appropriately. Psychotic symptoms including delusions and hallucinations occur in serious mental illnesses, such as depression, schizophrenia, bipolar disorders (manic depression), and some instances of substance abuse.

Psychotherapy: any purely psychological method of treatment for mental or emotional disorders.

Publication bias: negative experiments are less likely than positive ones to be published.

Pyoderma gangrenosa: deep skin ulcers sometimes associated with inflammatory bowel disease.

Quack: an untrained person who pretends to be a physician and dispenses medical advice and treatment; a charlatan; a mountebank.

Randomization: a method of selecting treatment groups for a clinical trial that are demographically equivalent.

Randomized controlled trial (RCT): a carefully and ethically designed experiment that includes the provision of adequate and appropriate controls by a process of randomization, so that precisely framed questions can be answered (Bulpitt).

Reductionism: a procedure or theory that reduces complex data or phenomena to simple terms.

Responder: an individual in a clinical trial judged to have responded to the therapy.

Scaling bias: biased results from an unbalanced ordinal or visual analogue scale (more positive than negative choices or vice versa).

Secondary care: care by specialists or consultants to whom the patient has been referred, usually by a primary-care physician.

Selection bias: selection of subjects into a clinical trial who, because of certain characteristics, might bias the outcome, or render it unsuitable for application to clinical practice.

Shaman: priest or priest-doctor among various northern Asian tribes and applied to similar personages elsewhere such as the Northwest American Indians.

Shamanism: the primitive religion of the Ural-Altaic people of Siberia in which all the good and evil of life are thought to be brought about by spirits that can be influenced only by shamans.

Single-blind: condition in a clinical trial where the trial subject does not know which treatment he is getting.

Somatic: affecting or characteristic of the body as opposed to the mind or spirit.

Somatizers: those with a propensity to experience and report somatic symptoms that have no pathophysiological explanation, to misattribute them to disease, and to seek medical attention for them.

Statistical significant difference: a difference in a measure between two groups that through statistical testing is determined to be probably true; that is, not due to chance. The probability is usually expressed as 0.95; that is, there is a 0.05% chance that the difference is not true. A statistically significant result is often expressed as $p < .05$ (or less). Statistical significance implies truth, not importance.

Subluxation: incomplete or partial dislocation of a bone in a joint. Subluxation of the spine is a basic tenet of chiropractic.

Synovium: the membrane lining a joint.

Systematic review: a summary of the medical literature that uses explicit methods to systematically search, critically appraise, and synthesize the literature on a specific topic.

Therapeutic gain: the effect on a patient's symptom or pathological abnormality of the treatment itself, which may be a drug, a diet, a device, a procedure, or a psychological treatment. Also called the *delta*, or *absolute benefit increase*.

Tort: damage, injury, or a wrongful act done willfully, negligently, or in circumstances involving strict liability, but not involving breach of contract, for which a civil suit can be brought.

Trialist: one who designs or conducts randomized clinical trials.

Type I error (α error): statistical demonstration of a difference between groups when none exists, e.g., a true null hypothesis is incorrectly rejected.

Type II error (β error): failure to demonstrate a difference between groups when one actually exists, e.g., a null hypothesis is incorrectly accepted.

Triple-blind: condition in a clinical trial where neither the trial subject, the investigator, nor the data manager knows which treatment the subject is getting.

Venesection: removal of blood from a vein, usually from the arm. Used for centuries to treat many diseases.

Visual analogue scale (VAS): a scale where subjects record quantitative responses on a measured line with the minimum at one end and the maximum on the other.

Voodoo: a body of superstitious beliefs including sorcery, serpent worship, and sacrificial rites current in Haiti, Africa, and the southern United States.

Voodoo death: people in primitive cultures killed after being subjected to a sorcerer's spell or hex (described by anthropologists).

White coat effect: transiently elevated blood pressure reading when taken by a professional in a white coat.

Within group: where the outcome measure in a clinical trial is the mean result in one group that can then be compared to the mean in another.

Within patient: where the outcome measure is applied to determine a responder (binary outcome).

NOTES

CHAPTER 1: WHAT IS A PLACEBO?

1. A. J. M. de Craen et al., "Placebos and Placebo Effects in Medicine: A Historical Overview," *Journal of the Royal Society of Medicine* 92 (1999): 511–14; W. G. Thompson, "Placebos: A Review of the Placebo Response," *American Journal of Gastroenterology* 95 (2000): 1637–43.

2. G. Chaucer, "The Parson's Tale," in *Chaucer: Complete Works*, ed. W. W. Skeat (London: Oxford University Press, 1967), pp. 674–717.

3. G. Chaucer, "The Merchant's Tale," in *Chaucer: Complete Works*, ed. W. W. Skeat (London: Oxford University Press, 1967).

4. S. Wolf, "The Pharmacology of Placebos," *Pharmacological Reviews* 11 (1959): 689–704.

5. Ibid.

6. A. K. Shapiro and E. Shapiro, "The Placebo: Is It Much Ado about Nothing?" in *The Placebo Effect*, ed. Anne Harrington (Cambridge, MA: Harvard University Press, 1999), pp. 12–36.

7. Ibid.; A. K. Shapiro and E. Shapiro, *The Powerful Placebo: From Ancient Priest to Modern Physician* (Baltimore: Johns Hopkins University Press, 1997).

8. Shapiro and Shapiro, "The Placebo: Is It Much Ado About Nothing?"; Shapiro and Shapiro, *The Powerful Placebo*.

9. W. Osler, *Principles and Practice of Medicine*, 1st ed. (London: Pentland, 1892).

10. W. G. Thompson and K. W. Heaton, *Irritable Bowel Syndrome*, 2nd ed. (Oxford: Health Press, 2003), p. 56.

11. E. Ernst and K. L. Resch, "Concept of True and Perceived Placebo Effects," *British Medical Journal* 311 (1995): 551–53.

12. Ibid.

13. J. M. Bland and D. G. Altman, "Regression Towards the Mean," *BMJ* 308, no. 6942 (1994): 1499.

14. P. C. Gotzsche, "Is There Logic in the Placebo?" *Lancet* 344 (1994): 925–26.

15. Shapiro and Shapiro, *The Powerful Placebo.*

16. H. Brody, "The Lie That Heals: The Ethics of Giving Placebos," *Annals of Internal Medicine* 97 (1982): 112–18.

CHAPTER 2: HISTORY OF PLACEBOS

1. A. K. Shapiro and E. Shapiro, "The Placebo: Is It Much Ado About Nothing?" in *The Placebo Effect*, ed. Anne Harrington (Cambridge, MA: Harvard University Press University Press, 1999), pp. 12–36.

2. Ibid.; A. J. M. de Craen et al., "Placebos and Placebo Effects in Medicine: A Historical Overview," *Journal of the Royal Society of Medicine* 92 (1999): 511–14; J. L. Maddox, *The Medicine Man* (New York: Macmillan, 1923); A. K. Shapiro and E. Shapiro, *The Powerful Placebo: From Ancient Priest to Modern Physician* (Baltimore: Johns Hopkins University Press, 1997), pp. 1–27.

3. Maddox, *The Medicine Man.*

4. Ibid.

5. De Craen et al., "Placebos and Placebo Effects in Medicine: A Historical Overview"; Shapiro and Shapiro, *The Powerful Placebo.*

6. K. B. Thomas, "The Placebo in General Practice," *Lancet* 344 (1994): 1066–67.

7. J. D. Levine, N. C. Gordon, and H. L. Fields, "The Mechanism of Placebo Analgesia," *Lancet* (1978): 654–57; D. J. Rowbotham, "Endogenous Opioids, Placebo Response and Pain," *Lancet* 357 (2001): 1901–1902.

8. W. G. Thompson, "Placebos: A Review of the Placebo Response," *American Journal of Gastroenterology* 95 (2000): 1637–43.

9. M. Fava et al., "The Problem of the Placebo Response in Clinical Trials for Psychiatric Disorders: Culprits, Possible Remedies, and a Novel Study Design Approach," *Psychother. Psychosom.* 72, no. 3 (2003): 115–27.

10. A. Holbrook and C. Goldsmith, "Innovation and Placebos in Research: A New Design of a Clinical Trial," *Lancet* 362 (2003): 2036–37.

11. P. C. Gotzsche, "Is There Logic in the Placebo?" *Lancet* 344 (1994): 925–26.

12. A. Harrington, "Introduction," in *The Placebo Effect*, ed. Anne Harrington (Cambridge, MA: Harvard University Press, 1997), 1–11.

13. Ibid.

CHAPTER 3: PLACEBO RESEARCH: SOME FACTS AND MYTHS

1. A. Ilnyckyj et al., "Quantitation of the Placebo Response in Ulcerative Colitis," *Gastroenterology* 112 (1997): 1854–58; C. Su et al., "A Meta-Analysis of the Placebo Rates of Remission and Response in Clinical Trials of Active Crohn's Disease," *Gastroenterology* 126, no. 5 (2004): 1257–69.

2. D. M. Owens, D. K. Nelson, and N. J. Talley, "The Irritable Bowel Syndrome: Long Term Prognosis and the Patient-Physician Interaction," *Annals of Internal Medicine* 122 (1995): 107–12.

3. S. P. Buckelew and K. E. Coffield, "An Investivation of Drug Expectancy as a Function of Capsule Colour, Size and Preparation Form," *Journal of Clinical Psychopharmacology* 2 (1982): 245–48.

4. B. Blackwell, S. Bloomfield, and C. R. Buncher, "Demonstration to Medical Students of Placebo Responses and Non-Drug Factors," *Lancet* 1 (1972): 1279–82.

5. Buckelew and Coffield, "An Investivation of Drug Expectancy."

6. K. Schapira et al., "Study on the Effects of Tablet Colour in the Treatment of Anxiety States," *British Medical Journal* 1, no. 707 (1970): 446–49.

7. J. D. Levine, N. C. Gordon, and H. L. Fields, "The Mechanism of Placebo Analgesia," *Lancet* (1978): 654–57; D. J. Rowbotham, "Endogenous Opioids, Placebo Response and Pain," *Lancet* 357 (2001): 1901–1902.

8. F. Benedetti and M. Amanzio, "The Neurobiology of Placebo Analgesia: From Endogenous Opioids to Cholecystokinin," *Prog.Neurobiol.* 52, no. 2 (1997): 109–25.

9. F. Benedetti et al., "Placebo-Responsive Parkinson Patients Show Decreased Activity in Single Neurons of Subthalamic Nucleus," *Nat.Neurosci.* 7, no. 6 (2004): 587–88.

10. T. D. Wager et al., "Placebo-Induced Changes in FMRI in the Anticipation and Experience of Pain," *Science* 303, no. 5661 (2004): 1162–67.

11. L. C. Park and L. Covi, "Nonblind Placebo Trial," *Archives of General Psychiatry* 12 (1965): 336–44.

12. L. D. Egbert et al., "Reduction of Postoperative Pain by Encouragement and Instruction of Patients," *New England Journal of Medicine* 270 (1964): 825–28.

13. F. Benedetti et al., "Open Versus Hidden Medical Treatments: The Patient's Knowledge About a Therapy Affects the Therapy Outcome," http://journals.apa.org/prevention/volume6/pre0060001a.html.

14. R. Ader, "The Role of Conditioning in Pharmacotherapy," in *The Placebo Effect*, ed. Anne Harrington (Cambridge, MA: Harvard University Press, 1997), pp. 138–65.

15. A. L. Suchman and R. Ader, "Classic Conditioning and Placebo Effects in Crossover Studies," *Clinical Pharmacology and Therapeutics* 52 (1992): 372–77.

16. B. A. Gould et al., "Does Placebo Lower Blood-Pressure?" *Lancet* 2, no. 8260–61 (1981): 1377–81.

17. W. B. Kannel and M. Feinleib, "Natural History of Angina Pectoris in the Framingham Study: Prognosis and Survival," *American Journal of Cardiology* 29, no. 2 (1972): 154–63.

18. T. A. Kerr, K. Schapira, and M. Roth, "Relationship Between Premature Death and Affective Disorders," *Psychiatry Digest* 31, no. 7 (1970): 19.

19. D. M. Tucker et al., "Dietary Fiber and Personality Factors as Determinants of Stool Output," *Gastroenterology* 81 (1981): 879.

20. "Psychotherapy: Effective Treatment or Expensive Placebo?" *Lancet* 1 (1984): 83–84.

21. H. Benson and D. P McCallie, "Angina Pectoris and the Placebo Effect," *New England Journal of Medicine* 3000 (1979): 1424–28.

22. W. Caryell and R Noyes, "Placebo Response in Panic Disorder," *American Journal of Psychiatry* 145 (1988): 1138–40.

23. Benson and McCallie, "Angina Pectoris and the Placebo Effect."

24. I. Kirsch, "Specifying Nonspecifics: Psychological Mechanisms of the Placebo Response," in *The Placebo Effect*, ed. Anne Harrington (Cambridge, MA: Harvard University Press, 1997), pp. 166–86.

25. A. R. Northcutt et al., "Persistant Placebo Response During a Year-Long Controlled Trial of IBS Treatment," *Gastroenterology* 124 (2003): A-640.

26. H. K. Beecher, "The Powerful Placebo," *Journal of the American Medical Association* 159 (1955): 1602–1606.

27. K. B. Thomas, "Temporarily Dependent Patient in General Practice," *British Medical Journal* 1 (1974): 625–26.

28. B. Rise, "The Hawthorne Defect: Persistence of a Flawed Theory," http://www.cs.unc.edu/~stotts/204/nohawth.html.

CHAPTER 4: THE PLACEBO EFFECT

1. J. N. Blau, "Clinician and Placebo," *Lancet* 1 (1985): 344.

2. A. K. Shapiro and E. Shapiro, "The Placebo: Is It Much Ado about Nothing?" in *The Placebo Effect*, ed. Anne Harrington (Cambridge, MA: Harvard University Press, 1999), pp. 12–36.

3. E. Ernst and K. L. Resch, "Concept of True and Perceived Placebo Effects," *British Medical Journal* 311 (1995): 551–53.

4. G. S. Kienle and H. Kiene, "The Powerful Placebo Effect: Fact or

Fiction?" *Journal of Clinical Epidemiology* 50 (1997): 1312–18; A. Hrobjartsson and P. C. Gotzsche, "Is the Placebo Powerless?" *New England Journal of Medicine* 344 (2001): 1594–1602.

5. H. K. Beecher, "The Powerful Placebo," *Journal of the American Medical Association* 159 (1955): 1602–1606.

6. Kienle and Kiene, "The Powerful Placebo Effect."

7. Ibid.

8. Hrobjartsson and Gotzsche, "Is the Placebo Powerless?"

9. Ibid.

10. Hrobjartsson and Gotzsche, "Is the Placebo Powerless? Update of a Systematic Review With 52 New Randomized Trials Comparing Placebo With No Treatment," *Journal of Internal Medicine* 256, no. 2 (2004): 91–100.

11. J. C. Bailar, "The Powerful Placebo and the Wizard of Oz," *New England Journal of Medicine* 344 (2001): 1630–32.

12. R. L. Koretz, "Is There a Place for Placebos?" *Gastroenterology* 121 (2001): 1251–53.

13. P. C. Gotzsche, "Is There Logic in the Placebo?" *Lancet* 344 (1994): 925–26.

14. K. B. Thomas, "General Practice Consultations: Is There Any Point in Being Positive?" *British Medical Journal* 294 (1987): 1200–1202.

15. Ibid.

16. G. N. Verne et al., "Reversal of Visceral and Cutaneous Hyperalgesia by Local Rectal Anesthesia in Irritable Bowel Syndrome (IBS) Patients," *Pain* 105, no. 1–2 (2003): 223–30; L. Vase et al., "The Contributions of Suggestion, Desire, and Expectation to Placebo Effects in Irritable Bowel Syndrome Patients: An Empirical Investigation," *Pain* 105, no. 1–2 (2003): 17–25.

17. Ernst and Resch, "Concept of True and Perceived Placebo Effects."

CHAPTER 5: ELEMENTS OF THE PLACEBO EFFECT

1. D. D. Price and H. L. Fields, "The Contribution of Desire and Expectation to Placebo Analgesia: Implications for New Research Strategies," in *The Placebo Effect*, ed. A. Harrington (Cambridge, MA: Harvard University Press, 1997), pp. 117–37.

2. L. H. Gliedman et al., "Some Implications of Conditional Reflex Studies for Placebo Research," *American Journal of Psychiatry* 113, no. 12 (1957): 1103–1107.

3. W. E. Whitehead et al., "Learned Illness Behavior in Patients with Irritable Bowel Syndrome and Peptic Ulcer," *Digestive Diseases and Sciences* 27 (1982): 202–208.

4. N. J. Voudouris, C. L. Peck, and G. Coleman, "Conditioned Response Models of Placebo Phenomena: Further Support," *Pain* 38 (1989): 109–16.

5. R. Ader, "The Role of Conditioning in Pharmacotherapy," in *The Placebo Effect*, ed. Anne Harrington (Cambridge, MA: Harvard University Press, 1997), pp. 138–65.

6. R. C. Batterman and W. R. Lower, "Placebo Responsiveness—Influence of Previous Therapy," *Journal of Current Therapy* 10 (1968): 136–43.

7. R. C. Batterman, "Persistance of Responsiveness With Placebo Therapy Following an Effective Drug Trial," *Journal of New Drugs* 6 (1966): 137–41.

8. A. L. Suchman and R. Ader, "Classic Conditioning and Placebo Effects in Crossover Studies," *Clinical Pharmacology and Therapeutics* 52 (1992): 372–77.

9. N. J. Voudouris, C. L. Peck, and G. Coleman, "The Role of Conditioning and Verbal Expectancy in the Placebo Response," *Pain* 43 (1990): 121–28.

10. Price and Fields, "The Contribution of Desire and Expectation to Placebo Analgesia."

11. I. Kirsch, "Specifying Nonspecifics: Psychological Mechanisms of the Placebo Response," in *The Placebo Effect*, ed. Anne Harrington (Cambridge, MA: Harvard University Press, 1997), pp. 166–86.

12. I. Kirsch and M. J. Rosadino, "Do Double Blind-Studies with Informed Consent Yield Externally Valid Results?" *Psychopharmacology* 110 (1993): 437–42.

13. D. A. Stone et al., "Patient Expectations in Placebo-Controlled Randomized Clinical Trials," *J.Eval.Clin.Pract.* 11, no. 1 (2005): 77–84.

14. A. Branthwaite and P. Cooper, "Analgesic Effects of Branding in Treatment of Headaches," *British Medical Journal (Clin.Res.Ed)* 282, no. 6276 (1981): 1576–78.

15. A. G. Johnson, "Surgery As a Placebo," *Lancet* 344 (1994): 1140–43.

16. F. Benedetti, C. Arduino, and M. Amanzio, "Somatic Activation of Opiod Systems by Target-Directed Expectations of Analgesia," *Journal of Neuroscience* 19 (1999): 3639–48.

17. D. M. Owens, D. K. Nelson, and N. J. Talley, "The Irritable Bowel Syndrome: Long Term Prognosis and the Patient-Physician Interaction," *Annals of Internal Medicine* 122 (1995): 107–112.

18. H. Brody, "The Lie That Heals: The Ethics of Giving Placebos," *Annals of Internal Medicine* 97 (1982): 112–18; H. Brody, "The Placebo Response: Recent Research and Implications for Family Practice," *Journal of Family Practice* 47 (2000): 649–54.

19. G. B. Shaw, *The Doctor's Dilemma* (New York: Penguin Books, 1911).

20. K. B. Thomas, "General Practice Consultations: Is There Any Point in Being Positive?" *British Medical Journal* 294 (1987): 1200–1202; K. B. Thomas, "The Placebo in General Practice," *Lancet* 344 (1994): 1066–67.

21. Brody, "The Placebo Response."

22. H. C. Sox Jr., I. Margulies, and C. H. Sox, "Psychologically Mediated Effects of Diagnostic Tests," *Annals of Internal Medicine* 95 (1981): 680–85.

23. Ibid.

24. D. E. Moerman and W. B. Jonas, "Deconstructing the Placebo Effect and Finding the Meaning Response," *Annals of Internal Medicine* 136 (2002): 471–76; D. E. Moerman, "The Meaning Response and the Ethics of Avoiding Placebos," *Evaluation of Health Professions* 25 (2002): 399–409.

25. W. G. Thompson et al., "Irritable Bowel Syndrome in General Practice: Prevalence, Management and Referral," *Gut* 46 (2000): 78–82.

26. Ibid.

CHAPTER 6: THE NOCEBO EFFECT

1. T. A. Brennan et al., "Incidence of Adverse Events and Negligence in Hospitalized Patients: Results of the Harvard University Press Medical Practice Study I," *New England Journal of Medicine* 324, no. 6 (1991): 370–76; R. M. Wilson et al., "The Quality in Australian Health Care Study," *Medical Journal of Australia* 163, no. 9 (1995): 458–71; G. R. Baker and P. G. Norton, "Adverse Events and Patient Safety in Canadian Health Care," *Canadian Medical Association Journal* 170, no. 3 (2004): 353–54.

2. R. A. Hahn, "The Nocebo Phenomenon, Scope and Foundations," in *The Placebo Effect*, ed. Anne Harrington (Cambridge, MA: Harvard University Press, 1997), pp. 56–76.

3. J. L. Maddox, *The Medicine Man* (New York: Macmillan, 1923).

4. R. A. Reminick, "The Evil Eye Belief Among the Amhara of Ethiopia," in *Culture, Disease and Healing*, ed. D. Landy (New York: Macmillan, 1977), pp. 218–30.

5. Maddox, *The Medicine Man*; B. A. Lex, "Voodoo Death: New Thoughts on an Old Explanation," in *Culture, Disease and Healing*, ed. D. Landy. (New York: Macmillan, 1977), pp. 327–31.

6. W. B. Cannon, "'Voodoo' Death," *American Antrhopologist* 44 (1942): 169–81.

7. Lex, "Voodoo Death."

8. E. M. Sternberg, "Walter B. Cannon and 'Voodoo' Death': A Perspective from 60 Years On," *American Journal of Public Health* 92, no. 10 (2002): 1564–66.

9. D. R. Morse, J. Martin, and J. Moshonov, "Psychosomatically Induced Death: Relative to Stress, Hypnosis, Mind Control, and Voodoo: Review and Possible Mechanisms," *Stress Medicine* 7 (1991): 213–32.

10. H. K. Beecher, "The Powerful Placebo," *Journal of the American Medical Association* 159 (1955): 1602–1606.

11. G. S. Kienl and H. Kiene, "The Powerful Placebo Effect: Fact or Fiction?" *Journal of Clinical Epidemiology* 50 (1997): 1312–18; D. M. Green, "Pre-Existing Conditions, Placebo Reactions and 'Side Effects,'" *Annals of Internal Medicine* 60 (1964): 255–64.

12. M. M. Reidenberg and D. T. Lowenthal, "Adverse Nondrug Reactions," *New England Journal of Medicine* 279 (1968): 678–79.

13. Green, "Pre-Existing Conditions."

14. Hahn, "The Nocebo Phenomenon."

15. Ibid.

16. R. Anda et al., "Depressed Affect, Hopelessness, and the Risk of Ischemic Heart Disease in a Cohort of U.S. Adults," *Epidemiology* 4, no. 4 (1993): 285–94.

17. H. Brody, "The Lie That Heals: The Ethics of Giving Placebos," *Ann Int Med* 97 (1982): 112–18; H. Brody, "The Placebo Response: Recent Research and Implications for Family Practice," *Journal of Family Practice* 47 (2000): 649–54.

18. H. C. Sox Jr., I. Margulies, and C. H. Sox, "Psychologically Mediated Effects of Diagnostic Tests," *Annals of Internal Medicine* 95 (1981): 680–85.

19. W. G. Thompson et al., "Irritable Bowel Syndrome in General Practice: Prevalence, Management and Referral," *Gut* 46 (2000): 78–82.

20. D. A. Drossman et al., *The Functional Gastrointestinal Disorders*, 2nd ed. (McLean, VA: Degnon, 2000).

21. Hahn, "The Nocebo Phenomenon."

22. C. K. Meador, "The Last Well Person," *New England Journal of Medicine* 330 (1994): 440–41.

23. S. Wessely, C. Mimnuan, and M. Sharpe, "Functional Somatic Syndromes: One or Many?" *Lancet* 354 (1999): 936–39.

24. Hahn, "The Nocebo Phenomenon."

25. J. S. McQuade, "The Medical Malpractice Crisis—Reflections on the Alleged Causes and Proposed Cures: Discussion Paper," *Journal of the Royal Society of Medicine* 84 (1991): 408–11.

26. W. Levinson et al., "Physician-Patient Communication: The Relationship With Malpractice Claims Among Primary Care Physicians and Surgeons," *Journal of the American Medical Association* 277 (1997): 553–59.

27. S. S. Entman et al., "The Relationship Between Malpractice Claims History and Subsequent Obstetrics Care," *Journal of the American Medical Association* 272 (1994): 1588–91.

28. G. B. Hickson et al., "Obstetricians' Prior Malpractice Experience and Patients' Satisfaction With Care," *Journal of the American Medical Association* 272 (1994): 1583–87.

29. J. T. Condon, "Medical Litigation: The Aetiological Role of Psychological and Interpersonal Factors," *Medical Journal of Australia* 157 (1992): 768–70.

30. N. Cousins, "The Physician as Communicator," *Journal of the American Medical Association* 248 (1982): 287–89.

31. A. Jain and J. Ogden, "General Practitioners' Experiences of Patients' Complaints: Qualitative Study," *British Medical Journal* 318 (1999): 1596–99; Wessely, Mimnuan, and Sharpe, "Functional Somatic Syndromes."

32. N. Summerton, "Positive and Negative Factors in Defensive Medicine: A Questionnaire Study of General Practitioners," *British Medical Journal* 310 (1995): 27–29.

33. Wessely, Mimnuan, and Sharpe, "Functional Somatic Syndromes."

34. D. Mechanic, "Introduction," in *Humanizing Health Care*, ed. H. Strauss (New York: Wiley, 1975), pp. 1–11.

35. D. A. Drossman, "Medicine Has Become a Business, but What Is the Cost?" *Gastroenterology* 126 (2004).

36. Hahn, "The Nocebo Phenomenon."

CHAPTER 7: RANDOMIZED CLINICAL TRIALS

1. W. G. Thompson, *The Ulcer Story: The Authoritative Guide to Ulcers, Dyspepsia and Heartburn* (New York: Plenum, 1996).

2. C. J. Bulpitt, *Randomised Controlled Clinical Trials* (Boston: Kluwer, 1996); A. K. Shapiro and E. Shapiro, *The Powerful Placebo: From Ancient Priest to Modern Physician* (Baltimore: Johns Hopkins University Press, 1997); A. Jadad, *Randomized Controlled Trials* (London: BMJ Books, 1998); A. J. M. de Craen et al., "Placebos and Placebo Effects in Medicine: A Historical Overview," *Journal of the Royal Society of Medicine* 92 (1999): 511–14.

3. Bulpitt, *Randomised Controlled Clinical Trials*.

4. J. Lind, *A Treatise of the Scurvey*, ed. C. P. Stewart and D. Guthrie (Edinburgh, UK: Edinburgh University Press, 1953).

5. E. Martini, "Treatment for Scurvy Not Discovered by Lind," *Lancet* 364, no. 9452 (2004): 2180.

6. P. J. Pead, "Benjamin Jesty: New Light in the Dawn of Vaccination," *Lancet* 362, no. 9401 (2003): 2104–2109.

7. Ibid.

8. Shapiro and Shapiro, *The Powerful Placebo*.

9. H. Gold, N. T. Kwit, and H. Otto, "The Xanthines (Theobromide

and Aminophylline) in the Treatment of Cardiac Pain," *Journal of the American Medical Association* 108 (1937): 2173–79.

10. A. B. Hill, "Suspended Judgement: Memories of the British Streptomycin Trial in Tuberculosis: The First Randomised Clinical Trial," *Clinical Trials Journal* 11 (1990): 77–79; P. D. Hart, "A Change in Scientific Approach: From Alternation to Randomized Allocation in Clinical Trials in the 1940s," *British Medical Journal* 319 (1999): 572–73.

11. Hart, "A Change in Scientific Approach."

12. J. Kleijnen et al., "Placebo Effect in Double-Blind Trials: A Review of Interactions and Medications," *Lancet* 340 (1994): 1347–49.

13. Bulpitt, *Randomised Controlled Clinical Trials*.

14. Ibid.

15. W. G. Thompson and K. W. Heaton, *Irritable Bowel Syndrome*, 2nd ed. (Oxford: Health Press, 2003).

16. K. F. Schulz, I. Chalmers, and D. G. Altman, "The Landscape and Lexicon of Blinding in Randomized Trials," *Annals of Internal Medicine* 136, no. 3 (2002): 254–59.

17. P. M. Rothwell, "External Validity of Randomized Controlled Trials: 'To Whom Do the Results of This Trial Apply?'" *Lancet* 365, no. 9453 (2005): 82–93.

18. Schulz, Chalmers, and Altman, "The Landscape and Lexicon of Blinding in Randomized Trials."

19. W. G. Thompson, *The Angry Gut* (Reading, MA: Perseus Books, 1993).

20. Ibid.

21. S. A. Muller-Lissner et al., "Tegaserod, a 5-HT4 Receptor Agonist, Relieves Symptoms in Irritable Bowel Syndrome Patients With Abdominal Pain, Bloating and Constipation," *Alimentary Pharmacology and Therapeutics* 15 (1999): 1655–66.

22. W. G. Thompson, "Tegaserod and IBS : A Perfect Match?" *Gut* 52 (2003): 621–22.

23. D. L. Sackett, "Why Randomized Controlled Trials Fail but Needn't: Failure to Employ Physiological Statistics, or the Only Formula a Clinician-Trialist Is Ever Likely to Need," *Canadian Medical Association Journal* 165 (2001): 1226–37.

24. F. M. Kovacs et al., "Effect of Firmness of Matress on Chronic, Non-Specific Low-Back Pain: Randomised, Dopuble-Blind, Controlled Multicentre Trial," *Lancet* 362 (2003): 1599–1604.

25. J. McConnell, "Mattresses for a Pain in the Back," *Lancet* 362 (2003): 1594–95.

CHAPTER 8: EVIDENCE-BASED MEDICINE

1. S. Wolf, "The Pharmacology of Placebos," *Pharmacological Reviews* 11 (1959): 689–704.

2. D. L. Sackett et al., "Evidence Based Medicine: What It Is and What It Isn't," *British Medical Journal* 312, no. 7023 (1996): 71–72.

3. C. Begg et al., "Improving the Quality of Reporting of Randomized Controlled Trials: The CONSORT Statement," *Journal of the American Medical Association* 276, no. 8 (1996): 637–39.

4. A. Harrington, "Introduction," in *The Placebo Effect*, ed. Anne Harrington (Cambridge, MA: Harvard University Press, 1997), pp. 1–11.

5. Wolf, "The Pharmacology of Placebos."

6. J. M. Ritter, "Placebo-Controlled, Double-Blind Clinical Trials Can Impede Medical Progress," *Lancet* 1, no. 8178 (1980): 1126–27.

7. M. Goozner, *The $800 Million Pill* (Berkeley and Los Angeles: University of California Press, 2004).

8. P. Wallace, "The Health of Nations: A Survey of Health-Care Finance," *Economist*, no. 17 (July 2004): 3–19.

9. P. C. Gotzsche, "Reference Bias in Reports of Drug Trials," *British Medical Journal* 295 (1987): 654–56.

10. A. D. Oxman, D. J. Cook, and G. Guyatt, "Users' Guide to the Medical Literature: How to Use an Overview," *Journal of the American Medical Association* 272 (1994): 1367–71.

11. A. Whitehead, *Meta–Analysis of Controlled Clinical Trials* (Chichester: John Wiley and Sons, 2002).

12. H. S. Sachs et al., "Meta-Analsis of Randomized Controlled Trials," *New England Journal of Medicine* 316 (1987): 450–55.

13. P. Crowley, "Prophylactic Corticosteroids for Preterm Birth (Cochrane Review)," http://www.cochrane.org/cochrane/ revabstr/ab000065.htm.

14. T. Poynard et al., "Meta-Analysis of Smooth Muscle Relaxants in the Treatment of Irritable Bowel Syndrome," *Alimentary Pharmacology and Therapeutics* 8 (1994): 499–510.

15. A. D. Oxman, "Checklists for Review Articles," *British Medical Journal* 309 (1994): 648–51.

16. W. G. Thompson, "Review Article: The Treatment of Irritable Bowel Syndrome," *Alimentary Pharmacology and Therapeutics* 16 (2002): 1395–1406.

17. R. Raine et al., "An Experimental Study of Determinants of Group Judgments in Clinical Guideline Development," *Lancet* 364, no. 9432 (2004): 429–37.

18. P. Villenueva et al., "Accuracy of Pharmaceutical Advertisement in Medical Journals," *Lancet* 261 (2003): 27–32.

19. M. S. Wilkes, B. H. Doblin, and M. F. Shapiro, "Pharmaceutical Advertisements in Leading Medical Journals: Experts' Assessments," *Annals of Internal Medicine* 116, no. 11 (1992): 912–19.

20. R. H. Fletcher, "Adverts in Medical Journals: Caveat Lector," *Lancet* 261 (2003): 10–11.

21. J. E. Rossouw et al., "Risks and Benefits of Estrogen Plus Progestin in Healthy Postmenopausal Women: Principal Results rrom the Women's Health Initiative Randomized Controlled Trial," *Journal of the American Medical Association* 288, no. 3 (2002): 321–33.

22. "US Estrogen Plus Progesterone Study Halted Due to Increased Risk of Breast Cancer, Stroke and Heart Attack.," *Canadian Medical Association Journal* 288 (2002): 294.

23. G. Sreenivasan, "Does Informed Consent to Research Require Comprehension?" *Lancet* 362, no. 9400 (2003): 2016–18.

24. D. A. Bennett and A. Jull, "FDA: Untapped Source of Unpublished Trials," *Lancet* 361 (2003): 1402–1403.

25. W. Kondro and B. Sibbald, "Drug Company Experts Advised Staff to Withhold Data about SSRI Use in Children," *Canadian Medical Association Journal* 170, no. 5 (2004): 783; J. S. G. Montaner, M. V. O'Shaughnessy, and M. T. Schechter, "Industry-Sponsored Clinical Research: A Double-Edged Sword," *Lancet* (2001): 1893–95.

26. P. A. Rochon et al., "Relation between Randomized Controlled Trials Published in Leading General Medical Journals and the Global Burden of Disease," *Canadian Medical Association Journal* 170, no. 11 (2004): 1673–77.

27. A. J. Munro, "Publishing the Findings of Clinical Research," *British Medical Journal* 307, no. 6915 (1993): 1340–41.

28. J. Lenzer, "Cochrane Collaboration's Stand versus Industry Funding," *Canadian Medical Association Journal* 171, no. 2 (2004): 122.

29. J. M. Drazen et al.,"Clinical Trial Registration: A Statement from the International Committee of Medical Journal Editors," *Canadian Medical Association Journal* 171 (2004): 606–607.

30. T. Komoto and N. Davis, "Evidence-Based CME," *American Family Physician* 66, no. 2 (2002): 200–202.

31. "Scientific Publishing: Access All Areas," *Economist*, no. 7 (August 2004): 64–65.

CHAPTER 9: CAN SURGERY BE A PLACEBO?

1. G. B. Shaw, *The Doctor's Dilemma* (New York: Penguin Books, 1911).

2. "George Washington Death by Malpractice," http://www.medical–malpractice–lawyers–attorneys.com/george_washington_death.html.

3. Ibid.

4. R. B. Nelson, "Are Clinical Trials Pseudoscience?" *Forum in Medicine* (September 1979): 594–600.

5. B. Bynum, "Autointixication," *Lancet* 357 (2001): 1717.

6. W. G. Thompson, *The Irritable Gut* (Baltimore: University Park Press, 1979).

7. A. G. Johnson, "Surgery as a Placebo," *Lancet* 344 (1994): 1140–43.

8. H. K. Beecher, "Surgery as Placebo," *Journal of the American Medical Association* 176 (1961): 1102–1107.

9. W. Osler, "Aequanimitas," in *Sir William Osler: A Selection*, ed. C. G. Roland (Toronto: Clarke & Irwin, 2004), pp. 1–8.

10. A. Pope, *An Essay on Criticism*, part 2 (1744).

11. Johnson, "Surgery as a Placebo."

12. H. Benson and D. P McCallie, "Angina Pectoris and the Placebo Effect," *New England Journal of Medicine* 3000 (1979): 1424–28.

13. Ibid.; W. B. Kannel and M. Feinleib, "Natural History of Angina Pectoris in the Framingham Study: Prognosis and Survival," *American Journal of Cardiology* 29, no. 2 (1972): 154–63.

14. Beecher, "Surgery as Placebo."

15. Johnson, "Surgery as a Placebo."

16. R. Adams, "Internal Mammary Artery Ligation for Coronory Insufficiency: An Evaluation," *New England Journal of Medicine* 258 (1958): 113–15.

17. E. G. Dimond, C. F. Kittle, and J. E. Crockett, "Evaluation of Internal Mammary Ligation and Sham Procedure in Angina Pectoris," *Circulation* 18 (1958): 712–13.

18. L. A. Cobb, "Internal Mammary Artery Ligation for Coronary Insufficiency: An Evaluation," *New England Journal of Medicine* 260 (1959): 1115–18.

19. S. M. Collins, T. Piche, and P. Rampal, "The Putative Role of Inflammation in the Irritable Bowel Syndrome," *Gut* 49 (2001): 743–45.

20. J. B. Moseley Jr. et al., "A Controlled Trial of Arthroscopic Surgery for Osteoarthritis of the Knee," *New England Journal of Medicine* 347 (2002): 81–88.

21. Ibid.

22. Ibid.

23. R. Macklin, "The Ethical Problems with Sham Surgery in Clinical Research," *New England Journal of Medicine* 341 (1999): 992–96; S. Horing and F. G. Miller, "Is Placebo Surgery Unethical?" *New England Journal of Medicine* 347 (2002): 137–39; D. T. Felson and J. Buckwalter, "Debridement and Lavage for Osteoarthritis of the Knee," *New England Journal of Medicine* 347 (2002): 132–33.

24. C. W. Olanow et al., "A Double-Blind Controlled Trial of Bilateral

Fetal Nigral Transplantation in Parkinson's Disease," *Annals of Neurology* 54, no. 3 (2003): 403–14.

25. C. McRae et al., "Effects of Perceived Treatment on Quality of Life and Medical Outcomes in a Double-Blind Placebo Surgery Trial," *Archives of General Psychiatry* 61, no. 4 (2004): 412–20; A. J. Stoessl and R. Fuente-Fernandez, "Willing Oneself Better on Placebo—Effective in Its Own Right," *Lancet* 364, no. 9430 (2004): 227–28.

26. T. B. Freeman et al., "Use of Placebo Surgery in Controlled Trials of a Cellular-Based Therapy for Parkinson's Disease," *New England Journal of Medicine* 341 (1999): 988–92.

27. Johnson, "Surgery as a Placebo."

28. J. J. T. Tate et al., "Laparoscopic Versus Open Appendectomy: Prospective Randomised Trial," *Lancet* 342 (1993): 633–37.

29. J. P. Nicholl et al., "Randomised Controlled Trial of Cost Effectiveness of Lithotrypsy and Open Cholecystectomy as Treatments for Gallbladder Stones," *Lancet* 340 (1992): 801–807.

30. A. J. M. de Craen et al., "Placebos and Placebo Effects in Medicine: A Historical Overview," *Journal of the Royal Society of Medicine* 92 (1999): 511–14.

31. W. Cumming, "Electro-Galvanism in a Peculiar Affliction of the Mucous Membrane of the Bowels," *London Medical Gazette* NS9 (1849): 969–73.

32. A. T. Barker et al., "Pulsed Magnetic Field Therapy for Tibial Non-Union," *Lancet* 1 (1984): 994–96.

33. R. L. Park, "Currents of fear: In Which Power Lines Are Suspected of Causing Cancer," in *Voodoo Science: The Road From Foolishness to Fraud*, ed. R. L. Park (Oxford: Oxford University Press, 2000), pp. 140–61.

CHAPTER 10: PLACEBO EFFECTS AND PSYCHOTHERAPY

1. "Psychotherapy: Effective Treatment or Expensive Placebo?" *Lancet* 1 (1984): 83–84.

2. R. Porter, *Madness: A Brief History* (Oxford: Oxford University Press, 2002).

3. "Psychotherapy: Effective Treatment or Expensive Placebo?"

4. American Psychiatric Association Task force for DSM IV, *Diagnostic and Statistical Manual of Mental Disorders*, test revision, 4th ed. (Washington, DC: American Psychiatric Association, 2000).

5. B. J. Cohen, "Psychotherapy," in *Theory and Practice of Psychiatry* (Oxford: Oxford University Press, 2003), pp. 467–81.

6. "Psychotherapy: Effective Treatment or Expensive Placebo?"

7. Cohen, "Psychotherapy."

8. "Psychotherapy: Effective Treatment or Expensive Placebo?"

9. Ibid.

10. Ibid.

11. I. Elkins et al., "National Institute of Mental Health Treatment of Depression Collaborative Research Program: General Effectiveness of Treatments," *Archives of General Psychiatry* 46 (1989): 971–82.

12. R. Michels and P. M. Marzuk, "Medical Progress: Progress in Psychiatry," *New England Journal of Medicine* 329, (1993): 552–60.

13. D. A. Drossman et al., "Cognitive-Behavioural Therapy Versus Education and Desipramine Versus Placebo for Moderate to Severe Functional Bowel Disorders," *Gastroenterology* 125 (2003): 19–31.

14. J. R. Laporte and A. Figuras, "Placebo Effects in Psychiatry," *Lancet* 340 (1994): 1206–1209.

15. J. Paris, *The Fall of an Icon: Psychoanalysis and Academic Psychiatry* (Toronto, Ontario: University of Toronto Press, 2005).

16. Ibid., p. 64.

17. Ibid., p. 94.

18. Ibid., p. 106.

19. Ibid., p. 46.

20. Ibid., p. 145.

CHAPTER 11: COMPLEMENTARY AND ALTERNATIVE MEDICINE

1. S. B. Clark, "Mark Twain and Medicine: 'Any Mummery Will Cure,'" *New England Journal of Medicine* 2350 (2005): 2529–30.

2. G. Bodeker and F. Kronenberg, "A Public Health Agenda for Traditional, Complementary and Alternative Medicine," *American Journal of Public Health* 92 (2002): 1582–90.

3. B. McFarland et al., "Complementary and Alternative Medicine in Canada and the United States," *American Journal of Public Health* 92 (2002): 1616–17.

4. L. Buske, "Looking for an Alternative," *Canadian Medical Association Journal* 161 (1999): 3.

5. S. Pappas and A. Perlman, "Complementary and Alternative Medicine: The Importance of Doctor-Patient Communication," *Med.Clin.North Am.* 86, no. 1 (2002): 1–10.

6. Bodeker and Kronenberg, "A Public Health Agenda."

7. Buske, "Looking for an Alternative."

8. McFarland et al., "Complementary and Alternative Medicine."

9. Holistic Online, "Classification of Alternative Systems of Medical Practice," available from www.holistic–online.com/Alt_Medicine/altmed _classification.htm.

10. J. Ezzo, B. M. Berman, and A. J. Vickers, "Complementary Medicine and the Cochrane Collaboration," *Journal of the American Medical Association* 280 (2004): 1628–30.

11. Cochrane Collaboration, "The Cochrane Library," http://www .cochrane.org/cochrane/revabstr/mainindex.htm.

12. T. J. Kaptchuk and D. M. Eisenberg, "Varieties of Healing: A Taxonomy of Unconventional Healing Practices," *Annals of Internal Medicine* 135 (2001): 196–204.

13. J. A. Astin et al., "A Review of the Incorporation of Complementary and Alternative Medicine by Mainstream Physicians," *Archives of Internal Medicine* 158, no. 21 (1998): 2303–10.

14. D. M. Eisenberg, "Advising Patients Who Seek Alternative Medical Therapies," *Annals of Internal Medicine* 127, no. 1 (1997): 61–69.

15. Pappas and Perlman, "Complementary and Alternative Medicine."

16. A. K. Shapiro and E. Shapiro, *The Powerful Placebo: From Ancient Priest to Modern Physician* (Baltimore: Johns Hopkins University Press, 1997).

17. G. R. Hamilton and T. F. Baslett, "Mandrake to Morphine: Anodynes of Antiquity," *Annals of the Royal College of Surgeons of Canada* 32 (1999): 403–406.

18. W. B. Fye, "Nitroglycerine: A Homeopathic Remedy," *Circulation* 73 (1986): 21–28.

19. G. Ritter, "The Herbal History of Digitalis: Lessons for Alternative Medicine," *Journal of the American Medical Association* 283 (2000): 885.

20. W. G. Thompson, "Constipation: A Physiological Approach," *Canadian Journal of Gastroenterology* 14, suppl D (2000): 155D–62D.

21. T. J. Kaptchuk and D. M. Eisenberg, "Varieties of Healing 1: Medical Pluralism in the United States," *Annals of Internal Medicine* 135 (2001): 189–95.

22. Ibid.

23. O. W. Holmes, *Homeopathy and Its Kindred Delusions* (Boston: Ticknor, 1842).

24. S. Barrett, Quackwatch, http://www.quackwatch .com.

25. K. Lewit, "Changes in Locomotor Function, Complementary Medicine and the General Practitioner," *Journal of the Royal Society of Medicine* 87 (1994): 2639.

26. R. Porter, *Madness: A Brief History* (Oxford: Oxford University Press, 2002).

27. G. L. Engel, "The Clinical Application of the Biopsychosocial Model," *American Journal of Psychiatry* 137 (1980): 535–44.

28. C. R. B. Joyce, "Placebos and Complementary Medicine," *Lancet* 340 (1994): 1279–81.

29. W. C. Meeker and S. Haldeman, "Chiropractic: A Profession at the Crossroads of Mainstream and Alternative Medicine," *Annals of Internal Medicine* 136, no. 3 (2002): 216–27.

30. E. Ernst, "Chiropractic Care: Attempting a Risk–Benefit Analysis," *American Journal of Public Health* 92 (2002): 1603–1604.

31. W. Evans, "Chiropractic Care: Attempting a Risk-Benefit Analysis," *American Journal of Public Health* 93, no. 4 (2003): 522–23.

32. Meeker and S. Haldeman, "Chiropractic."

33. D. C. Cherkin et al., "A Comparison of Physical Therapy, Chiropractic Manipulation, and Provision of an Educational Booklet for the Treatment of Patients with Low Back Pain," *New England Journal of Medicine* 339, no. 15 (1998): 1021–29.

34. Evans, "Chiropractic Care"; E. Ernst et al., "Chiropractic," *Annals of Internal Medicine* 137, no. 8 (2002): 701–702.

35. J. D. Childs et al., "A Clinical Prediction Rule to Identify Patients with Low Back Pain Most Likely to Benefit From Spinal Manipulation: A Validation Study," *Annals of Internal Medicine* 141, no. 12 (2004): 920–28.

36. R. A. Deyo, "Treatments for Back Pain: Can We Get Past Trivial Effects?" *Annals of Internal Medicine* 141, no. 12 (2004): 957–58.

37. E. Fee et al., "Exploring Acupuncture:Ancient Ideas, Modern Techniques," *American Journal of Public Health* 92 (2002): 1592.

38. L. C. Jenkins and W. E. Spoerel, "Acupuncture: Canadian Anaesthetists Report on Visit to China," *Canadian Medical Association Journal* 111 (1974): 1123–29.

39. Bodeker and Kronenberg, "A Public Health Agenda."

40. J. Ezzo et al., "Is Acupuncture Effective for the Treatment of Chronic Pain? A Systematic Review," *Pain* 86 (2000): 217–25.

41. Cochrane Collaboration, "The Cochrane Library."

42. J. Ezzo et al., "Is Acupuncture Effective?"

43. P. White et al., "Acupuncture versus Placebo for the Treatment of Chronic Mechanical Neck Pain: A Randomized, Controlled Trial," *Annals of Internal Medicine* 141, no. 12 (2004): 911–19; B. M. Berman et al., "Effectiveness of Acupuncture as Adjunctive Therapy in Osteoarthritis of the Knee: A Randomized, Controlled Trial," *Annals of Internal Medicine* 141, no. 12 (2004): 901–10.

44. R. B. Bausell et al., "Is Acupuncture Analgesia an Expectancy Effect?: Preliminary Evidence Based on Participants' Perceived Assignments in Two Placebo-Controlled Trials," *Eval.Health Prof.* 28, no. 1 (2005): 9–26.

45. D. So, "Acupuncture Outcomes, Expectations, Patient-Provider Relationship, and the Placebo Effect: Implications for Health Promotion," *American Journal of Public Health* 92 (2002): 1662–67.

46. H. Yamashita et al., "Adverse Events Related to Acupuncture," *Journal of the American Medical Association* 280 (1998): 1563–64.

47. W. B. Jonas, T. J. Kaptchuk, and K. Linde, "A Critical Overview of Homeopathy," *Annals of Internal Medicine* 138, no. 5 (2003): 393–99.

48. J. P. Vandenbroucke and A. J. de Craen, "Alternative Medicine: A 'Mirror Image' for Scientific Reasoning in Conventional Medicine," *Annals of Internal Medicine* 135, no. 7 (2001): 507–13.

49. Jonas, Kaptchuk, and Linde, "A Critical Overview of Homeopathy."

50. Vandenbroucke and de Craen, "Alternative Medicine."

51. P. Lokken et al., "Effect of Homoeopathy on Pain and Other Events after Acute Trauma: Placebo Controlled Trial with Bilateral Oral Surgery," *British Medical Journal* 310, no. 6992 (1995): 1439–42.

52. P. A. De Smet, "Herbal Remedies," *New England Journal of Medicine* 347 (2002): 2046–56.

53. De Smet, "Herbal Medicine in Europe—Relaxing Regulatory Standards," *New England Journal of Medicine* 352, no. 12 (2005): 1176–78.

54. De Smet, "Herbal Remedies."

55. E. Ernst, "The Risk-Benefit Profile of Commonly Used Herbal Therapies: Ginko, St. John's Wort, Ginseng, Eccinacea, Saw Palmetto, and Kava," *Annals of Internal Medicine* 136 (2002): 42–53.

56. H. S. Boon and A. H. C. Wong, "Kava: A Test Case for Canada's New Approach to Natural Health Products," *Journal of the Canadian Medical Association* 169 (2003): 1163–64.

57. R. B. Turner, "Echinacea for the Common Cold: Can Alternative Medicine Be Evidence-Based Medicine?" *Annals of Internal Medicine* 137 (2002): 1001–1002.

58. Cochrane Collaboration, "The Cochrane Library."

59. Ernst, "The Risk-Benefit Profile."

60. B. P. Barrett et al., "Treatment of the Common Cold with Unrefined Echinacea: A Randomized, Double-Blind, Placebo-Controlled Trial," *Ann.Intern.Med.* 137, no. 12 (2002): 939–46.

61. Turner, "Echinacea for the Common Cold."

62. Ernst, "The Risk-Benefit Profile."

63. De Smet, "Herbal Remedies."

64. Cochrane Collaboration, "The Cochrane Library."

65. Ernst, "The Risk-Benefit Profile."

66. Cochrane Collaboration, "The Cochrane Library."

67. Ibid.

68. T. A. Barringer et al., "Effect of a Multivitamin and Mineral Supplement on Infection and Quality of Life: A Randomized, Double-Blind, Placebo-Controlled Trial," *Annals of Internal Medicine* 138, no. 5 (2003): 365–71.

69. W. Fawzi and M. J. Stumpfer, "A Role for Multivitimins in Infection," *Annals of Internal Medicine* 138 (2003): 430–31.

70. Barringer et al., "Effect of a Multivitamin."

71. G. Bjelakovic et al., "Antioxidant Supplements for Prevention of Gastrointestinal Cancers: A Systematic Review and Meta-Analysis," *Lancet* 364, no. 9441 (2004): 1219–28.

72. E. R. Miller III et al., "Meta-Analysis: High-Dosage Vitamin E Supplementation May Increase All-Cause Mortality,"*Annals of Internal Medicine* 142, no. 1 (2005): 37–46.

73. R. L. Park, "Placebos Have Side Effects," in *Voodoo Science: The Road from Foolishness to Fraud* (Oxford: Oxford University Press, 2001), pp. 46–68.

74. H. Ogilvie, "The Large Bowel and Its Functions," *Proceedings of the Royal Society of Medicine* 44 (1951): 200–206.

75. "Colonic Lavage," http://www.colovage.com/ ColLavageNeed.htm.

76. A. M. Smith, *The No. 1 Ladies' Detective Agency* (New York: Anchor Books, 2003), p. 195.

77. K. F. Schulz, I. Chalmers, and D. G. Altman, "The Landscape and Lexicon of Blinding in Randomized Trials," *Annals of Internal Medicine* 136, no. 3 (2002): 254–59.

78. A. Margolin, S. K. Avants, and H. D. Kleber, "Investigating Alternative Medicine Therapies in Randomized Controlled Trials," *Journal of the American Medical Association* 280, no. 18 (1998): 1626–28; P. B. Fontanarosa and G. D. Lundberg, "Alternative Medicine Meets Science," *Journal of the American Medical Association* 280, no. 18 (1998): 1618–19.

79. S. Bondurant and H. C. Sox, "Mainstream and Alternative Medicine: Converging Paths Require Common Standards," *Annals of Internal Medicine* 142, no. 2 (2005): 149–50.

80. C. Weze, H. L. Leathard, and G. Stevens, "Evaluation of Healing by Gentle Touch for the Treatment of Musculoskeletal Disorders," *American Journal of Public Health* 94, no. 1 (2004): 50–52; C. Weze, H. L. Leathard, and G. Stevens, "Weze et al. Responds," *American Journal of Public Health* 94 (2004): 1074.

81. E. Ernst, "The Need for Scientific Rigor in Studies of Complementary and Alternative Medicine," *American Journal of Public Health* 94, no. 7 (2004): 1074–75.

82. Weze, Leathard, and Stevens, "Weze et al. Responds."

83. Joyce, "Placebos and Complementary Medicine."

84. P. C. Gotzsche, "Is There Logic in the Placebo?" *Lancet* 344 (1994): 925–26.

85. L. J. Hoffer, "Complementary or Altenative Medicine: The Need for Plausibility," *Journal of the Canadian Medical Association* 268 (2003): 180–82.

86. P. Knipschild, "Alternative Treatments: Do They Work?" *Lancet* 237 (2000): s4.

87. R. J. Huxtable, "The Myth of Beneficent Nature: The Risks of Herbal Preparations," *Annals of Internal Medicine* 117, no. 2 (1992): 165–66.

88. Ibid.; "Hepatitis Induced by Traditional Chinese Herbs: Possible Toxic Components," *Gut* 36 (1995): 146–47.

89. Huxtable, "The Myth of Beneficent Nature."

90. T. J. Kaptchuk, "The Placebo Effect in Alternative Medicine: Can the Performance of a Healing Ritual Have Clinical Significance?" *Annals of Internal Medicine* 136, no. 11 (2002): 817–25.

CHAPTER 12: THE DOCTOR AS PLACEBO

1. F. W. Peabody, "The Care of the Patient," *Journal of the American Medical Association* 88 (1927): 877–82.

2. C. Chantler, "The Second Greatest Benefit to Mankind?" *Lancet* 360 (2002): 1870–77.

3. "The Modern Scientific Physician: Theory of Medicine," *Canadian Medical Association Journal* 165 (2001): 1327–28.

4. D. E. Moerman, "The Meaning Response and the Ethics of Avoiding Placebos," *Evaluation of Health Professions* 25 (2002): 399–409.

5. H. Brody, "The Placebo Response: Recent Research and Implications for Family Practice," *Journal of Family Practice* 47 (2000): 649–54.

6. D. W. Blumhagen, "The Doctor's White Coat: The Image of the Physician in Modern America," *Annals of Internal Medicine* 91, no. 1 (1979): 111–16.

7. B. T. Chan, "The Declining Comprehensiveness of Primary Care," *Canadian Medical Association Journal* 166, no. 4 (2002): 429–34.

8. L. Sanders, "The End of Primary Care," *New York Times Magazine*, April 18, 2004, pp. 52–55; B. Wright et al., "Career Choice of New Medical Students at Three Canadian Universities: Family Medicine versus Specialty Medicine," *Canadian Medical Association Journal* 170, no. 13 (2004): 1920–24.

9. Peabody, "The Care of the Patient."

10. W. Osler, *Principles and Practice of Medicine*, 1st ed. (London: Pentland, 1892).

11. W. Osler, "Aequanimitas," in *Sir William Osler: A Selection*, ed. C. G. Roland (Toronto, Ontario: Clarke & Irwin, 2004), pp. 1–8.

12. S. Wolf, "The Pharmacology of Placebos," *Pharmacological Reviews* 11 (1959): 689–704.

13. Osler, "Aequanimitas."

14. Ibid.

15. S. L. Gryll and M. Katahn, "Situational Factors Contributing to the

Placebo Effect," *Psychopharmacology (Berl)* 57, no. 3 (1978): 253–61; A. K. Shapiro and E. Shapiro, "Predicting Placebo Response," in *The Powerful Placebo: From Anient Priest to Modern Physician*, ed. A. K. Shapiro and E. Shapiro (Baltimore: Johns Hopkins University Press, 1997).

16. K. B. Thomas, "The Consultation and the Therapeutic Illusion," *British Medical Journal* 1 (1978): 1327–28.

17. K. B. Thomas, "General Practice Consultations: Is There Any Point in Being Positive?" *British Medical Journal* 294 (1987): 1200–1202.

18. L. D. Egbert et al., "Reduction of Postoperative Pain by Encouragement and Instruction of Patients," *New England Journal of Medicine* 270 (1964): 825–28.

19. Gryll and M. Katahn, "Situational Factors."

20. R. H. Gracely et al., "Clinician's Expectations Influence Placebo Analgesia," *Lancet* 1 (1985): 43.

21. D. M. Chaput de Saintonge and A. Herxheimer, "Harnessing Placebo Effects in Health Care," *Lancet* 344 (1994): 995–98.

22. T. J. Kaptchuk, "The Placebo Effect in Alternative Medicine: Can the Performance of a Healing Ritual Have Clinical Significance?" *Annals of Internal Medicine* 136, no. 11 (2002): 817–25.

23. Coronory Drug Study Research Group, "Influence of Adherance to Treatment and Response to Cholesterol on Mortality in the Coronory Drugs Project," *New England Journal of Medicine* 303 (1980): 1038–41.

24. K. B. Thomas, "Temporarily Dependent Patient in General Practice," *British Medical Journal* 1 (1974): 625–26.

25. G. L. Engel, "The Clinical Application of the Biopsychosocial Model," *American Journal of Psychiatry* 137 (1980): 535–44; D. A. Drossman, "Gastrointestinal Illness and the Biopsychosocial Model," *Journal of Clinical Gastroenterology* 22 (1996): 252–54.

26. Thomas, "Temporarily Dependent Patient."

27. I. G. McDonald et al., "Opening Pandora's Box: The Unpredictability of Reassurance by a Normal Test Result," *British Medical Journal* 313 (1996): 329–32.

28. N. Cousins, "The Physician as Communicator," *Journal of the American Medical Association* 248 (1982): 287–89.

29. Ibid.

30. J. A. Balint, "Brief Encounters: Speaking with Patients," *Annals of Internal Medicine* 131, no. 3 (1999): 231–34.

31. E. McColl et al., "Assessing Symptoms in Gastroesophageal Reflux Disease: How Well Do Clinicians' Assessments Agree with Those of Their Patients?" *American Journal of Gastroenterology* 100, no. 1 (2005): 11–18.

32. M. A. Stewart, "Effective Physician-Patient Communication and Health Outcomes: A Review," *Canadian Medical Association Journal* 152 (2004): 1423–33.

33. F. Davidoff, "Time," *Annals of Internal Medicine* 127, no. 6 (1997): 483–85.

34. C. T. Lin et al., "Is Patients' Perception of Time Spent with the Physician a Determinant of Ambulatory Patient Satisfaction?" *Archives of Internal Medicine* 161, no. 11 (2001): 1437–42.

35. A. D. Wilson, "Consultation Length: General Practitioners' Attitudes and Practices," *British Medical Journal (Clin.Res.Ed)* 290, no. 6478 (1985): 1322–24; D. Wilkin and D. H. Metcalfe, "List Size and Patient Contact in General Medical Practice," *British Medical Journal (Clin.Res.Ed)* 289, no. 6457 (1984): 1501–1505.

36. D. C. Morrell et al., "The 'Five Minute' Consultation: Effect of Time Constraint on Clinical Content and Patient Satisfaction," *British Medical Journal (Clin.Res.Ed)* 292, no. 6524 (1986): 870–73.

37. L. Buske, "Younger Physicians Providing Less Direct Patient Care," *Canadian Medical Association Journal* 170, no. 8 (2004): 1217.

38. D. Mechanic, D. D. McAlpine, and M. Rosenthal, "Are Patients' Office Visits With Physicians Getting Shorter?" *New England Journal of Medicine* 344, no. 3 (2001): 198–204.

39. W. B. Jonas, T. J. Kaptchuk, and K. Linde, "A Critical Overview of Homeopathy," *Annals of Internal Medicine* 138, no. 5 (2003): 393–99.

40. Chantler, "The Second Greatest Benefit to Mankind?"

41. Morrell et al., "The 'Five Minute' Consultation."

42. M. O. Roland et al., "The 'Five Minute' Consultation: Effect of Time Constraint on Verbal Communication," *British Medical Journal (Clin.Res.Ed)* 292, no. 6524 (1986): 874–76.

43. Wilson, "Consultation Length."

44. J. G. Howie, A. M. Porter, and J. F. Forbes, "Quality and the Use of Time in General Practice: Widening the Discussion," *British Medical Journal* 298, no. 6679 (1989): 1008–10.

45. J. G. Howie et al., "Long to Short Consultation Ratio: A Proxy Measure of Quality of Care for General Practice," *British Journal of General Practice* 41, no. 343 (1991): 48–54.

46. D. M. Owens, D. K. Nelson, and N. J. Talley, "The Irritable Bowel Syndrome: Long Term Prognosis and the Patient-Physician Interaction," *Annals of Internal Medicine* 122 (1995): 107–12.

47. Wilkin and D. H. Metcalfe, "List Size and Patient Contact."

48. Peabody, "The Care of the Patient."

49. H. Brody, *The Healer's Power* (New Haven, CT: Yale University Press, 1992).

CHAPTER 13: THE PLACEBO RESPONDER

1. S. Wolf, "The Pharmacology of Placebos," *Pharmacological Reviews* 11 (1959): 689–704.

2. E. Ernst and K. L. Resch, "Concept of True and Perceived Placebo Effects," *British Medical Journal* 311 (1995): 551–53.

3. T. J. Kaptchuk, "The Placebo Effect in Alternative Medicine: Can the Performance of a Healing Ritual Have Clinical Significance?" *Annals of Internal Medicine* 136, no. 11 (2002): 817–25.

4. Ernst and Resch, "Concept of True and Perceived Placebo Effects."

5. J. M. Bland and D. G. Altman, "Regression towards the Mean," *British Medical Journal* 308, no. 6942 (1994): 1499.

6. Ernst and Resch, "Concept of True and Perceived Placebo Effects."

7. H. K. Beecher, "The Powerful Placebo," *Journal of the American Medical Association* 159 (1955): 1602–1606.

8. L. Lasagna et al., "A Study of the Placebo Response," *American Journal of Medicine* 16 (1954): 770–79.

9. A. K. Shapiro and E. Shapiro, "Predicting Placebo Response," in *The Powerful Placebo: From Anient Priest to Modern Physician*, ed. A. K. Shapiro and E. Shapiro (Baltimore: Johns Hopkins University Press, 1997).

10. W. A. Brown, M. F. Johnson, and M. G. Chen, "Clinical Features of Depressed Patients Who Do and Do Not Improve with Placebo," *Psychiatry Res.* 41, no. 3 (1992): 203–14.

11. R. J. Bailik et al., "A Comparison of Placebo Responders and Non-responders in Subgroups of Depressive Disorders," *Journal of Psychiatry and Neuroscience* 20 (1994): 265–70.

12. C. G. Moertel et al., "Who Responds to Sugar Pills?" *Mayo Clinic Proceedings* 51, no. 2 (1976): 96–100.

13. J. A. Astin, "Why Patients Use Alternative Medicine: Results of a National Study," *Journal of the American Medical Association* 279, no. 19 (1998): 1548–53.

14. Shapiro and Shapiro, "Predicting Placebo Response."

15. Moertel et al., "Who Responds to Sugar Pills?"

16. S. L. Gryll and M. Katahn, "Situational Factors Contributing to the Placebo Effect," *Psychopharmacology* 57, no. 3 (1978): 253–61.

17. D. So, "Acupuncture Outcomes, Expectations, Patient-Provider Relationship, and the Placebo Effect: Implications for Health Promotion," *American Journal of Public Health* 92 (2002): 1662–67.

18. A. Branthwaite and P. Cooper, "Analgesic Effects of Branding in Treatment of Headaches," *British Medical Journal (Clin.Res.Ed)* 282, no. 6276 (1981): 1576–78.

19. M. H. Cohen and D. M. Eisenberg, "Potential Physician Malprac-

tice Liability Associated With Complementary and Integrative Medical Therapies," *Annals of Internal Medicine* 136, no. 8 (2002): 596–603.

20. A. Ilnyckyj et al., "Quantitation of the Placebo Response in Ulcerative Colitis," *Gastroenterology* 112 (1997): 1854–58.

21. Gryll and Katahn, "Situational Factors."

22. Ilnyckyj et al., "Quantitation of the Placebo Response."

23. R. I. Horowitz and S. M. Horowitz, "Adherance to Treatment and Health Outcome," *Archives of Internal Medicine* 153 (1993): 1863–68.

24. Coronary Drug Study Research Group, "Influence of Adherance to Treatment and Response to Cholesterol on Mortality in the Coronary Drugs Project," *New England Journal of Medicine* 303 (1980): 1038–41.

25. R. I. Horwitz et al., "Treatment Adherence and Risk of Death after a Myocardial Infarction," *Lancet* 336, no. 8714 (1990): 542–45.

26. Horowitz and Horowitz, "Adherance to Treatment and Health Outcome."

27. Astin, "Why Patients Use Alternative Medicine."

28. J. S. Goodwin, J. M. Goodwin, and A. V. Vogel, "Knowledge and Use of Placebos by House Officers and Nurses," *Annals of Internal Medicine* 91, no. 1 (1979): 106–10.

29. Wolf, "The Pharmacology of Placebos."

30. S. Lee et al., "Does Elimination of Placebo Responders in a Placebo Run-in Increase the Treatment Effect in Randomized Clinical Trials? A Meta-Analytic Evaluation," *Depress.Anxiety.* 19, no. 1 (2004): 10–19.

CHAPTER 14: THE ETHICS OF USING PLACEBOS

1. D. Mechanic, "Introduction," in *Humanizing Health Care*, ed. H. Strauss (New York: Wiley, 1975), pp. 1–11.

2. D. J. Rothman, *Strangers at the Bedside* (New York: Basic Books, 1991), p. 84.

3. Ibid.

4. "The Nuremberg Code," http://www.ohsr.od.nih.gov/nuremberg.php3.

5. A. B. Hill, "Medical Ethics and Controlled Trials," *British Medical Journal* 5337 (1963): 1043–49.

6. H. K. Beecher, "Ethics and Clinical Research," *New England Journal of Medicine* 274, no. 24 (1966): 1354–60.

7. Ibid.

8. A. K. Shapiro and E. Shapiro, *Ethical Controversies about the Use of Placebos, the Double-Blind and Controlled Cinical Trials* (Cambridge, MA: Harvard University Press, 1997), pp. 175–89; S. Bok, "The Ethics of Giving Placebos," *Scientific American* 231, no. 5 (1974): 17–23.

9. "The Nuremberg Code."

10. R. Temple and S. S. Ellenberg, "Placebo-Controlled Trials and Active Control Trials in the Evaluation of New Treatments—Part 1: Ethical and Scientific Issues," *Annals of Internal Medicine* 133 (2004): 455–63; W. Fawzi and M. J. Stumpfer, "A Role for Multivitimins in Infection," *Annals of Internal Medicine* 138 (2003): 430–31.

11. K. J. Rothman and K. M. Michels, "The Continuing Unethical Use of Placebo Controls," *New England Journal of Medicine* 331 (1994): 394–97.

12. Temple and Ellenberg, "Placebo-Controlled Trials—Part1"; Temple and Ellenberg, "Placebo-Controlled Trials and Active-Control Trials in the Evaluation of New Treatments—Part 2: Practical Issues and Specific Cases," *Annals of Internal Medicine* 133, no. 6 (2000): 464–70.

13. E. J. Emanual and F. G. Miller, "The Ethics of Placebo-Controlled Trials—A Middle Ground," *New England Journal of Medicine* 345 (2001): 916–18.

14. L. Hirsch, "Randomized Clinical Trials: What Gets Published, and When?" *Canadian Medical Association Journal* 170, no. 4 (2004): 481–83.

15. H. P. Forster, E. Emanuel, and C. Grady, "The 2000 Revision of the Declaration of Helsinki: A Step Forward or More Confusion?" *Lancet* 358, no. 9291 (2001): 1449–53.

16. G. Sreenivasan, "Does Informed Consent to Research Require Comprehension?" *Lancet* 362, no. 9400 (2003): 2016–18.

17. "Consent: How Informed?" *Lancet* 1, no. 8392 (1984): 1445–47.

18. Hirsch, "Randomized Clinical Trials"; "Consent: How Informed?"

19. "The 'File Drawer' Phenomenon: Suppressing Clinical Evidence," *Canadian Medical Association Journal* 170, no. 4 (2004): 437; A. J. Munro, "Publishing the Findings of Clinical Research," *British Medical Journal* 307, no. 6915 (1993): 1340–41.

20. Shapiro and Shapiro, *Ethical Controversies*; Bok, "The Ethics of Giving Placebos"; T. J. Kaptchuk, "Powerful Placebo: The Dark Side of the Randomised Controlled Trial," *British Medical Journal* 351 (1998): 1722–25; H. Brody, "The Lie That Heals: The Ethics of Giving Placebos," *Annals of Internal Medicine* 97 (1982): 112–18.

21. Bok, "The Ethics of Giving Placebos"; "Drug or Placebo?" available from *PM:4113900*.

22. U. Nitzan and P. Lichtenberg, "Questionnaire Survey on Use of Placebo," *British Medical Journal* 329, no. 7472 (2004): 944–46.

23. J. Hill, "Placebos in Clinical Care: For Whose Pleasure," *Lancet* 262 (2003): 254.

24. K. B. Thomas, "General Practice Consultations: Is There Any Point in Being Positive?" *British Medical Journal* 294 (1987): 1200–1202.

25. D. M. Chaput de Saintonge and A. Herxheimer, "Harnessing Placebo Effects in Health Care," *Lancet* 344 (1994): 995–98.

26. Brody, "The Lie That Heals"; Brody, "The Placebo Response: Recent Research and Implications for Family Practice," *Journal of Family Practice* 47 (2000): 649–54.

CHAPTER 15: STRANGERS IN THE CONSULTING ROOM

1. D. J. Rothman, *Strangers at the Bedside* (New York: Basic Books, 1991).
2. A. K. Shapiro and E. Shapiro, *The Powerful Placebo: From Ancient Priest to Modern Physician* (Baltimore: Johns Hopkins University Press, 1997).
3. Rothman, *Strangers at the Bedside*.
4. Ibid.
5. Ibid.
6. L. Sanders, "The End of Primary Care," *New York Times Magazine*, April 18, 2004, pp. 52–55.
7. B. Kralj, "Physician Human Resources in Ontario: The Crisis Continues," *Ontario Medical Review* (October 2001): 19–27.
8. Ibid.; L. Gagnon, "Medicine's Feminine Side," *Globe and Mail*, April 18, 2004; K. Burton, "A Force to Contend With: The Gender Gap Closes in Canadian Medical Schools," *Canadian Medical Association Journal* 170 (2004): 1385–86.
9. L. Buske, "Younger Physicians Providing Less Direct Patient Care," *Canadian Medical Association Journal* 170, no. 8 (2004): 1217.
10. Rothman, *Strangers at the Bedside*.
11. H. K. Beecher, "Ethics and Clinical Research," *New England Journal of Medicine* 274, no. 24 (1966): 1354–60.
12. World Medical Association, "The Declaration of Helsinki," available from http://www.wma.net/e/policy/b3.htm.
13. Rothman, *Strangers at the Bedside*.
14. Translation from the Greek by Ludwig Edelstein—*The Hippocratic Oath* (Baltimore: Johns Hopkins University Press, 1943).
15. W. G. Thompson et al., "Irritable Bowel Syndrome in General Practice: Prevalence, Management and Referral," *Gut* 46 (2000): 78–82.
16. W. G. Patterson et al., "Recommendations for the Management of Irritable Bowel Syndrome in Family Practice," *Canadian Medical Association Journal* 161 (1999): 154–60; "Pushing Pills," *Economist*, no. 15 (March 2003): 61.
17. E. R. Berndt, "To Inform or Persuade? Direct-to-Consumer Advertising of Prescription Drugs," *New England Journal of Medicine* 352, no. 4 (2005): 325–28; R. Steinbrook, "Commercial Support and Continuing Medical Education," *New England Journal of Medicine* 352, no. 6 (2005): 534–35; D. Blumenthal, "Doctors and Drug Companies," *New England Journal of*

Medicine 351, no. 18 (2004): 1885–90; D. M. Studdert, M. M. Mello, and T. A. Brennan, "Financial Conflicts of Interest in Physicians' Relationships with the Pharmaceutical Industry: Self–Regulation in the Shadow of Federal Prosecution," *New England Journal of Medicine* 351, no. 18 (2004): 1891–1900; M. Angell, "Excess in the Pharmaceutical Industry," *Canadian Medical Association Journal.* 171, no. 12 (2004): 1451–53; "Pushing Pills," *Economist*, March 15, 2003, p. 61; C. Elliott, "You Scratch My Back and I'll Scratch Yours," *Ottawa Citizen*, Jan. 2, 2004, p. A17.

18. Blumenthal, "Doctors and Drug Companies."

19. "Drug Marketing: Unsafe at Any Dose?" *Canadian Medical Association Journal* 167 (2002): 981.

20. D. L. Sackett, "The Arrogance of Preventive Medicine," *Canadian Medical Association Journal* 167, no. 4 (2002): 363–64.

21. A. D. Feld and D. Walta, "Malpractice, Tort Reform and You: An Introduction to Risk Management," *American Journal of Gastroenterology* 99 (2004): 192–93.

22. M. M. Mello, D. M. Studdert, and T. A. Brennan, "The New Medical Malpractice Crisis," *New England Journal of Medicine* 348, no. 23 (2003): 2281–84.

23. J. S. McQuade, "The Medical Malpractice Crisis—Reflections on the Alleged Causes and Proposed Cures: Discussion Paper," *Journal of the Royal Society of Medicine* 84 (1991): 408–11.

24. N. Summerton, "Positive and Negative Factors in Defensive Medicine: A Questionnaire Study of General Practitioners," *British Medical Journal* 310 (1995): 27–29.

25. H. P. Forster, J. Schwartz, and E. DeRenzo, "Reducing Legal Risk by Practicing Patient-Centered Medicine," *Archives of Internal Medicine* 162, no. 11 (2002): 1217–19.

26. A. R. Localio et al., "Relation Between Malpractice Claims and Adverse Events Due to Negligence: Results of the Harvard University Press Medical Practice Study III," *New England Journal of Medicine* 325, no. 4 (1991): 245–51; T. A. Brennan, C. M. Sox, and H. R. Burstin, "Relation between Negligent Adverse Events and the Outcomes of Medical-Malpractice Litigation," *New England Journal of Medicine* 335, no. 26 (1996): 1963–67.

27. McQuade, "The Medical Malpractice Crisis."

28. Feld and Walta, "Malpractice, Tort Reform and You."

29. A. D. Feld, "Informed Consent: Not Just for Procedures Anymore," *American Journal of Gastroenterology* 99, no. 6 (2004): 977–80.

CHAPTER 16: THE BURDEN OF PROOF

1. A. C. Doyle, "The Sign of the Four (Quoting Winwood Reade)," in *The Complete Sherlock Holmes* (New York: Doubleday, 1892), 89–158.

2. S. R. Maxwell and D. J. Webb, "COX-2 Selective Inhibitors: Important Lessons Learned," *Lancet* 365, no. 9458 (2005): 449–51.

3. "Safety Concerns at the FDA," *Lancet* 365, no. 9461 (2005): 727–28.

4. M. Camilleri et al., "Efficacy and Safety of Alosetron in Women With Irritable Bowel Syndrome: A Randomised, Placebo-Controlled Trial," *Lancet* 355 (2000): 1035–39.

5. G. Bodeker and F. Kronenberg, "A Public Health Agenda for Traditional, Complementary and Alternative Medicine," *American Journal of Public Health* 92 (2002): 1582–90.

6. American Psychiatric Association Task force for DSM IV, *Diagnostic and Statistical Manual of Mental Disorders*, text revision, 4th ed. (Washington, DC: American Psychiatric Association, 2000).

7. R. L. Park, "Placebos Have Side Effects," in *Voodoo Science: The Road from Foolishness to Fraud* (Oxford: Oxford University Press, 2001), pp. 46–68.

8. W. G. Thompson, "Review Article: The Treatment of Irritable Bowel Syndrome," *Alimentary Pharmacology and Therapeutics* 16 (2002): 1395–1406.

9. Ibid.

10. W. G. Thompson and K. W. Heaton, *Irritable Bowel Syndrome*, 2nd ed. (Oxford: Health Press, 2003).

11. R. Asher, *Richard Asher Talking Sense* (Edinburgh, UK: Churchill Livingstone, 1972), p 104

12. A. J. Wakefield et al., "Ileal-Lymphoid-Nodular Hyperplasia, Non-Specific Colitis, and Pervasive Developmental Disorder in Children," *Lancet* 351, no. 9103 (1998): 637–41.

13. R. Horton, "A Statement by the Editors of The Lancet," *Lancet* 363, no. 9411 (2004): 820–21.

14. "More Clinical Judgment, Fewer 'Clinical' Judges," *Lancet* 351, no. 9099 (1998): 303; G. Bertelli, "Di Bella Therapy," Quackwatch, http://www.quackwatch.org/01QuackeryRelatedTopics/Cancer/dibella.htm.

15. Park, "Placebos Have Side Effects."

16. "Evaluation of an Unconventional Cancer Treatment (the Di Bella Multitherapy): Results of Phase II Trials in Italy; Italian Study Group for the Di Bella Multitherapy Trails," *British Medical Journal* 318, no. 7178 (1999): 224–28.

17. B. Simini, "Italian 'Wonder' Cure for Cancer Is Ineffective," *Lancet* 252 (2004): 207.

18. B. Wilson, "The Rise and Fall of Laetrile," Quackwatch, http://www.quackwatch.org/01QuackeryRelatedTopics/Cancer/laetrile.htm.

19. C. G. Moertel et al., "A Clinical Trial of Amygdalin (Laetrile) in the Treatment of Human Cancer," *New England Journal of Medicine* 306, no. 4 (1982): 201–206.

20. Ibid.

21. J. S. G. Montaner, M. V. O'Shaughnessy, and M. T. Schechter, "Industry-Sponsored Clinical Research: A Double-Edged Sword," *Lancet* (2001): 1893–95.

22. E. Borst-Eilers, "Availability of Pharmaceutical Drugs," *Economist* December 2000, p.56.

23. "Fixing the Drugs Pipeline," *Economist*, no. 13 (March 2004): 37.

24. R. Nelson, "Antibiotic Development Pipeline Runs Dry: New Drugs to Fight Resistant Organisms Are Not Being Developed, Experts Say," *Lancet* 362, no. 9397 (2003): 1726–27.

25. P. A. Rochon et al., "Relation Between Randomized Controlled Trials Published in Leading General Medical Journals and the Global Burden of Disease," *Canadian Medical Association Journal* 170, no. 11 (2004): 1673–77.

26. Montaner, O'Shaughnessy, and Schechter, "Industry-Sponsored Clinical Research."

27. G. Farrell, "Pfizer Settles Fraud Case for US$430 Million," *USA Today* (2004).

28. J. P. Vandenbroucke, "When Are Observational Studies as Credible as Randomised Trials?" *Lancet* 363, no. 9422 (2004): 1728–31.

29. D. A. Lawlor et al., "Those Confounded Vitamins: What Can We Learn from the Differences Between Observational versus Randomised Trial Evidence?" *Lancet* 363, no. 9422 (2004): 1724–27.

30. Ibid.

31. Ibid.

32. J. Concato and R. I. Horwitz, "Beyond Randomised versus Observational Studies," *Lancet* 363, no. 9422 (2004): 1660–61.

33. J. Ryan, J. Piercy, and P. James, "Assessment of NICE Guidance on Two Surgical Procedures," *Lancet* 363, no. 9420 (2004): 1525–26.

34. "Drug Marketing: Unsafe at Any Dose?" *Canadian Medical Association Journal* 167 (2002): 981; "Whats Wrong With CME," *Canadian Medical Association Journal* 170, (2004): 917.

35. "Educating, With Evidence," *Lancet* 363, no. 9420 (2004): 1485.

36. Borst-Eilers, "Availability of Pharmaceutical Drugs"; M. Goozner, *The $800 Million Pill* (Berkeley and Los Angeles: University of California Press, 2004); "Pushing Pills," *Economist*, no. 15 (March 2003): 61.

37. Goozner, *The $800 Million Pill*.

38. "An Overdose of Bad News: Can Big Drug Companies Recover from Bad News?" *Economist*, 2005, pp. 73–75.

39. D. A. Davis, "CME and the Pharmaceutical Industry: Two Worlds, Three Views, Four Steps," *Canadian Medical Association Journal* 171, no. 2 (2004): 149–50; B. Marlow, "The Future Sponsorship of CME in Canada: Industry, Government, Physicians or a Blend?" *Canadian Medical Association Journal* 171, no. 2 (2004): 150–51.

40. A. Picard, "How Can We Improve Medical Reporting? Let Me Count the Ways," *Globe and Mail*, Dec. 30, 2004, p. A10.

41. T. H. Lee, "Quiet in the Library," *New England Journal of Medicine* 352, no. 11 (2005): 1068.

42. D. A. Lindberg and B. L. Humphreys, "2015: The Future of Medical Libraries," *New England Journal of Medicine* 352, no. 11 (2005): 1067–70.

43. Doyle, "The Sign of the Four."

44. P. Wallace, "The Health of Nations: A Survey of Health-Care Finance," *Economist*, no. 17 (July 2004): 3–19.

CHAPTER 17: HEALTH-CARE SYSTEMS AND THE PLACEBO EFFECT

1. D. A. Matcha, *Health Care Systems of the Developed World: How the United States' System Remains an Outlier* (Westport, CT: Praeger, 2003); P. Wallace, "The Health of Nations: A Survey of Health-Care Finance," *Economist*, no. 17 (July 2004): 3–19.

2. J. Miller and M. Miller, "Singled Out," *New York Times Magazine*, April 18, 2004, pp. 48–51.

3. Matcha, *Health Care Systems*; M. I. Roemer, "National Health Systems throughout the World," *Annual Review of Public Health* 14 (1993): 335–53.

4. C. Orellana, "German Patients Angered by New Charges for Consultations: Health-Care Reforms Aim to Increase Efficiency by Making Patients Think Twice about Visiting a Doctor," *Lancet* 363, no. 9409 (2004): 630; C. Orellana, "Germany's New User Fee Cuts Doctor Visits," *Canadian Medical Association Journal* 171, no. 3 (2004): 226.

5. "The Sound of Iron Dropping," *Economist*, July 24, 2004, p. 50.

6. Ibid.

7. World Bank Web site, http://www.worldbank.org/.

8. H. R. Clinton, "Now Can We Talk about Health Care?" *New York Times Magazine*, April 18, 2004, pp. 26–31.

9. Matcha, *Health Care Systems*.

10. World Bank Web site.

11. Ibid.

12. Ibid.

13. World Health Organization Web site, http://www.who.int/ whosis/.

14. World Bank Web site.

15. W. Beveridge, *Social and Allied Services* (New York: Macmillan, 1942).

16. W. G. Thompson, "Contemporary English Health Care: What Lessons Can We Learn from It?" *Canadian Medical Association Journal* 155, no. 5 (1996): 581–84.

17. Z. Kmietowicz, "GP Dossier Says Patients Getting 'Second Rate' Service," *British Medical Journal* 322, no. 7296 (2001): 1197.

18. R. Horton, "Why Is Ian Kennedy's Healthcare Commission Damaging NHS Care?" *Lancet* 364 (2004): 401–402.

19. S. Harrison, "Bill 8 and Opted Out Physicians," *Ontario Medical Review* (July/August 2004): 63.

20. L. Gagnon, "Stats Can: 14% of Canadians Have No Family Doctor," *Canadian Medical Association Journal* 171, no. 2 (2004): 124; L. Sanders, "The End of Primary Care," *New York Times Magazine*, April 18, 2004, pp. 52–55.

21. P. Comeau, "Crisis in Orthopedic Care: Surgeon and Resource Shortage," *Canadian Medical Association Journal* 171, no. 3 (2004): 223.

22. Matcha, *Health Care Systems*.

23. S. R. Leeder, "Achieving Equity in the Australian Healthcare System," *Medical Journal of Australia* 179, no. 9 (2003): 475–78.

24. J. Oberlander, "The US Health Care System: On a Road to Nowhere," *Canadian Medical Association Journal* 167 (2002): 163–71.

25. J. Shapiro and S. Smith, "Lessons for the NHS From Kaiser Permanente," *British Medical Journal* 327, no. 7426 (2003): 1241–42; R. G. A. Feachem, N. K. Sekhri, and K. L. White, "Getting More for Their Dollar: A Comparison of the NHS with California's Kaiser Permanente," *British Medical Journal* 324, no. 7330 (2002): 135–41; D. Light and M. Dixon, "Making the NHS More Like Kaiser Permanente," *British Medical Journal* 328, no. 7442 (2004): 763–65.

26. Feachem, Sekhri, and White, "Getting More for Their Dollar."

27. D. Lawrence, "Gatekeeping Reconsidered," *New England Journal of Medicine* 345, no. 18 (2001): 1342–43.

28. Shapiro and Smith, "Lessons for the NHS."

29. P. J. Devereaux et al., "A Systematic Review and Meta-Analysis of Studies Comparing Mortality Rates of Private For-Profit and Private Not-For-Profit Hospitals," *Canadian Medical Association Journal* 166, no. 11 (2002): 1399–1406; E. Ginzberg and M. Ostow, "Managed Care: A Look Back and a Look Ahead," *New England Journal of Medicine* 336, no. 14 (1997): 1018–20.

30. J. K. Iglehart, "Revisiting the Canadian Health Care System," *New England Journal of Medicine* 342, no. 26 (2000): 2007–12.

31. Miller and Miller, "Singled Out."

32. D. U. Himmelstein et al., "MarketWatch: Illness and Injury as Contributors to Bankruptcy," *Health Aff.(Millwood.)*, 2005.

33. S. Woolhandler, T. Campbell, and D. U. Himmelstein, "Costs of Health Care Administration in the United States and Canada," *New England Journal of Medicine* 349, no. 8 (2003): 768–75; Clinton, "Now Can We Talk about Health Care?"

34. S. R. Leeder and I. A. McAuley, "The Future of Medicare and Health Service Financing," *Medical Journal of Australia* 173, no. 1 (2000): 48–51.

35. G. York, "In New China, Millions Can't Afford Doctors," *Globe and Mail*, May 17, 2004, p. A10.

36. Matcha, *Health Care Systems*.

37. C. Van Weel, "How General Practice Is Funded in the Netherlands," *Medical Journal of Australia* 181, no. 2 (2004): 110–11.

38. D. P. Weller and A. Maynard, "How General Practice Is Funded in the United Kingdom," *Medical Journal of Australia* 181, no. 2 (2004): 109–10.

39. C. Van Weel and C. B. Del Mar, "How Should GPs Be Paid?" *Medical Journal of Australia* 181, no. 2 (2004): 98–99.

40. L. A. Green, "How Family Physicians Are Funded in the United States," *Medical Journal of Australia* 181, no. 2 (2004): 113–14.

41. Van Weel and Del Mar, "How Should GPs Be Paid?"

42. C. M. Martin and W. E. Hogg, "How Family Physicians Are Funded in Canada," *Medical Journal of Australia* 181, no. 2 (2004): 111–12.

43. Green, "How Family Physicians Are Funded."

44. Van Weel and Del Mar, "How Should GPs Be Paid?"

45. Ibid.

46. Weller and Maynard, "How General Practice Is Funded."

47. Martin and Hogg, "How Family Physicians Are Funded."

48. Weller and Maynard, "How General Practice Is Funded."

49. Van Weel and Del Mar, "How Should GPs Be Paid?"

50. P. Nisselle, "Managing Medical Indemnity: Must We Choose Between Quality Assurance and Risk Management?" *Medical Journal of Australia* 181, no. 2 (2004): 64–65.

51. J. C. MacKinnon, "The Arithmetic of Health Care," *Canadian Medical Association Journal* 171, no. 6 (2004): 603–604.

52. A. K. Cohen, "Medibank and the Physician," *Medical Journal of Australia* 173, no. 1 (2000): 33–34.

53. F. C. Cunningham, "Medicare: Diagnosis and Prognosis," *Medical Journal of Australia* 173, no. 1 (2000): 52–55.

54. R. Klein, "Britain's National Health Service Revisited," *New England Journal of Medicine* 350, no. 9 (2004): 937–42.

55. Orellana, "German Patients Angered by New Charges"; T. Sper-

schneider and S. Kleinert, "Germany's Sick Health Care System," *Lancet* 360 (2002): 1758.

56. X. Bosch, "French Health System on Verge of Collapse, Says Report," *Lancet* 363 (2004): 376.

57. "French Medicine: The Price of Popping Pills," *Economist*, May 15, 2004, p. 51.

58. Bosch, "French Health System on Verge of Collapse"; "French Medicine: The Price of Popping Pills"; Bosch, "French Government Approves Unpopular Health Reforms," *Lancet* 363, no. 9427 (2004): 2148.

59. "Jacques Chirac and the Politics of the Past," *Economist*, 2005, pp. 45–46; V. G. Rodwin and C. Le Pen, "Health Care Reform in France: The Birth of State-Led Managed Care," *New England Journal of Medicine* 351, no. 22 (2004): 2259–62.

60. Rodwin and Le Pen, "Health Care Reform in France."

61. Ginzberg and Ostow, "Managed Care."

62. T. Bodenheimer, "The HMO Backlash—Righteous or Reactionary?" *New England Journal of Medicine* 335, no. 21 (1996): 1601–1604.

63. A. S. Kesselheim and T. A. Brennan, "Overbilling vs. Downcoding: The Battle between Physicians and Insurers," *New England Journal of Medicine* 352, no. 9 (2005): 855–57.

64. Sanders, "The End of Primary Care."

65. Ibid.; Oberlander, "The US Health Care System"; Ginzberg and Ostow, "Managed Care."

66. Lawrence, "Gatekeeping Reconsidered."

67. Bodenheimer, "The HMO Backlash."

68. Ginzberg and Ostow, "Managed Care."

69. Horton, "Why Is Ian Kennedy's Healthcare Commission?"

70. T. G. Ferris et al., "Leaving Gatekeeping Behind—Effects of Opening Access to Specialists for Adults in a Health Maintenance Organization," *New England Journal of Medicine* 345, no. 18 (2001): 1312–17; C. B. Forrest et al., "Self-Referral in Point-of-Service Health Plans," *Journal of the American Medical Association* 285, no. 17 (2001): 2223–31.

71. Ginzberg and Ostow, "Managed Care"; Bodenheimer, "The HMO Backlash."

72. J. J. Mongan and T. H. Lee, "Do We Really Want Broad Access to Health Care?" *New England Journal of Medicine* 352, no. 12 (2005): 1260–63; W. H. Frist, "Shattuck Lecture: Health Care in the 21st Century," *New England Journal of Medicine* 352, no. 3 (2005): 267–72.

73. Clinton, "Now Can We Talk about Health Care?"

74. A. Enthoven and R. Kronick, "A Consumer-Choice Health Plan for the 1990s: Universal Health Insurance in a System Designed to Promote Quality and Economy (1)," *New England Journal of Medicine* 320, no. 1 (1989): 29–37.

75. Bodenheimer, "The HMO Backlash."

76. Clinton, "Now Can We Talk about Health Care?"

77. Woolhandler, Campbell, and Himmelstein, "Costs of Health Care Administration"; Clinton, "Now Can We Talk about Health Care?"

78. Oberlander, "The US Health Care System"; E. S. Fisher, "Medical Care—Is More Always Better?" *New England Journal of Medicine* 349, no. 17 (2003): 1665–67.

79. Fisher, "Medical Care."

80. L. Buske, "Younger Physicians Providing Less Direct Patient Care," *Canadian Medical Association Journal* 170, no. 8 (2004): 1217.

81. B. Kralj, "Physician Human Resources in Ontario: The Crisis Continues," *Ontario Medical Review* (October 2001): 19–27.

82. Sanders, "The End of Primary Care"; B. Wright et al., "Career Choice of New Medical Students at Three Canadian Universities: Family Medicine versus Specialty Medicine," *Canadian Medical Association Journal* 170, no. 13 (2004): 1920–24.

83. B. T. Chan, "The Declining Comprehensiveness of Primary Care," *Canadian Medical Association Journal* 166, no. 4 (2002): 429–34; R. Dawes et al., "Why Ontario Physicians Are Leaving Hospital Work," *Ontario Medical Review* (March 2002): 21–29.

84. "More Doctors Needed, Without Discrimination," *Lancet* 364, no. 9434 (2004): 555–56.

85. L. Gagnon, "Medicine's Feminine Side," *Globe and Mail*, 2004, p. A11; K. Burton, "A Force to Contend With: The Gender Gap Closes in Canadian Medical Schools," *Canadian Medical Association Journal* 170 (2004): 1385–86.

86. Gagnon, "Medicine's Feminine Side."

87. Buske, "Younger Physicians"; A. Laupacis, "Inclusion of Drugs in Provincial Drug Benefit Programs: Who Is Making These Decisions, and Are They the Right Ones?" *Canadian Medical Association Journal* 166 (2002): 44–47.

88. A. Zuger, "Dissatisfaction with Medical Practice," *New England Journal of Medicine* 350, no. 1 (2004): 69–75.

89. Ibid.

90. Sanders, "The End of Primary Care"; P. Sullivan, "Students Still Ambivalent about Family Medicine," *Canadian Medical Association Journal* 170 (2004): 1380.

91. M. Angell, "Is Academic Medicine for Sale?" *New England Journal of Medicine* 342, no. 20 (2000): 1516–18.

92. Zuger, "Dissatisfaction with Medical Practice."

93. Ibid.

94. "OMA Membership Survey," *Ontario Medical Review* (February 2004): 18.

95. G. Carpenter, "Italian GPs Strike Over Long-Awaited Contract," *Lancet* 362, no. 9399 (2003): 1903.

96. Orellana, "German Patients Angered by New Charges."

97. L. Culliford, "Why Are Doctors So Unhappy? Healing and Happiness Go Together," *British Medical Journal* 322, no. 7298 (2001): 1273–74.

98. Kmietowicz, "GP Dossier"; "Why Are Doctors So Unhappy?" *British Medical Journal* 322 (2001): 1361–65.

99. M. Chew, "Battling Red Tape," *Medical Journal of Australia* 181, no. 2 (2004): 60.

100. Zuger, "Dissatisfaction with Medical Practice."

101. D. M. Chaput de Saintonge and A. Herxheimer, "Harnessing Placebo Effects in Health Care," *Lancet* 344 (1994): 995–98.

102. K. B. Thomas, "Temporarily Dependent Patient in General Practice," *British Medical Journal* 1 (1974): 625–26.

103. S. R. Leeder and L. Rychetnik, "Ethics and Evidence-Based Medicine," *Medical Journal of Australia* 175, no. 3 (2001): 161–64; "Evidence-Based Medicine in Its Place," *Lancet* 346 (1995): 785.

104. D. L. Sackett et al., "Evidence Based Medicine: What It Is and What It Isn't," *British Medical Journal* 312, no. 7023 (1996): 71–72.

105. Lawrence, "Gatekeeping Reconsidered."

106. Klein, "Britain's National Health Service Revisited."

107. Lawrence, "Gatekeeping Reconsidered."

108. A. I. Mushlin, H. S. Ruchlin, and M. A. Callahan, "Cost-effectiveness of Diagnostic Tests," *Lancet* 358, no. 9290 (2001): 1353–55.

109. E. C. Mansley and M. T. McKenna, "Importance of Perspective in Economic Analyses of Cancer Screening Decisions," *Lancet* 358, no. 9288 (2001): 1169–73.

110. H. C. Sox Jr., I. Margulies, and C. H. Sox, "Psychologically Mediated Effects of Diagnostic Tests," *Annals of Internal Medicine* 95 (1981): 680–85; L. Rabeneck et al., "Impact of Upper Endoscopy on Satisfaction in Patients With Previously Uninvestigated Dyspepsia," *Gastrointest.Endosc.* 57, no. 3 (2003): 295–99.

111. B. Jonsson, "Economics of Drug Treatment: For Which Patients Is It Cost-effective to Lower Cholesterol?" *Lancet* 358, no. 9289 (2001): 1251–56.

112. Green, "How Family Physicians Are Funded."

113. E. A. McGlynn et al., "The Quality of Health Care Delivered to Adults in the United States," *New England Journal of Medicine* 348, no. 26 (2003): 2635–45.

114. B. Jonsson et al., "Remembering Fractures: Fracture Registration and Proband Recall in Southern Sweden," *Journal of Epidemiology and Community Health* 48 (1995): 489–90.

115. T. Evans, M. Gulmezoglu, and T. Pang, "Registering Clinical Trials: An Essential Role for WHO," *Lancet* 363, no. 9419 (2004): 1413–14.

116. Clinton, "Now Can We Talk about Health Care?"

CHAPTER 18: PHYSICIANS, HEAL YOURSELVES

1. D. Loxterkamp, "Being There: On the Place of the Family Physician," *J.Am.Board Fam.Pract.* 4, no. 5 (1991): 354–60.

2. uger, "Dissatisfaction With Medical Practice," *New England Journal of Medicine* 350, no. 1 (2004): 69–75.

3. L. Sanders, "The End of Primary Care," *New York Times Magazine*, April 18, 2004, pp. 52–55.

4. J. Nauwelaers, "Eraritjaritjaka," *Lancet* 356, no. 9248 (2000): 2169–70.

5. C. Chantler, "The Second Greatest Benefit to Mankind?" *Lancet* 360 (2002): 1870–77.

6. "Academic Medicine: Resuscitation in Progress," *Canadian Medical Association Journal* 170, no. 3 (2004): 309–11.

7. L. Culliford, "Why Are Doctors So Unhappy? Healing and Happiness Go Together," *British Medical Journal* 322, no. 7298 (2001): 1273–74.

8. L. Sanders, "The End of Primary Care" ; L. Gagnon, "Medicine's Feminine Side," *Globe and Mail*, 2004, p. A11; P. Sullivan, "Students Still Ambivalent about Family Medicine," *Canadian Medical Association Journal* 170 (2004): 1380.

9. S. Wells and G. Taylor, eds., *William Shakespeare: The Complete Works* (Oxford: Oxford University Press, 1988), p. 754.

10. Zuger, "Dissatisfaction with Medical Practice."

11. D. J. Rothman, "Medical Professionalism—Focusing on the Real Issues," *New England Journal of Medicine* 342, no. 17 (2000): 1283–86.

12. D. Irvine, "Doctors in the UK: Their New Professionalism and Its Regulatory Framework," *Lancet* 358, no. 9295 (2001): 1807–10.

13. Rothman, "Medical Professionalism."

14. S. R. Leeder, C. A. Silagy, and G. L. Rubin, "Sceptical Medicine," *Medical Journal of Australia* 170, no. 3 (1999): 99–100.

15. S. Wessely, C. Mimnuan, and M. Sharpe, "Functional Somatic Syndromes: One or Many?" *Lancet* 354 (1999): 936–39.

16. P. Wallace, "The Health of Nations: A Survey of Health-Care Finance," *Economist*, no. 17 (July 2004): 3–19.

17. R. M. Wachter, "Hospitalists in the United States—Mission Accomplished or Work in Progress?" *New England Journal of Medicine* 350, no. 19 (2004): 1935–36.

18. J. D. Birkmeyer et al., "Variation Profiles of Common Surgical Procedures," *Surgery* 124, no. 5 (1998): 917–23.

19. W. L. Hasler and P. Schoenfeld, "Systematic Review: Abdominal and Pelvic Surgery in Patients with Irritable Bowel Syndrome," *Aliment.Pharmacol.Ther.* 17, no. 8 (2003): 997–1005.

20. G. C. Harewood and D. A. Lieberman, "Colonoscopy Practice Patterns Since Introduction of Medicare Coverage for Average-Risk Screening," *Clin.Gastroenterol.Hepatol.* 2, no. 1 (2004): 72–77.

21. P. Schoenfeld et al., "Accuracy of Polyp Detection by Gastroenterologists and Nurse Endoscopists during Flexible Sigmoidoscopy: A Randomized Trial," *Gastroenterology* 117, no. 2 (1999): 312–18; S. Pathmakanthan et al., "Nurse Endoscopists in United Kingdom Health Care: A Survey of Prevalence, Skills and Attitudes," *J.Adv.Nurs.* 36, no. 5 (2001): 705–710.

22. S. Smale et al., "Upper Gastrointestinal Endoscopy Performed by Nurses: Scope for the Future?" *Gut* 52, no. 8 (2003): 1090–94.

23. L. Rabeneck and L. F. Parzat, "Colorectal Cancer Screening in Canada: Why Not Consider Nurse Endoscopists?" *Canadian Medical Association Journal* 169 (2003): 206–207.

24. P. Schoenfeld et al., "Flexible Sigmoidoscopy by Nurses: State of the Art 1999," *Gastroenterol.Nurs.* 22, no. 6 (1999): 254–61.

25. Nauwelaers, "Eraritjaritjaka."

26. D. A. Drossman, "Medicine Has Become a Business, but What Is the Cost?" *Gastroenterology* 126 (2004): 952–53.

27. "Academic Medicine: Resuscitation in Progress."

28. "The Soft Science of Medicine," *Lancet* 363, no. 9417 (2004): 1247.

29. "Hearts and Minds," *Globe and Mail*, April 17, 2004.

30. "The Soft Science of Medicine."

31. W. Osler, "Aequanimitas," in *Sir William Osler: A Selection*, ed. C. G. Roland (Toronto, Ontario: Clarke & Irwin, 2004), pp. 1–8.

32. G. R. Baker and P. G. Norton, "Adverse Events and Patient Safety in Canadian Health Care," *Canadian Medical Association Journal* 170, no. 3 (2004): 353–54; T. A. Brennan et al., "Incidence of Adverse Events and Negligence in Hospitalized Patients: Results of the Harvard University Press Medical Practice Study," *New England Journal of Medicine* 324, no. 6 (1991): 370–76.

33. R. Horton, "Sacred Trust, Why American Medicare Hasn't Been Fixed," *New England Journal of Medicine* 344 (2001): 2032.

34. Ibid.

35. H. R. Clinton, "Now Can We Talk about Health Care?" *New York Times Magazine*, April 18, 2004, pp. 26–31.

36. R. Steinbrook, "Public Registration of Clinical Trials," *New England Journal of Medicine* 351, no. 4 (2004): 315–17.

37. B. Meier, "AMA Urges Disclosure of Drug Trials," *New York Times* June 16, 2004.

38. J. M. Drazen et al., "Clinical Trial Registration: A Statement From the International Committee of Medical Journal Editors," *Canadian Medical Association Journal* 171 (2004): 606–607.

39. Ibid.

40. M. M. Mello, D. M. Studdert, and T. A. Brennan, "The New Medical Malpractice Crisis," *New England Journal of Medicine* 348, no. 23 (2003): 2281–84.

41. C. Condit, "Science Reporting to the Public: Does the Message Get Twisted?" *Canadian Medical Association Journal* 170 (2004): 1415–16.

42. "Academic Medicine: Resuscitation in Progress"; Drossman, "Medicine Has Become a Business."

INDEX